Thoracic Infections

Editor

LOREN KETAI

RADIOLOGIC CLINICS
OF NORTH AMERICA

www.radiologic.theclinics.com

Consulting Editor
FRANK H. MILLER

May 2022 • Volume 60 • Number 3

ELSEVIER

1600 John F. Kennedy Boulevard • Suite 1800 • Philadelphia, Pennsylvania, 19103-2899

http://www.theclinics.com

RADIOLOGIC CLINICS OF NORTH AMERICA Volume 60, Number 3
May 2022 ISSN 0033-8389, ISBN 13: 978-0-323-89764-8

Editor: John Vassallo (j.vassallo@elsevier.com)
Developmental Editor: Karen Solomon

Radiologic Clinics of North America (ISSN 0033-8389) is published bimonthly by Elsevier Inc., 360 Park Avenue South, New York, NY 10010-1710. Months of issue are January, March, May, July, September, and November. Periodicals postage paid at New York, NY and additional mailing offices. Subscription prices are USD 529 per year for US individuals, USD 1335 per year for US institutions, USD 100 per year for US students and residents, USD 624 per year for Canadian individuals, USD 1362 per year for Canadian institutions, USD 717 per year for international individuals, USD 1362 per year for international institutions, USD 100 per year for Canadian students/residents, and USD 315 per year for international students/residents. To receive student and resident rate, orders must be accompanied by name of affiliated institution, date of term and the signature of program/residency coordinatior on institution letterhead. Orders will be billed at individual rate until proof of status is received. Foreign air speed delivery is included in all *Clinics* subscription prices. All prices are subject to change without notice. **POSTMASTER:** Send address changes to *Radiologic Clinics of North America*, Elsevier Health Sciences Division, Subscription Customer Service, 3251 Riverport Lane, Maryland Heights, MO63043. **Customer Service: Telephone: 1-800-654-2452** (U.S. and Canada); **1-314-447-8871** (outside U.S. and Canada). **Fax: 1-314-447-8029. E-mail: journalscustomerservice-usa@elsevier.com (for print support); journalsonlinesupport-usa@elsevier.com (for online support)**.

Reprints. For copies of 100 or more of articles in this publication, please contact the Commercial Reprints Department, Elsevier Inc., 360 Park Avenue South, New York, New York 10010-1710. Tel.: +1-212-633-3874; Fax: +1-212-633-3820; E-mail: reprints@elsevier.com.

Radiologic Clinics of North America also published in Greek Paschalidis Medical Publications, Athens, Greece.

Radiologic Clinics of North America is covered in *MEDLINE/PubMed (Index Medicus), EMBASE/Excerpta Medica, Current Contents/Life Sciences, Current Contents/Clinical Medicine, RSNA Index to Imaging Literature, BIOSIS, Science Citation Index,* and *ISI/BIOMED.*

Contributors

CONSULTING EDITOR

FRANK H. MILLER, MD, FACR
Lee F. Rogers MD Professor of Medical
Education, Chief, Body Imaging Section and
Fellowship Program, Medical Director, MRI,
Department of Radiology, Northwestern
Memorial Hospital, Northwestern University,
Feinberg School of Medicine, Chicago, Illinois,
USA

EDITOR

LOREN KETAI, MD
Professor Emeritus, Department of Radiology,
University of New Mexico, Albuquerque,
New Mexico, USA

AUTHORS

ADAM BERNHEIM, MD
Department of Diagnostic, Molecular and
Interventional Radiology, Icahn School of
Medicine at Mount Sinai, Mount Sinai Hospital,
New York, New York, USA

ANUPAMA GUPTA BRIXEY, MD
Department of Diagnostic Radiology, Section
of Cardiothoracic Imaging, Oregon Health &
Science University, Portland, Oregon, USA

JORGE CARRILLO, MD
Universidad Nacional de Colombia, Bogotá,
Colombia

JARED D. CHRISTENSEN, MD, MBA
Associate Professor, Department of Radiology,
Duke University Medical Center, Durham,
North Carolina, USA

MICHAEL CHUNG, MD
Department of Diagnostic, Molecular and
Interventional Radiology, Icahn School of
Medicine at Mount Sinai, Mount Sinai Hospital,
New York, New York, USA

PERE DOMINGO, MD, PhD
Department of Infectious Diseases, Hospital de
la Santa Creu i Sant Pau, Barcelona,
Universidad Autónoma de Barcelona, Institut
de Recerca Biomèdica del Hospital de Sant
Pau, Barcelona, Spain

JENNIFER FEBBO, MD
Assistant Professor, University of New Mexico,
Albuquerque, New Mexico, USA

HANNA R. FERREIRA DALLA PRIA, MD
Imaging Research Specialist, Department of
Thoracic Imaging, The University of Texas MD
Anderson Cancer Center, Houston, Texas, USA

MARK FINKELSTEIN, MD
Department of Diagnostic, Molecular and
Interventional Radiology, Icahn School of
Medicine at Mount Sinai, Mount Sinai Hospital,
New York, New York, USA

TOMÁS FRANQUET, MD, PhD
Department of Diagnostic Radiology, Hospital
de la Santa Creu i Sant Pau, Universidad
Autónoma de Barcelona, Barcelona, Spain

SHEWIT P. GIOVANNI, MD, MS
Assistant Professor of Medicine, Department of Pulmonary and Critical Care, Oregon Health & Science University, Portland, Oregon, USA

MYRNA C.B. GODOY, MD, PhD
Professor, Department of Thoracic Imaging, The University of Texas MD Anderson Cancer Center, Houston, Texas, USA

MARK M. HAMMER, MD
Department of Radiology, Brigham and Women's Hospital, Boston, Massachusetts, USA

MICHELLE HERSHMAN, MD
Assistant Professor of Clinical Radiology, Cardiothoracic Imaging Division, University of Pennsylvania, Philadelphia, Pennsylvania, USA

FAISAL JAMAL, MBBS
Department of Radiology, Brigham and Women's Hospital, Boston, Massachusetts, USA

JEFFREY P. KANNE, MD
Professor of Radiology, Chief of Thoracic Imaging, Vice Chair of Quality and Safety, Department of Radiology, University of Wisconsin School of Medicine and Public Health, Madison, Wisconsin, USA

LOREN KETAI, MD
Professor Emeritus, Department of Radiology, University of New Mexico, Albuquerque, New Mexico, USA

ANA SANTOS LIMA, MD
Department of Diagnostic Radiology, Oregon Health & Science University, Portland, Oregon, USA

EDITH M. MAROM, MD
Professor, Department of Diagnostic Radiology, The Chaim Sheba Medical Center, Affiliated with the Tel Aviv University, Tel Aviv, Israel

H. PAGE MCADAMS, MD
Professor, Department of Radiology, Duke University Medical Center, Durham, North Carolina, USA

GUSTAVO S.P. MEIRELLES, MD
Chief Medical Officer Alliar Group, Rua Ernesto Nazaré, São Paulo, São Paulo, Brazil

BRYAN O'SULLIVAN-MURPHY, MD, PhD
Medical Instructor, Department of Radiology, Duke University Medical Center, Durham, North Carolina, USA

CHING CHING ONG, FRCR
Senior Consultant, Department of Diagnostic Imaging, National University Hospital, Singapore

RAJU REDDY, MD
Assistant Professor of Medicine, Department of Pulmonary and Critical Care, Oregon Health & Science University, Portland, Oregon, USA

CARLOS S. RESTREPO, MD
Professor of Radiology and Director, Cardiothoracic Imaging, Vice-Chairman, Department of Radiology, The University of Texas Health Science Center at San Antonio

JONATHAN REVELS, DO
Assistant Professor, University of New Mexico, Albuquerque, New Mexico, USA

ROLANDO REYNA, MD
Hospital Santo Tomás, Panama

SEBASTIAN ROSSINI, MD
Instituto Radiológico Mar del Plata, Buenos Aires, Argentina

CHARA E. RYDZAK, MD, PhD
Associate Professor of Radiology, Department of Diagnostic Radiology, Oregon Health & Science University, Portland, Oregon, USA

GIRISH S. SHROFF, MD
Professor, Department of Thoracic Imaging, The University of Texas MD Anderson Cancer Center, Houston, Texas, USA

SCOTT SIMPSON, DO
Assistant Professor of Clinical Radiology, Cardiothoracic Imaging Division, University of Pennsylvania, Philadelphia, Pennsylvania, USA

AYUSHI P. SINGH, DO
Department of Diagnostic, Molecular and Interventional Radiology, Icahn School of Medicine at Mount Sinai, Mount Sinai Hospital, New York, New York, USA

FORTUNATO SUAREZ, MD
Instituto Nacional de Enfermedades
Respiratórias Ismael Cosio Villegas, Ciudad de
México, México

LYNETTE L.S. TEO, FRCR
Senior Consultant, Department of Diagnostic
Imaging, National University Hospital,
Assistant Professor, Department of
Diagnostic Radiology, Yong Loo Lin School of
Medicine, National University of Singapore,
Singapore

MYLENE T. TRUONG, MD
Professor and Department Chair, Department of
Thoracic Imaging, The University of Texas MD
Anderson Cancer Center, Houston, Texas, USA

DANIEL ANDRES VARGAS ZAPATA, MD
The University of Texas Health Science Center
at San Antonio

LACEY WASHINGTON, MD
Associate Professor, Department of Radiology,
Duke University Medical Center, Durham,
North Carolina, USA

FORTUNATO SUÁREZ, MD
Instituto Nacional de Enfermedades Respiratorias Ismael Cosío Villegas, Ciudad de México, México

LYNETTE L.S. TEO, FRCR
Senior Consultant, Department of Diagnostic Imaging, National University Hospital
Assistant Professor, Department of Diagnostic Radiology, Yong Loo Lin School of Medicine, National University of Singapore, Singapore

MYLENE T. TRUONG, MD
Professor and Department Chair, Department of Thoracic Imaging, The University of Texas MD Anderson Cancer Center, Houston, Texas, USA

DANIEL ANDRES VARGAS ZAPATA, MD
The University of Texas Health Science Center at San Antonio

LACEY WASHINGTON, MD
Associate Professor, Department of Radiology, Duke University Medical Center, Durham, North Carolina, USA

Contents

Severe acute respiratory syndrome coronavirus 2 (SARS-CoV-2) is an easily transmissible coronavirus that emerged in late 2019 and has caused a global pandemic characterized by acute respiratory disease named coronavirus disease 2019 (COVID-19). Diagnostic imaging can be helpful as a complementary tool in supporting the diagnosis of COVID-19 and identifying alternative pathology. This article presents an overview of acute and postacute imaging findings in COVID-19.

The chest radiograph is the most common imaging examination performed in most radiology departments, and one of the more common indications for these studies is suspected infection. Radiologists must therefore be aware of less common radiographic patterns of pulmonary infection if they are to add value in the interpretation of chest radiographs for this indication. This review uses a case-based format to illustrate a range of imaging findings that can be associated with acute pulmonary infection and highlight findings that should prompt investigation for diseases other than community-acquired pneumonia to prevent misdiagnosis and delays in appropriate management.

Viral pneumonia is usually community acquired and caused by influenza, parainfluenza, respiratory syncytial virus, human metapneumovirus, and adenovirus. Many of these infections are airway centric and chest imaging demonstrates bronchiolitis and bronchopneumonia, With the exception of adenovirus infections, the presence of lobar consolidation usually suggests bacterial coinfection. Community-acquired viral pathogens can cause more severe pneumonia in immunocompromised hosts, who are also susceptible to CMV and varicella infection. These latter 2 pathogens are less likely to manifest the striking airway-centric pattern. Airway-centric pattern is distinctly uncommon in Hantavirus pulmonary syndrome, a rare environmentally acquired infection with high mortality.

Mycobacterial species other than Mycobacterium tuberculosis and Mycobacterium leprae constitute nontuberculous mycobacteria (NTM). NTM infections are on the rise, particularly in the Western world. They cause a wide range of pulmonary and systemic manifestations. The 2 most common types are as follows: classical cavitary type, seen with preexisting lung disease, and the nonclassical bronchiectatic type, seen in elderly women without preexisting lung disease. Disseminated infections by the hematogenous route are common in immunocompromised patients including those with HIV. Imaging plays a key role in the diagnosis and monitoring of NTM infection.

Histoplasmosis, blastomycosis, and coccidioidomycosis are endemic fungal infections in North America. Many infections are subclinical, and many symptomatic infections are mild. Pneumonia is the most common clinical manifestation. All can occur in immunocompetent and immunocompromised patients, with the latter at greater risk for disseminated and more severe disease. As with other acute respiratory illness, imaging can play a role in diagnosis. Knowledge of the acute and chronic imaging findings of endemic fungal infections is important for radiologists so that they can assist in establishing these often-elusive diagnoses, recognize normal evolution of imaging findings of infection, and identify complications.

Infectious diseases, including parasitic diseases, which are commonly associated with poverty and poor sanitation, continue to cause significant morbidity, disability, and mortality in Latin America and the Caribbean region. This article reviews the epidemiology, pathophysiology, and cardiothoracic imaging manifestation of several communicable diseases endemic to this region.

Southeast Asia lies between the tropics with generally warm temperatures all year round and heavy rainfall during the monsoon season. This hot and humid weather, together with climate change, massive globalization, urbanization, and increased population density in Southeast Asian cities including Singapore, provide an ideal environment for pathogenic organisms to flourish and accelerate the spread of contagious diseases. This review highlights the viral, bacterial, fungal, and parasitic infections that are endemic in Southeast Asia, with particular focus on pulmonary tuberculosis that has distinct radiological patterns.

Although many of the thoracic infections endemic to Africa are also present around the world, this article focuses on entities that are emerging or disproportionately affect populations living in sub-Saharan Africa. Important emerging or reemerging viral and bacterial diseases that commonly affect the lung include dengue fever, plague, leptospirosis, and rickettsioses. Most parasitic infections endemic to Africa can also manifest within the thorax, including malaria, amebiasis, hydatid disease, schistosomiasis, paragonimiasis, ascariasis, strongyloidiasis and cysticercosis. Level of sanitation, interaction between humans and host animals, climate change,

Solid organ transplantations (SOT) continue to increase in number, and infections remain one of, if not the most important factor affecting patient morbidity and mortality. The number of possible pulmonary infections in SOT is vast, which include community-acquired, nosocomial, and opportunistic pathogens. Incorporating additional information, such as characteristic imaging appearances, time from transplantation, and an approach to imaging features, the radiological differential diagnosis can be narrowed, allowing imaging to remain central in SOT patient management.

Fungal pneumonia is the most frequent presentation of invasive fungal infections (IFIs) in patients with hematologic malignancies (HM) and hematopoietic stem cell transplantation (HSCT) recipients. The most common causes include Aspergillus, Mucor, Fusarium, and Candida species. The high incidence and high morbidity and mortality rate of fungal pneumonias in HM/HSCT populations arise from severe immune dysfunction that may be caused by both the underlying disease and/or its treatment. CT is routinely used when pulmonary complications are suspected after HSCT. Appropriate image interpretation of the posttransplant patient requires a combination of pattern recognition and knowledge of the clinical setting. In this article, we provide an overview of the clinical manifestations and CT imaging features of the most common invasive fungal pneumonias (IFPs) seen in severely immunosuppressed hosts.

Despite the development of combination antiretroviral therapy (cART) infections continue to cause significant morbidity and mortality among people living with HIV (PLWH). Pulmonary infections with Streptococcus pneumoniae, Haemophilus influenza, and Staphylococcus aureus remain common. One-third of PLWH worldwide are infected with tuberculosis and the infection manifests at any stage of HIV infection. Fungal infection is usually confined to PLWH unaware of their HIV infection until immunosuppression is advanced or those choosing to discontinue cART. The importance of viral infections has diminished since wide availability of cART; however, mortality from COVID-19 in PLWH may remain greater than in the non-HIV population.

This article reviews the various nonimaging diagnostic tests available for the diagnosis of pneumonia including the methods by which specimens are obtained and the speed with which certain tests are available. Because tests results may be available at the time of radiologic image interpretation, it is important for the radiologist to be aware of the type of specimens and diagnostic tests to search for in the electronic medical record in order to provide a more refined imaging report. Diagnostic tests for the most common bacterial, fungal, viral, and parasitic infections are discussed.

PROGRAM OBJECTIVE

The objective of the *Radiologic Clinics of North America* is to keep practicing radiologists and radiology residents up to date with current clinical practice in radiology by providing timely articles reviewing the state of the art in patient care.

TARGET AUDIENCE

Practicing radiologists, radiology residents, and other healthcare professionals who provide patient care utilizing radiologic findings.

LEARNING OBJECTIVES

Upon completion of this activity, participants will be able to:

1. Describe the epidemiology of endemic thoracic infections, as well as their current and potential consequences in various global populations.
2. Discuss the use of non-imaging and radiologic imaging as diagnostic techniques in the diagnosis and management of endemic thoracic infections in various patient populations.
3. Recognize the clinical presentation of endemic thoracic infections to promote a systematic approach to assessment, diagnosis, identification of potential consequences, and timely treatment.

ACCREDITATION

The Elsevier Office of Continuing Medical Education (EOCME) is accredited by the Accreditation Council for Continuing Medical Education (ACCME) to provide continuing medical education for physicians.

The EOCME designates this journal-based CME activity for a maximum of 12 *AMA PRA Category 1 Credit*(s)™. Physicians should claim only the credit commensurate with the extent of their participation in the activity.

All other healthcare professionals requesting continuing education credit for this enduring material will be issued a certificate of participation.

DISCLOSURE OF CONFLICTS OF INTEREST

The EOCME assesses conflict of interest with its instructors, faculty, planners, and other individuals who are in a position to control the content of CME activities. All relevant conflicts of interest that are identified are thoroughly vetted by EOCME for fair balance, scientific objectivity, and patient care recommendations. EOCME is committed to providing its learners with CME activities that promote improvements or quality in healthcare and not a specific proprietary business or a commercial interest.

The planning committee, staff, authors, and editors listed below have identified no financial relationships or relationships to products or devices they or their spouse/life partner have with commercial interest related to the content of this CME activity:

Adam Bernheim, MD; Anupama Gupta Brixey, MD; Jorge Carrillo, MD; Jared D. Christensen, MD, MBA; Michael Chung, MD; Pere Domingo, MD, PhD; Jennifer Febbo, MD; Hanna R. Ferreira Dalla Pria, MD; Mark Finkelstein, MD; Tomás Franquet, MD, PhD; Shewit P. Giovanni, MD, MS; Myrna C. B. Godoy, MD, PhD; Mark M. Hammer, MD; Michelle Hershman, MD; Faisal Jamal, MBBS; Jeffrey P. Kanne, MD; Loren Ketai, MD; Pradeep Kuttysankaran; Ana Santos Lima, MD; Edith M. Marom, MD; H. Page McAdams, MD; Bryan O'Sullivan-Murphy, MD, PhD; Ching Ching Ong, FRCR; Raju Reddy, MD; Carlos S. Restrepo, MD; Jonathan Revels, DO; Rolando Reyna, MD; Sebastian Rossini, MD; Chara E. Rydzak, MD, PhD; Girish S. Shroff, MD; Scott Simpson, DO; Ayushi P. Singh, DO; Fortunato Suarez, MD; Lynette L.S. Teo, FRCR; Doreen Thomas-Payne, MSN, BSN, RN, PMHNP-BC; Mylene T. Truong, MD; Daniel Andres Vargas Zapata, MD; John Vassallo; Lacey Washington, MD

The planning committee, staff, authors, and editors listed below have identified financial relationships or relationships to products or devices they or their spouse/life partner have with commercial interest related to the content of this CME activity:

Gustavo S. P. Meirelles, MD: *Executive*: Alliar Group, Ambra Saude, Datalife.ai and Bright Photomedicine, I2A2; *Speaker and Advisor*: Boehringer-Ingelheim

UNAPPROVED/OFF-LABEL USE DISCLOSURE

The EOCME requires CME faculty to disclose to the participants:

1. When products or procedures being discussed are off-label, unlabelled, experimental, and/or investigational (not US Food and Drug Administration [FDA] approved); and
2. Any limitations on the information presented, such as data that are preliminary or that represent ongoing research, interim analyses, and/or unsupported opinions. Faculty may discuss information about pharmaceutical agents that is outside of FDA-approved labelling. This information is intended solely for CME and is not intended to promote off-label use of these medications. If you have any questions, contact the medical affairs department of the manufacturer for the most recent prescribing information.

TO ENROLL

To enroll in the *Radiologic Clinics of North America* Continuing Medical Education program, call customer service at 1-800-654-2452 or sign up online at http://www.theclinics.com/home/cme. The CME program is available to subscribers for an additional annual fee of USD 356.00.

METHOD OF PARTICIPATION

In order to claim credit, participants must complete the following:

1. Complete enrolment as indicated above.
2. Read the activity.
3. Complete the CME Test and Evaluation. Participants must achieve a score of 70% on the test. All CME Tests and Evaluations must be completed online.

CME INQUIRIES/SPECIAL NEEDS

For all CME inquiries or special needs, please contact elsevierCME@elsevier.com.

RADIOLOGIC CLINICS OF NORTH AMERICA

RELATED SERIES

Advances in Clinical Radiology
Available at: https://www.advancesinclinicalradiology.com/
Magnetic Resonance Imaging Clinics
Available at: https://www.mri.theclinics.com/
Neuroimaging Clinics
Available at: www.neuroimaging.theclinics.com
PET Clinics
Available at: www.pet.theclinics.com

THE CLINICS ARE AVAILABLE ONLINE!
Access your subscription at:
www.theclinics.com

RADIOLOGIC CLINICS OF NORTH AMERICA

Preface
Thoracic Infections and the International Radiology Community

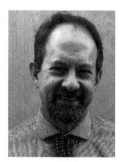

Loren Ketai, MD
Editor

As the twenty-first century unfolds, humankind's shared destiny will be shaped by our responses to changing political constructs, changing climate, and changing diseases. The current pandemic is a daily reminder that no country stands in isolation with respect to infectious diseases. COVID-19 has reshaped our personal and professional lives and has generated a vast medical literature, which is expertly synopsized by Ayushi and colleagues in this issue. COVID-19 is unlikely, however, to be the last pathogen that focuses our attention on the global scope of thoracic infections. Over the coming decades, the world's interconnectivity will be accentuated by global patterns of travel and migration.

Accordingly, this issue of *Radiology Clinics of North America* emphasizes the international scope of infectious disease in addition to updating conventional aspects of imaging thoracic infections. Foundational articles address community-acquired pneumonia (Washington and colleagues) and specific classes of organisms, including viral (Febbo and colleagues), mycobacterial (Hammer and colleagues), and fungal pathogens (Kanne and colleagues and Godoy and colleagues). Comprehensive reviews also address patients with immune defects, specifically, solid organ transplant (Simpson and colleagues) and HIV infection (Franquet and colleagues). An overview of the most current laboratory methods for the diagnosis of thoracic infections (Brixey and colleagues) complements these articles. Augmenting these important conventional topics, this issue of *Radiology Clinics of North America* addresses geographic consideration in the approach to thoracic infections.

In order to offset the medical literature's frequent focus on North America and Europe, separate articles address infectious thoracic diseases endemic to Southeast Asia (Teo and colleagues), Latin and South America (Restrepo and colleagues), and Africa (Rydzak and colleagues).

Radiol Clin N Am 60 (2022) xv–xvi
https://doi.org/10.1016/j.rcl.2022.02.002
0033-8389/22/© 2022 Published by Elsevier Inc.

Some of the thoracic infections of these regions are common to multiple regions (eg, Stronglyodiasis), their prevalence abetted by challenges to national public health systems in many countries around the world. Other infections, such as tuberculosis, are distributed globally, but their diagnosis is confounded by infectious mimics (eg, melioidosis and paracoccidioidomycosis) endemic to specific regions.

An outstanding roster of international contributors has worked together to provide a global perspective to this issue of *Radiology Clinics of North America*. I am profoundly grateful to both the international and North American authors who have spent long hours at work on this project and have been consistently gracious in their response to editorial suggestions. Should any of them choose to be guest editors in the future, I can only hope that they have the good fortune to work with such a talented group of contributors.

Loren Ketai, MD
Department of Radiology
MSC 10 5530, 1 University of New Mexico
Albuquerque, NM 87131-0001, USA

E-mail address:
lketai@unm.edu

Review of Thoracic Imaging Manifestations of COVID-19 and Other Pathologic Coronaviruses

Ayushi P. Singh, DO*, Mark Finkelstein, MD, Michael Chung, MD, Adam Bernheim, MD

KEYWORDS

- Coronavirus disease 2019 (COVID-19)
- Severe acute respiratory syndrome coronavirus 2 (SARS-CoV-2) • Computed tomography
- Severe acute respiratory syndrome coronavirus (SARS-CoV)
- Middle East respiratory syndrome coronavirus (MERS-CoV)

KEY POINTS

- Chest radiography (CXR) is often used as an initial diagnostic imaging tool in patients presenting with respiratory complaints.
- Computed tomography (CT) is more sensitive and specific than radiography for identifying lung abnormalities in patients with COVID-19.
- Common early imaging manifestations of COVID-19 on CT include ground-glass opacities, sometimes with a rounded morphology, and often with a peripheral and lower lobe predominant distribution.
- Several scoring methods have been proposed to evaluate the severity of lung disease on CXR and CT, and reporting guidelines have been produced by societies to assist in standardizing radiology reporting and guiding imaging in the postacute stage.

INTRODUCTION

Severe acute respiratory syndrome coronavirus 2 (SARS-CoV-2) is an easily transmissible coronavirus that emerged in late 2019 and has caused a global pandemic characterized by acute respiratory disease named coronavirus disease 2019 (COVID-19).[1] Although COVID-19 was first reported in the city of Wuhan, the capital city of central China's Hubei Province, it rapidly spread throughout the world and became one of the greatest global health crises of this century.[2] To date, there are more than 235 million people worldwide with documented SARS-CoV-2 infection and more than 4.8 million deaths.[3,4]

SARS-CoV-2 belongs to a family of viruses known as coronaviridae. To date, 7 coronaviruses that infect humans have been identified,[5] which include severe acute respiratory syndrome coronavirus (SARS-CoV) and Middle East respiratory syndrome coronavirus (MERS-CoV).[6] SARS-CoV emerged in 2002 and led to an epidemic in southeast China, which ultimately resulted in 774 deaths out of 8098 total cases.[7] MERS originated in Saudi Arabia in 2012 and ultimately resulted in 858 deaths out of 2494 infected individuals.[8] The SARS outbreak of 2002 was eradicated and has never resurfaced, with the last case being reported in 2003. MERS, however, continues to have

Nothing to disclose; The authors have no commercial or financial conflicts of interest. No funding sources.
Department of Diagnostic, Molecular and Interventional Radiology, Icahn School of Medicine at Mount Sinai, Mount Sinai Hospital, New York, NY 10029, USA
* Corresponding author.
E-mail address: ayushi.singh@mountsinai.org

Radiol Clin N Am 60 (2022) 359–369
https://doi.org/10.1016/j.rcl.2022.01.004
0033-8389/22/Published by Elsevier Inc.

episodic small outbreaks, often clustered in families or hospitals but usually limited to a single geographic location. The number of people infected with COVID-19 has far surpassed both SARS and MERS, but COVID-19 has a much lower mortality rate than both diseases.[9] The remaining coronaviruses known to infect humans are (HCoV)-229E, HCoV-NL63, HCoV-OC43, and HCoV-HKU1.[5] These are relatively benign respiratory pathogens in humans (often children), typically causing upper respiratory tract disease and common cold symptoms.[5]

Most of the COVID-19 diagnostic assays available to date require the collection of nasopharyngeal swab to assess for SARS-CoV-2 viral RNA.[2] Although diagnosis of COVID-19 is definitively made through laboratory testing, diagnostic imaging can be helpful as a complementary tool in supporting the diagnosis or identifying alternative pathology. In this article, the authors aim to review the thoracic imaging manifestations of COVID-19.

CLINICAL MANIFESTATIONS

SARS-CoV-2 infection has been estimated to have a mean incubation period of 5.1 to 6.4 days, with most of the patients (97.5%) developing symptoms within 11.5 days.[2] SARS-CoV-2 typically affects the lower respiratory tract. It can present clinically with a multitude of symptoms, with the most common including fever, cough, and dyspnea. Patients with COVID-19 may be asymptomatic or show symptoms ranging from mild to severe. In severe cases, symptoms can escalate into acute respiratory distress syndrome (ARDS), and this can develop in 17% to 29% of patients.[10,11] Complicated COVID-19 infection can result in multiorgan dysfunction characterized by respiratory failure, encephalopathy, coagulopathy and vasculopathy, acute cardiac injury and cardiac failure, renal failure, and other end-organ damage.[2,11] Studies suggest that most of the COVID-19 mortalities occur among patients with ARDS in the intensive care unit (ICU).[12]

DIAGNOSTIC CONFIRMATION OF COVID-19

Current detection methods rely on real-time reverse transcription polymerase chain reaction (RT-PCR) to test mucosal swabs of suspected patients. However, some false-negative RT-PCR results were reported in the early stages of the disease, possibly because of inadequate viral material in the sample or technical issues during nucleic acid extraction.[13] In the early stages of the pandemic, there was limited availability of RT-PCR in some locations because of a lack of testing kits and reagents. Turnaround times for test results were (and continue to be) variable, ranging from hours to days.[14]

The role of radiology in COVID-19 is evolving and may vary depending on local disease prevalence and availability of laboratory testing.

THE ROLE OF IMAGING

Chest computed tomography (CT) findings have proved to be diagnostic in several cases with an initial false-negative RT-PCR screening test.[13] The positive and negative predictive value of chest CT for COVID-19 are estimated at 92% and 42%, respectively, in a population with high pretest probability for the disease (eg, 85% prevalence by RT-PCR).[15] The potential value of CT is that it is widely available and can be performed rapidly. However, findings on chest imaging in COVID-19 are somewhat nonspecific in many cases and may overlap with other pulmonary infections.[16] In addition, there are concerns regarding time management in the CT scanner, given that scan rooms must be thoroughly cleaned after imaging a suspected COVID-19 patient, and the air needs to be recirculated.[2] Currently, the Centers for Disease Control and Prevention (CDC), the American College of Radiology (ACR), the Society of Thoracic Radiology (STR), and the American Society of Emergency Radiology (ASER) have all recommended against the use of CT for routine screening and diagnosis of COVID-19 pneumonia, reserving CT for cases in which there is clinical suspicion of a complication of the disease or another diagnosis.[17,18]

Several scoring methods have been proposed to evaluate the severity of lung inflammation on chest radiography (CXR) and CT. One chest CT severity score proposed by Yang and colleagues calculated individual scores from 20 lung regions; scores of 0, 1, and 2 were assigned for each region if parenchymal opacification involved 0%, less than 50%, or equal to or more than 50% of each region, respectively. The CT severity score was higher in patients with severe COVID-19 in comparison to patients with mild disease.[19]

ACUTE IMAGING MANIFESTATIONS
Chest Radiography

CXR is often used as an initial diagnostic imaging tool in patients presenting with respiratory complaints. Radiography in patients with COVID-19 can vary from normal to hazy pulmonary opacities with a peripheral and lower lung distribution to frank diffuse pulmonary opacification depending on the severity of illness (Fig. 1). These findings

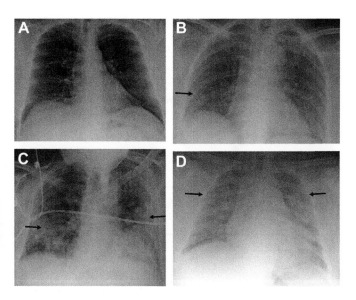

Fig. 1. Spectrum severity of COVID-19 on chest radiography. (*A*) No acute consolidation or other radiographic findings. (*B*) Mild bilateral ill-defined hazy opacities (*arrow*) in a peripheral and lower lobe distribution. (*C*) Moderate multifocal patchy opacities (*arrows*) in a predominately peripheral distribution. (*D*) Severe bilateral diffuse patchy opacities (*arrows*).

may be nonspecific and can overlap with imaging findings in other diseases such as influenza, organizing pneumonia, and other acute lung injuries.[20] Radiography is less sensitive than CT, with a reported baseline CXR sensitivity of 69%.[21] CXR is an effective way to assess progress/resolution of disease over time while minimizing radiation dose (**Fig. 2**).

Prognostic Value of Chest Radiography

It has been suggested that imaging in the acute phase can help predict disease severity in COVID-19. One study performed in patients aged 21 to 50 years with COVID-19 presenting to the emergency department demonstrated that a CXR severity score was predictive of risk for hospital admission and intubation.[22] Another study performed by Schalekamp and colleagues evaluated patients requiring hospitalization due to COVID-19 in the Netherlands. They found that patients who developed critical illness more often had higher initial chest radiography scores and bilateral involvement at admission.[23]

Computed Tomography

CT is more sensitive and specific than radiography for identifying lung abnormalities in patients with COVID-19 (**Fig. 3**).[20] Investigators have demonstrated that COVID-19 on CT most commonly produces a pattern of bilateral ground-glass opacities

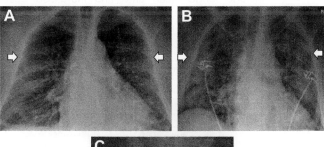
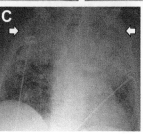

Fig. 2. A 75-year-old man with fever and cough. (*A*) CXR on admission shows mild multifocal hazy and patchy opacities in a peripheral distribution (*arrows*). (*B*) Follow-up CXR performed 5 days later shows worsening now moderate multifocal peripheral opacities (*arrow*). (*C*) Repeat CXR 14 days later shows interval worsening large consolidations in the upper to mid-lungs (*arrows*).

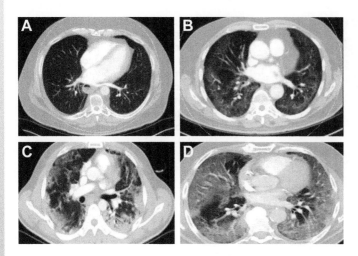

Fig. 3. Severity of COVID-19 on CT. (*A*) No acute pulmonary findings. (*B*) Mild bilateral ground-glass and reticular densities in a peripheral distribution. (*C*) Moderate bilateral peripheral consolidative and ground-glass opacities. (*D*) Severe diffuse peripheral ground-glass opacities.

(GGO), sometimes with a rounded morphology or with a "crazy paving" pattern (which is defined as GGO with superimposed interlobular septal thickening and visible intralobular lines) (**Fig. 4**).[24] The opacities often have a peripheral distribution, mainly in the lower lobes, with the right middle lobe typically being the least involved (**Fig. 5**). Additional less common imaging findings include interlobular septal thickening, bronchial dilatation, pleural thickening, and pleural effusions (**Figs. 6 and 7**).[12] Consolidation is considered an indication of disease progression.[25] A study by Pan and colleagues in China showed that the most severe lung abnormalities on CT in patients with COVID-19 were obtained approximately 10 days after symptom onset[25] (**Fig. 8**).

Chest CT findings in COVID-19 evolve as the illness progresses, similar to other causes of acute lung injury. In one study from the beginning of the pandemic, imaging findings related to disease progression were separated into phases based on the number of days from symptom onset to initial CT—early (0–2 days); intermediate (3–5 days); late (6–12 days); absorption stage/fourth stage (>14 days). Patients imaged in the early stage often had a negative chest CT (56%), with the remaining patients having GGO or consolidation that were often unilateral. Most patients in the intermediate, late, and absorption stage had bilateral GGO and consolidation (55%) with a peripheral lung distribution.[26] Bao and colleagues found that the right lower lobe and left lower lobe were the most commonly involved lobes in COVID-19 (**Fig. 9**).[27]

Additional Imaging Modalities

To date, there are limited data on the pulmonary MR imaging manifestations of COVID-19. Limitations to thoracic MR imaging implementation include longer scan time and increased cost

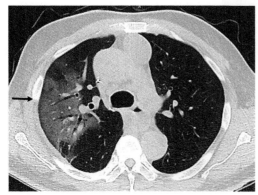

Fig. 4. A 60-year-old positive man with COVID-19 with focal ground-glass exhibiting a "crazy paving" pattern (*arrow*).

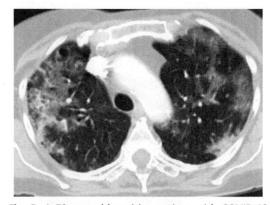

Fig. 5. A 70-year-old positive patient with COVID-19 with bilateral ground-glass opacities in a peripheral distribution.

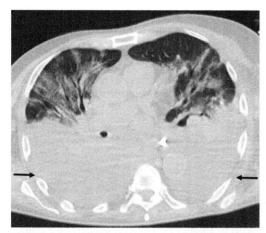

Fig. 6. A 74-year-old positive man with COVID-19 with large bilateral pleural effusions (*arrows*).

compared with CXR and CT. Nonetheless, MR imaging performed for unrelated indications such as cardiac, vascular, and musculoskeletal indications can demonstrate incidental findings related to COVID-19 in the lungs. The pulmonary distribution of COVID-19 on MR imaging mirrors CT and CXR, featuring basilar and peripheral predominant disease (**Fig. 10**). On MR imaging, the parenchymal changes of COVID-19 pneumonia seem as regions of abnormal increased signal intensity on both T1- and T2-weighted sequences, corresponding to the ground-glass or consolidative opacities seen on CXR and CT.[28,29]

The literature on imaging manifestations of COVID-19 on PET with fludeoxyglucose F 18 integrated with computed tomography (18F-FDG PET/CT) is currently limited to mostly case reports in which patients were incidentally found to have COVID-19 during a PET/CT scan for oncologic staging.[30] These reports demonstrate elevated FDG avidity in areas of pulmonary opacity[30,31] (**Fig. 11**). Reported maximum standardized uptake

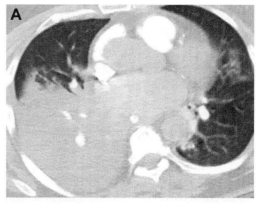

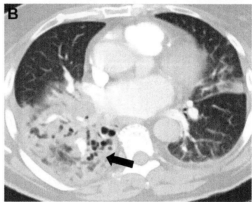

Fig. 8. Necrotizing pneumonia in a 69-year-old woman with RT-PCR-test–proven COVID-19. (*A*) Admission CT shows a large dense right lower lobe consolidation. (*B*) Follow-up CT performed 10 days later due to worsening respiratory symptoms shows new numerous air-filled cystic lucencies (*arrow*) within the consolidation, which suggests necrotizing pneumonia.

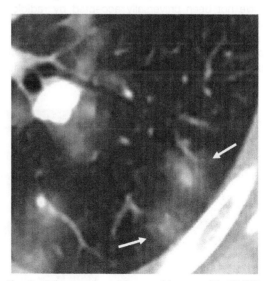

Fig. 9. Halo sign in a 31-year-old man with RT-PCR-test–proven COVID-19. Axial chest CT images show rounded dense consolidations surrounded by ground-glass opacities (*arrows*) in the left lower lobe, findings consistent with the halo sign.

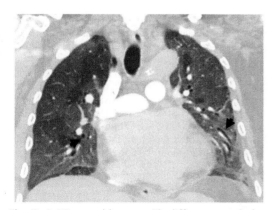

Fig. 7. A 79-year-old man with diffuse ground-glass opacification and mild bibasilar predominant bronchial dilatation (*arrows*).

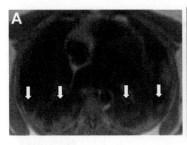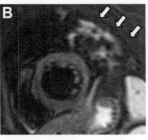

Fig. 10. Cardiac MR imaging performed in a 38-year-old woman with new-onset cardiomyopathy in the setting of COVID-19. (*A*) Axial T2-weighted sequence demonstrates multifocal areas of increased signal intensity (*arrows*) in a peripheral distribution. (*B*) Short-axis STIR sequence shows increased STIR signal in the corresponding areas of abnormality (*arrows*). STIR, short tau inversion recovery.

values have ranged from 4.6 to 12.2.[30,32] There may be some utility in monitoring disease severity on PET/CT. A study by Qin and colleagues found that patients with higher FDG uptake in lung lesions take longer to heal and are positively correlated with erythrocyte sedimentation rate.[33]

IMAGING REPORTING

In early 2020, globally increasing rates of COVID-19 necessitated the development of an organized, systematic, and reproducible approach for radiologists to report COVID-related findings and improve communication with referring clinicians.[33] An expert consensus panel assembled by the Radiological Society of North America (RSNA) developed guidelines for reporting chest CT findings potentially attributable to COVID-19 pneumonia. Four categories for standardized COVID-19 reporting were proposed, which include "typical appearance," "indeterminate appearance," "atypical appearance," and "negative for pneumonia" (**Fig. 12**).[18] The RSNA guidelines have not been universally accepted by radiologists, given differences in practice patterns across institutions. In addition, categorizing patients into a specific category can be difficult or somewhat subjective in patients who have mixed imaging

findings that include both typical and atypical features for COVID-19.

The COVID-19 Reporting and Data System (CO-RADS) is another categorical assessment system proposed in 2020. CO-RADS assesses the suspicion for pulmonary involvement of COVID-19 on a scale from 1 (very low) to 5 (very high).[34,35] The CO-RADS scaling is similar to other frequently used standardized reporting systems in radiology such as Lung Imaging Reporting and Data System, Prostate Imaging Reporting and Data System, and Breast Imaging Reporting and Data System. CO-RADS has been helpful in some settings, but in practice its widespread adoption in the United States has been limited. Some radiologists believe they can adequately identify and communicate findings without the formal structure of a recently introduced reporting system that many clinicians are unfamiliar with. In addition, the accuracy of the CO-RADS system depends on the prevalence of the disease in the population at any given point in time in addition to the prevalence of other diseases with overlapping CT morphology.

PULMONARY EMBOLISM IN COVID-19

Although the causes of mortality due to COVID-19 are multifactorial, respiratory failure from pneumonia

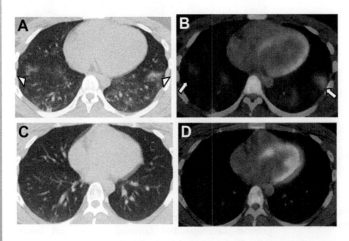

Fig. 11. A 19-year-old man with metastatic alveolar rhabdomyosarcoma presenting for follow-up PET/CT after radiation therapy. Incidentally found to be COVID positive. (*A, B*) CT demonstrates mild multifocal bibasilar ground-glass opacities (*arrowheads*) with corresponding FDG uptake (*arrows*) on the fused PET image. (*C, D*) Follow-up PET/CT performed 4 months later shows resolution of ground-glass opacity and FDG uptake.

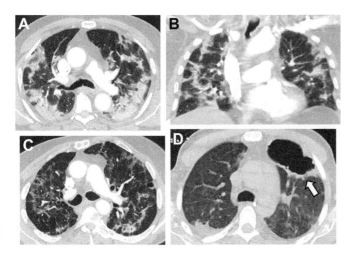

Fig. 12. Examples of COVID-19 categorization endorsed by the RSNA. (*A, B*) Axial and coronal views of a patient exhibiting commonly reported imaging features of COVID-19 pneumonia including peripheral, bilateral, ground-glass opacities. (*C*) Indeterminate appearance showing bilateral reticular and ground-glass opacities lacking typical COVID features. (*D*) Atypical appearance showing uncommonly or not reported features of COVID-19 pneumonia such as cavitation (*arrow*).

and subsequent ARDS is a primary contributor.[36] In addition, there is growing evidence of coagulopathy related to COVID-19, which may predispose patients to thromboembolic complications including deep venous thrombosis, pulmonary embolism (PE), limb ischemia, stroke, and myocardial infarction (**Fig. 13**).[37] A study performed by Suh and colleagues found the PE incidence was higher in patients with COVID-19 than in patients with non–COVID-19 viral pneumonia who were admitted to the ICU, patients with acute respiratory distress syndrome, or patients with H1N1 influenza (swine flu).[38] The presence of thromboembolic disease seems to be an added factor in worsened patient outcomes.[39]

APPROACH TO EVALUATION OF PULMONARY EMBOLISM IN PATIENTS WITH COVID

Deciding whether or not to image a patient for a PE can be challenging, given that the symptoms of PE and COVID overlap significantly.[39] Moreover, many patients infected with COVID-19 have an elevated D-dimer.[37] Overall, the clinical index of suspicion should dictate decision-making on whether to pursue chest CT angiography (CTA) based on evaluation of symptoms and risk factors. Clinicians can consider ordering lower extremity duplex ultrasonography first to rule out deep venous thrombosis if the clinical suspicion is relatively low. If the decision is made to perform a chest CTA, some advocate performing the study as a dual-energy CT if available because it can help characterize pulmonary blood volume and patterns of pulmonary perfusion (**Fig. 14**).[40]

POSTACUTE SEQUELAE OF COVID-19

Radiologic changes in patients who have recovered from COVID-19 comprise an active area of continued research efforts. Some patients have complete resolution of pulmonary findings

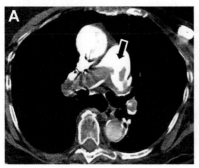
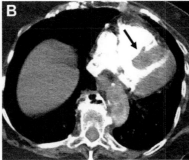
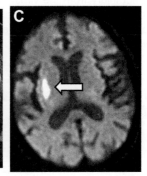

Fig. 13. CTA chest radiography in a 98-year-old man with dyspnea in the setting of COVID-19. (*A*) Large saddle pulmonary embolism (*arrow*) extending to the lobar branches. (*B*) There is mild right ventricular enlargement with flattening of the interventricular septum (*arrow*), which suggests right heart strain. (C) Brain MR imaging performed concurrently shows a small area of infarct (*arrow*) in the right middle cerebral artery (MCA) territory.

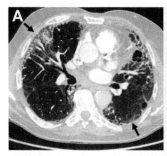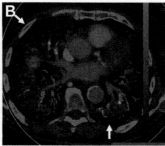

Fig. 14. A 50-year-old man presenting 1 month after recovering from COVID-19. (*A*) Chest CT shows moderate multifocal peripheral reticular opacities (*arrows*) with scattered areas of traction bronchiectasis. (*B*) DECT images obtained concurrently show perfusion defects (*arrows*) in the corresponding areas of lung involvement. DECT, dual-energy CT.

(Fig. 15). A subset of patients has CT abnormalities that persist 3 months after acute infection. The most commonly reported CT abnormalities at 3 months include GGO and subpleural bands (Fig. 16).[41] A study of 3-month scans in 48 survivors of severe COVID-19 who required mechanical ventilation found that 89% of patients had GGO and 67% had signs of fibrosis. At 6 months after acute infection, some patients have resolution of GGOs and development of fibrotic-like changes.[42] Fibrotic-like changes are described as coarse fibrous bands either with or without obvious parenchymal distortion, bronchiectasis, and bronchiolectasis[41] (Fig. 17). A study by Han and colleagues evaluated 6-month follow-up CT scans in 114 patients who recovered from severe COVID-19 pneumonia. Thirty-five percent of the patients had follow-up CTs showing fibrotic-like changes in the lungs.[43] A recent study performed by Caruso and colleagues found similar results. In their cohort of 118 patients with a history of moderate-to-severe COVID-19 pneumonia, 72% of patients showed fibrotic-like changes months after recovery.[44] Several studies suggest that older age is a potential predictor of 6-month fibrotic-like changes.[44,45] It is unclear if postacute changes are the sequelae of acute lung injury/ARDS, the effects of mechanical ventilation, or direct injury from the virus. Whether or not these fibrotic-like changes reflect permanent, irreversible change in the lungs remains to be known with certainty.

APPROACH TO LONG-TERM FOLLOW-UP IMAGING IN PATIENTS WITH COVID-19

There is no clear consensus at this time regarding the recommended frequency of follow-up imaging in patients who have recovered from COVID-19. Currently, follow-up imaging is dictated by the clinical symptoms of each individual patient. Recent studies have shown that in patients who had severe disease and recovered or had milder disease with lingering respiratory symptoms, CT surveillance can provide helpful information.[43] Radiologists can assess for evolution and organization of abnormality with time and quantify the amount of fibrosis. Evaluating the degree of fibrosis is of particular interest, given that there is ongoing research about the potential utility of antifibrotic therapies in attenuating profibrotic pathways in SARS-CoV-2 infection.[46]

IMAGING FOLLOWING COVID-19 VACCINATION

Vaccines have emerged as a vital tool in the battle against COVID-19. Thoracic lymphadenopathy ipsilateral to the injected deltoid muscle has become an important radiologic finding postvaccine that may present as a diagnostic dilemma on imaging studies performed in the oncology population[47] (Fig. 18). Some radiology consensus groups recommend scheduling routine imaging examinations such as those for oncologic screening at least 6 weeks after the final

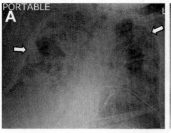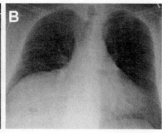

Fig. 15. A 64-year-old COVID-19 positive male. (*A*) Portable CXR on admission shows severe bilateral patchy opacities (*arrows*). (*B*) Follow-up CXR 1 year later shows complete resolution of pulmonary findings.

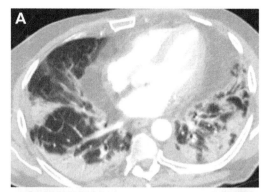

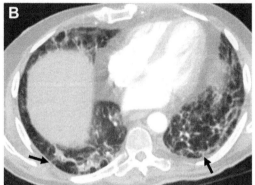

Fig. 16. A 71-year-old COVID-19 positive patient showing evolution of pathology over the span of 3 months. (*A*) CT in the acute phase shows severe bilateral dense peripheral consolidations. (*B*) Follow-up scan 3 months later shows resolution of ground-glass and consolidative densities with evolution into moderate mostly peripheral subpleural reticulation (*arrows*) and scarring with regions of bronchiectasis, findings consistent with fibrosis.

vaccination dose to allow for any reactive adenopathy to resolve.[48]

IMAGING OF OTHER CORONAVIRUSES

COVID-19 is related to the same family of coronaviruses that caused the SARS and MERS outbreaks during 2003 and 2012, respectively.[49]

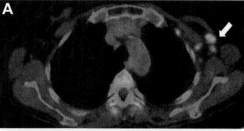

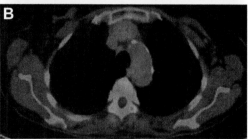

Fig. 18. PET/CT in a patient with a history of squamous cell carcinoma of the pharynx. (*A*) PET/CT performed 1 week following administration of the COVID vaccine in the left arm shows multiple enlarged and hypermetabolic left axillary lymph nodes (*arrow*). (*B*) Follow-up PET performed 2 months later shows decrease in size and FDG avidity within these lymph nodes.

Some CT features of patients with confirmed COVID-19 are similar to those described in SARS and MERS, including peripheral and lower lobe predominant GGO, interlobular septal thickening, and air trapping. In addition, all 3 of these related viruses rarely cause pneumothorax, lung cavitation, or lymphadenopathy.[14] In contrast to COVID-19, SARS tends to be unilateral and focal in distribution (50%). In addition, patients with MERS have been reported to develop pleural effusions more commonly (33%).[6,50] Both SARS and MERS are associated with constriction of the pulmonary vasculature, whereas enlargement of the vasculature has been reported in COVID-19.[51]

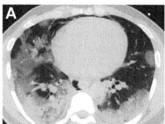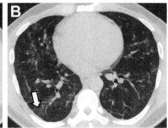

Fig. 17. A 38-year-old man with shortness of breath found to be COVID-19 positive on PCR. (*A*) Scan performed on admission demonstrates severe bilateral multifocal dense and ground-glass opacities in a peripheral distribution. (*B*) Follow-up CT scan performed 1 year later demonstrates mild fibrotic-like changes including mild reticular opacities (*arrow*) with traction bronchiectasis.

SUMMARY

With widespread global health implications related to COVID-19, a comprehensive understanding of the diagnostic thoracic imaging hallmarks is essential for effective diagnosis and management.

CLINICS CARE POINTS

- Chest radiography is an effective way to assess progression/resolution of COVID pneumonia over time while minimizing radiation dose.
- CT is more sensitive and specific than radiography for identifying lung abnormalities.
- Imaging findings in COVID-19 evolve as the illness progresses.
- A subset of patients will have CT abnormalities that persist after acute infection.

REFERENCES

1. Hu B, Guo H, Zhou P, et al. Characteristics of SARS-CoV-2 and COVID-19. Nat Rev Microbiol 2021;19(3): 141–54.
2. Stawicki SP, Jeanmonod R, Miller AC, et al. The 2019-2020 Novel Coronavirus (Severe Acute Respiratory Syndrome Coronavirus 2) Pandemic: A Joint American College of Academic International Medicine-World Academic Council of Emergency Medicine Multidisciplinary COVID-19 Working Group Consensus Paper. J Glob Infect Dis 2020; 12(2):47–93.
3. Johns Hopkins Coronavirus Resource Center. Available at: https://coronavirus.jhu.edu/map.html. Accessed October 6, 2021.
4. Centers for Disease Control. CDC Coronavirus Disease 2019 (COVID 2019) Basics. 2020. Available at: www.cdc.gov. Accessed September 10, 2021.
5. Chen B, Tian EK, He B, et al. Overview of lethal human coronaviruses. Signal Transduct Target Ther 2020;5(1):89.
6. Hosseiny M, Kooraki S, Gholamrezanezhad A, et al. Radiology perspective of COVID-19: lessons from Severe Acute Respiratory Syndrome and Middle East Respiratory Syndrome. AJR Am J Roentgenol 2020;214(5):1078–82.
7. World Health Organization. Summary of probable SARS cases with onset of illness. 2003. Available at: www.who.int/csr/sars/country/table2004_04_21/en/. Accessed October 9, 2020.
8. World Health Organization. Middle east respiratory syndrome coronavirus (MERS-CoV). 2019. Available at: www.who.int/emergencies/mers-cov/en/. Accessed October 9, 2020.
9. De Wit E, van Doremalen N, Falzarano D, et al. SARS and MERS: recent insights into emerging coronaviruses. Nat Rev Microbiol 2016;14(8):523–34.
10. Fan E, Beitler JR, Brochard L, et al. COVID-19-associated acute respiratory distress syndrome: is a different approach to management warranted? Lancet Respir Med 2020;8(8):816–21.
11. Chen N, Zhou M, Dong X, et al. Epidemiological and clinical characteristics of 99 cases of 2019 novel coronavirus pneumonia in Wuhan, China: a descriptive study. Lancet 2020;395:507–13.
12. Salehi S, Abedi A, Balakrishnan S, et al. Coronavirus disease 2019 (COVID 19): a systematic review of imaging findings in 919 patients. AJR Am J Roentgenol 2020;215(1):87–93.
13. Fang Y, Zhang H, Xie J, et al. Sensitivity of chest CT for COVID-19: comparison to RT-PCR. Radiology 2020;296(2):E115–7.
14. Li Y, Xia L. Coronavirus Disease 2019 (COVID-19): Role of Chest CT in Diagnosis and Management. AJR Am J Roentgenol 2020;214(6):1280–6.
15. Wen Z, Chi Y, Zhang L, et al. Coronavirus Disease 2019: Initial Detection on Chest CT in a Retrospective Multicenter Study of 103 Chinese Subjects. Radiol Cardiothorac Imaging 2020;2(2):1–6.
16. American College of Radiology. ACR recommendations for the use of chest radiography and computed tomography (CT) for suspected COVID-19 infection. Available at: www.acr.org/Advocacy-and-Economics/ACR-Position-Statements/Recommendations-for-Chest-Radiography-and-CT-for-Suspected-COVID19-Infection. Accessed October 30, 2020.
17. Raptis C, Hammer M, Short RG, et al. Chest CT and Coronavirus Disease (COVID-19): A Critical Review of the Literature to Date. AJR Am J Roentgenol 2020;215(4):839–42.
18. Simpson S, Kay FU, Abbara S, et al. Radiology Society of North America expert consensus statement on reporting Chest CT findings related to COVID-19. Endorsed by the Society of Thoracic Radiology, the American College of Radiology and RSNA. Cardiothorac Imaging 2020;2(2):1–2.
19. Yang R, Li X, Liu H, et al. Chest CT severity score: an imaging tool for assessing severe COVID-19. Radiol Cardiothorac Imaging 2020;2:e200047.
20. Goyal N, Chung M, Bernheim A. Computed Tomography Features of Coronavirus Disease 2019. J Thorac Imaging 2020;35(4):211–7.
21. Wong YFH, Lam HYS, Fong AH. Frequency and distribution of chest radiographic findings in COVID-19 positive patients. Radiology 2019;296(2):201160.
22. Toussie D, Voutsinas N, Finkelstein M. Clinical and chest radiography features determine patient outcomes in young and middle age adults with COVID-19. Radiology 2020;297(1):201754.
23. Schalekamp S, Huisman M, van Dijk RA, et al. Model-based Prediction of Critical Illness in

Hospitalized Patients with COVID-19. Radiology 2020;298(1):202723.

24. Chung M, Bernheim A, Mei X, et al. CT Imaging Features of 2019 Novel Coronavirus (2019-nCoV). Radiology 2020;295(1):202–7.

25. Pan F, Ye T, Sun P, et al. Time course of lung changes on chest CT during recovery from 2019 novel coronavirus (COVID-19) pneumonia. Radiology 2020;295:715–21.

26. Bernheim A, Mei X, Huang M. Chest CT findings in coronavirus disease-19 (COVID-19): relationship to duration of infection. Radiology 2020;295(3):200463.

27. Bao C, Liu X, Zhang H, et al. Coronavirus Disease 2019 (COVID-19) CT Findings: A Systematic Review and Meta-analysis. J Am Coll Radiol 2020;17(6):701–9.

28. Manna S, Wruble J, Maron SZ, et al. COVID-19: A Multimodality Review of Radiologic Techniques, Clinical Utility, and Imaging Features. Radiol Cardiothorac Imaging 2020;2(3):e200210.

29. Inciardi RM, Lupi L, Zaccone G, et al. Cardiac Involvement in a Patient With Coronavirus Disease 2019 (COVID-19). JAMA Cardiol 2020;5(7):819–24.

30. Kim IC, Kim JY, Kim HA, et al. COVID-19-related myocarditis in a 21-year-old female patient. Eur Heart J 2020;41(19):1859.

31. Albano D, Bertagna F, Bertoli M, et al. Incidental Findings Suggestive of COVID-19 in Asymptomatic Patients Undergoing Nuclear Medicine Procedures in a High-Prevalence Region. J Nucl Med 2020;61(5):632–6.

32. Zou S, Zhu X. FDG PET/CT of COVID-19. Radiology 2020;296(2):E118.

33. Qin C, Liu F, Yen TC, et al. 18F-FDG PET/CT findings of COVID-19: a series of four highly suspected cases. Eur J Nucl Med Mol Imaging 2020;47(5):1281–6.

34. Sharma A, Eisen JE, Shepard JO. Case 25-2020: A 47-Year-Old Woman with a Lung Mass. N Engl J Med 2020;383:665–74.

35. Prokop M, van Everdingen W, van Rees Vellinga T, et al. COVID-19 Standardized Reporting Working Group of the Dutch Radiological Society. CORADS: A Categorical CT Assessment Scheme for Patients Suspected of Having COVID-19-Definition and Evaluation. Radiology 2020;296(2):E97–104.

36. Danzi GB, Loffi M, Galeazzi G, et al. Acute pulmonary embolism and COVID-19 pneumonia: a random association? Eur Heart J 2020;41(19):1858.

37. Abou-Ismail MY, Diamond A, Kapoor S, et al. The hypercoagulable state in COVID-19: Incidence, pathophysiology, and management. Thromb Res 2020;194:101–15.

38. Suh Y, Hong H, Ohana M, et al. Pulmonary Embolism and Deep Vein Thrombosis in COVID-19: A Systematic Review and Meta-Analysis. Radiology 2021;298:E70–80.

39. Woodard PK. Pulmonary Thromboembolism in COVID-19. Radiology 2021;298:E107–8.

40. Ridge CA, Desai SR, Jeyin N, et al. Dual-Energy CT Pulmonary Angiography (DECTPA) Quantifies Vasculopathy in Severe COVID-19 Pneumonia. Radiol Cardiothorac Imaging 2020;2(5):e200428.

41. Solomon JJ, Heyman B, Ko JP, et al. CT of Postacute Lung Complications of COVID-19. Radiology 2021;301:E383–95.

42. Van Gassel RJJ, Bels JLM, Raafs A, et al. High Prevalence of Pulmonary Sequelae at 3 Months after Hospital Discharge in Mechanically Ventilated Survivors of COVID-19. Am J Respir Crit Care Med 2021;203(3):371–4.

43. Han X, Fan Y, Alwalid O, et al. Six Month Follow-up Chest CT Findings After Severe COVID-19 Pneumonia. Radiology 2021;299(1):E177–86.

44. Caruso D, Guido G, Zerunian M, et al. Postacute Sequelae of COVID-19 Pneumonia: 6 Month Chest CT Follow Up. Radiology 2021;301(2):E396–405.

45. Yu M, Liu Y, Xu D, et al. Prediction of the Development of Pulmonary Fibrosis Using Serial Thin-Section CT and Clinical Features in Patients Discharged after Treatment for COVID-19 Pneumonia. Korean J Radiol 2020;21(6):746–55.

46. George PM, Wells AU, Jenkins RG. Pulmonary fibrosis and COVID-19: the potential role for antifibrotic therapy. Lancet Respir Med 2020;8:807–15.

47. Mehta N, Sales RM, Babagbemi K, et al. Unilateral axillary Adenopathy in the setting of COVID-19 vaccine. Clin Imaging 2021;75:12–5.

48. Becker AS, Perez-Johnston R, Chikarmane SA, et al. Multidisciplinary Recommendations Regarding Post-Vaccine Adenopathy and Radiologic Imaging. Radiology 2021;300:E323–7.

49. Ortiz-Prado E, Simbaña-Rivera K, Gómez-Barreno L, et al. Clinical, molecular, and epidemiological characterization of the SARS-CoV-2 virus and the Coronavirus Disease 2019 (COVID-19), a comprehensive literature review. Diagn Microbiol Infect Dis 2020;98(1):115094.

50. Das KM, Lee EY, Langer RD, et al. Middle East Respiratory Syndrome Coronavirus: What Does a Radiologist Need to Know? AJR Am J Roentgenol 2016;206(6):1193–201.

51. Albarello F, Pianura E, Di Stefano F, et al. COVID 19 INMI Study Group. 2019-novel Coronavirus severe adult respiratory distress syndrome in two cases in Italy: An uncommon radiological presentation. Int J Infect Dis 2020;93:192–7.

Radiographic Imaging of Community-Acquired Pneumonia: A Case-Based Review

Lacey Washington, MD*, Bryan O'Sullivan-Murphy, MD, PhD,
Jared D. Christensen, MD, MBA, H. Page McAdams, MD

KEYWORDS

- Community-acquired pneumonia • Infection • Radiograph • Diagnosis • Differential

KEY POINTS

- Awareness of the multiple chest radiographic patterns of community-acquired pneumonia, including subtle bronchopneumonia and interstitial patterns and round pneumonia, facilitates diagnosis of infection but is not useful in identifying specific infectious agents.
- Pleural fluid and multilobar opacities may influence treatment decisions and should be reported when present.
- Because there are no guidelines that recommend universal follow-up radiography, it is important to correlate with clinical presentation and recommend follow-up radiographs in any patient with a discordant clinical presentation.
- Imaging findings that should prompt immediate consideration of alternative diagnoses include lymphadenopathy visible on radiography and the presence of multiple pulmonary nodules.
- Tuberculosis should be considered in patients with atypical, subacute symptom onset particularly when cavitation is present or when opacities involve the upper lobes.

INTRODUCTION

Chest radiography remains the most common imaging study performed both worldwide and in the United States. Although indications for chest radiography are numerous, many of these studies are performed for the evaluation of suspected infection. According to data from the 2019 Global Burden of Disease from before the coronavirus disease 2019 (COVID-19) pandemic, lower respiratory tract infections are the leading cause of mortality from infectious disease worldwide.[1] These infections are divided into community-acquired pneumonia (CAP) and hospital-acquired infections, and also between those in immunocompetent and immunocompromised patients. In the outpatient setting, a single radiograph may be the only imaging study performed and therefore may have a large impact on patient management. Unfortunately, the nonspecific radiographic manifestations of infection lead many radiologists to take a nihilistic approach to the interpretation of radiographs in this setting.

Although it is true that there are limitations of radiographic imaging for CAP, radiologists can still make important contributions to patient care in the setting of suspected acute pulmonary infection. The radiologist who is aware of the broad range of radiographic manifestations of infection may suggest the diagnosis on the basis of findings that are subtle or confusing to clinicians. Radiologic interpretation may identify findings that may alter treatment in the setting of suspected pneumonia. Finally, the radiologist should be alert for findings that are inconsistent with acute CAP or nonspecific enough to call into question a diagnosis of pneumonia in the acute setting, particularly when the clinical presentation is atypical, so as to prevent important misdiagnoses.

Department of Radiology, Duke University Medical Center, 2301 Erwin Road, DUMC Box 3808, Durham, NC 27710, USA
* Corresponding author.
E-mail address: lacey.washington@duke.edu

Radiol Clin N Am 60 (2022) 371–381
https://doi.org/10.1016/j.rcl.2022.01.011
0033-8389/22/© 2022 Elsevier Inc. All rights reserved.

This article reviews the indications for radiographic imaging of patients with suspected community-acquired pulmonary infection and discusses the imaging findings that are most important to current clinical guidelines for patient care. The range of radiographic manifestations of acute CAP and principles of image interpretation are presented in a case-based format. COVID-19 is not addressed, because there is an abundance of literature devoted to that specific diagnosis, and coronavirus pneumonias are discussed elsewhere in this issue (see article by Ayushi and colleagues).

INDICATIONS FOR RADIOGRAPHY IN SUSPECTED INFECTION

Very little research has been performed to assess whether obtaining a radiograph has an effect on clinical outcomes of patients with suspected pulmonary infection. A systematic literature review reveals only 2 such studies—one in a pediatric and one in an adult population. In both, the conclusions were confined to an ambulatory population, and neither of these studies showed a demonstrable effect on the primary end points, which were overall clinical outcomes for pediatric patients and length of illness for the adult population, although in the subgroup of adult patients with abnormal radiographs, duration of illness improved, presumably because of a higher rate of antibiotic use.[2]

These findings are in keeping with the results of studies looking at the impact of chest radiographs on patient management. In one series, among 300 patients in whom pneumonia was suspected, clinicians ordered radiographs in only 19%.[3] Radiographs were performed for only 61% of patients in whom a diagnosis of pneumonia was made. The investigators observed that clinicians who have a sufficiently high clinical suspicion of infection will treat patients regardless of imaging findings, making the chest radiograph superfluous. Another study of 2706 patients hospitalized with a diagnosis of pneumonia found that approximately one-third of patients (911) had negative radiographs, indicating that the diagnosis of pneumonia was not made on the basis of radiographic findings alone.[4] There was no difference in the rates of positive sputum or blood cultures between patients with radiographs interpreted as positive or negative for pneumonia, suggesting that significant lower respiratory tract infection may be found in patients with negative radiographs (false negatives). Studies comparing radiography with computed tomography (CT) suggest that radiography is inferior. A multicenter trial of patients in the emergency department observed that radiography was only 43.5%

sensitive for the detection of opacities compared with CT,[5] concluding that CT is more accurate in identifying pulmonary infection in this setting. Another study also in the emergency department setting found that almost one-third (29.8%) of patients with chest radiographs interpreted as positive for pneumonia had subsequently negative CTs, and one-third (33.3%) of patients with radiographs interpreted as negative had subsequently positive CTs.[6]

These studies notwithstanding, the 2007 American Thoracic Society and Infectious Disease Society of America (ATS/IDSA) criteria state that a diagnosis of pneumonia requires a "demonstrable infiltrate by chest radiograph or other imaging technique."[7] The 2019 update to these criteria limits the discussion of pneumonia to "studies that used radiographic criteria for defining CAP, given the known inaccuracy of clinical signs and symptoms alone for CAP diagnosis."[8] British Thoracic Society guidelines recommend radiography in selected outpatients and all patients admitted with CAP.[9] Furthermore, the use of radiography leads to detection of many more cases of pneumonia than clinical judgment alone, with general practitioners' clinical judgment having a sensitivity of only 29% when compared with radiography in one study.[10] Diagnostic radiographs will therefore continue to be performed in this setting, and interpretations should be focused on optimizing the usefulness of these studies.

Clinical guidelines with respect to appropriate radiographic follow-up have varied, with some suggesting that all patients should have follow-up radiographs to establish "a new radiographic baseline,"[11] whereas others implying that radiographic follow-up was unnecessary for patients with a good clinical response to treatment.[12] Major reasons that have been proposed for radiographic follow-up include assessment for improvement, assessment for progression of disease and complications, and the exclusion of malignancy either masquerading as infection or as a cause of postobstructive infection. Lung cancer diagnoses, however, have been reported to be relatively uncommon after a diagnosis of pneumonia.[13,14] As a consequence, the current ATS/IDSA guidelines do not recommend routine follow-up, and the initial radiograph should be interpreted with attention to any findings for which follow-up should be recommended.

Chest radiography may be useful beyond the confirmation of possible infection. Updated ATS/IDSA guidelines give a strong recommendation for the use of the pneumonia severity index (PSI) to identify those patients in need of hospitalization.[8] This index is a scoring system that confers points for parameters on a large number of clinical and laboratory findings; unlike other less well-validated criteria used in assessment of pneumonia severity, PSI includes a radiographic parameter (the presence of a pleural effusion on imaging) as an indicator of severity.[15] The 2007 ATS/IDSA guidelines also set forth additional criteria for severe pneumonia to identify patients early who would ultimately require intensive care unit (ICU) admission, because delayed transfer to the ICU rather than direct ICU admission is associated with increased mortality.[7] In addition to clinical and laboratory values, these criteria include "multilobar infiltrates" as an indication of severe infection (**Fig. 1**). The 2019 ATS/IDSA guidelines expand the use of these criteria, so that the score on this assessment is now one indication for intensive investigation for infectious agents (including sputum gram stain and cultures, blood cultures, and urinary antigen tests for *Legionella* and *Streptococcus pneumoniae*) and in some circumstances the score may influence antibiotic choice (see article by Brixey and colleagues in this issue).[8] Radiography may also be useful to assess for complications of infection, particularly the presence of pleural fluid requiring drainage or the presence of hydropneumothorax.

RADIOGRAPHIC PATTERNS IN ACUTE INFECTION

Classically, the thoracic manifestations of pneumonia are divided into 3 distinct patterns: lobar (also known as focal or airspace) pneumonia, bronchopneumonia, and interstitial pneumonia.[16–18]

Lobar Pneumonia

Lobar or air-space pneumonia (**Fig. 2**) is probably the most familiar of the 3 radiographic patterns of pneumonia. This radiographic abnormality is classically confined to a portion of the lungs subtended by a single lobar or segmental bronchus

or group of segmental bronchi and therefore can be described as having an anatomic distribution. The radiographic appearance is a function of the pathophysiology: the acini are filled first with fluid, which spreads easily throughout the collateral ventilatory pathways in the lung, limited only by the pleura of the fissures. Fluid carries organisms throughout the involved portions of the lungs, spreading from the periphery to the more central portions. The large bronchi remain patent, resulting in an air bronchogram sign. Classically, this radiographic appearance is described in bacterial infections such as those caused by *S pneumoniae*, *Klebsiella pneumoniae*, and *Legionella pneumophila*.

Bronchopneumonia

The second radiographic pattern of pneumonia is the bronchopneumonia pattern (**Fig. 3**). This pattern is characterized by multifocal opacities, predominantly nodules, which tend to become confluent, producing areas of consolidation up to the size of a pulmonary segment. This pattern is thought to be caused by infection originating in the bronchi, with a robust immune response confining the infection to smaller regions of the lungs in the immediate peribronchial parenchyma. The result is a heterogeneous pattern, with areas of opacity interposed with areas of normally aerated lung. The infectious agents classically associated with this pattern include *Staphylococcus aureus*, *Haemophilus influenzae*, and anaerobic bacteria. Bronchopneumonia is the pattern classically associated with the development of pulmonary abscesses.

Interstitial Pneumonia

The third, most subtle, radiographic pattern is that of acute infectious interstitial pneumonia (**Fig. 4**). The primary radiographic features include diffuse reticular opacities corresponding to infection involving the bronchial and bronchiolar walls and

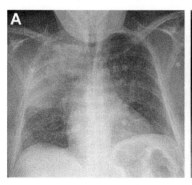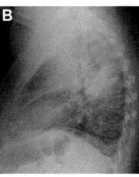

Fig. 1. Infection with findings of severity. Frontal (*A*) and lateral (*B*) views of the chest demonstrating multilobar pneumonia with opacities in the right upper and lower lobes and left lower lobe, and with small bilateral pleural effusions.

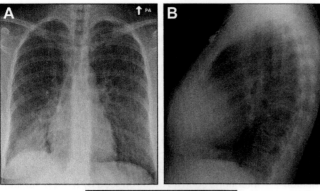

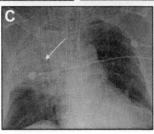

Fig. 2. Lobar pneumonia. (A, B) Opacity in a segmental distribution in the right lower lobe. Lateral radiograph shows faint opacity over the lower thoracic spine (spine sign). (C) Right upper lobar pneumonia with near-complete opacification of the right upper lobe with air bronchograms (yellow arrow).

the pulmonary interstitium; the alveoli are spared resulting in relatively little air-space abnormality. The acute interstitial pneumonia pattern is classically associated with *Mycoplasma*, *Pneumocystis jirovecii*, and a variety of viral pneumonias; due to the association with *Mycoplasma* infection, this radiographic pattern does not exclude bacterial pneumonia.

Limitations of the Pattern Approach

Although helpful conceptually in identifying pneumonia on chest radiography, these descriptions cannot reliably diagnose specific infectious pathogens and are therefore limited in directing management. There is little research on the correlation between patterns and infectious agents, perhaps at least in part due to infrequent isolation of a specific infectious pathogen. According to ATS/IDSA guidelines, outpatients and many inpatients who present with pulmonary opacities

and symptoms and signs of pulmonary infection are treated empirically rather than being investigated for specific agents.[8] In addition, sputum gram stains and cultures are notoriously often inadequate, with results commonly showing only upper airway flora. Patients are therefore more likely to receive a definitive diagnosis if they have urine antigen test results positive for *S pneumoniae* or *Legionella* or have positive cultures from bronchoscopy, blood, or pleural fluid specimens, leading to a biased distribution of patients who receive definitive diagnoses.

Studies attempting to establish correlations of patterns with agents have met with little success. A study of radiographs in 192 patients with hospital admissions for CAP showed very poor interreader agreement for radiographic pattern (with kappa < 0.4) among 2 radiologists and a pulmonary physician.[19] In this study *Mycoplasma pneumoniae* was not associated with an interstitial pattern (which was seldom described by the

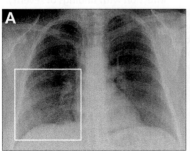

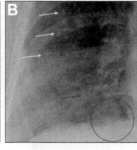

Fig. 3. Bronchopneumonia. (A) Nodular opacities with bronchial wall thickening and focal consolidative opacities in the right mid to lower lung, findings associated with bronchopneumonia. (B) Magnified right lower hemithorax (white box inset from A) highlighting the nodular opacities (yellow arrows), bronchial wall thickening (blue arrow), and developing confluent opacities (red circle).

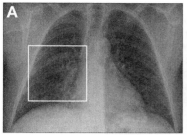
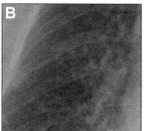
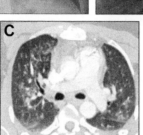

Fig. 4. Interstitial pneumonia. (*A*) Bilateral patchy peribronchovascular and reticular opacities representative of acute interstitial pneumonia. Magnified insert from (*A*) (*B*) and chest CT at the level of the pulmonary artery (*C*) highlight peribronchovascular and centrilobular nodular opacities with limited involvement of intervening parenchyma.

observers) but was associated with a "patchy alveolar pattern," and not a lobar pattern. In contrast, in another study of *M pneumoniae*, 48% of patients presented with a pattern of segmental or lobar consolidation.[20] Another study that looked at patients with *Chlamydia pneumoniae* and *S pneumoniae* infections found no radiographic features that distinguished between the 2 agents.[5] For this reason, identifying any possible infection rather than a particular pattern should be the goal of radiographic interpretation.

Principles guiding the interpretation of radiographs in suspected pneumonia are illustrated in a series of cases.

CASES
Case 1

A 50-year-old woman presented to the emergency department with cough and fever. A radiograph showed a moderately well-defined mass in the superior segment of the right lower lobe, measuring approximately 5 cm in diameter (**Fig. 5A**).

The radiograph was interpreted as suggestive of malignancy, and the patient's symptoms were attributed to an upper respiratory tract infection. The patient was therefore discharged from the emergency department with a recommendation for follow-up with her primary care provider; antibiotic treatment was not initiated. The patient, however, returned to the emergency department after 3 days with increasing respiratory symptoms. Repeat chest radiograph showed that the mass had nearly doubled in size and the margins were less well defined (**Fig. 5B**).

Diagnosis: Round Pneumonia

The diagnosis of round pneumonia should be considered in any patient who presents with a pulmonary mass at radiography and clinically with symptoms of respiratory tract infection; this is particularly true if the patient is at low risk for lung carcinoma, for example, a young, nonsmoker. If there is a recent normal chest radiograph, the finding of a new mass in a patient with clinical signs of infection is considered "virtually pathognomonic for round pneumonia."[21] Round pneumonia has classically been thought to occur primarily in children and attributed to incomplete development of collateral ventilation pathways. However, round pneumonia is also found occasionally in adults, where it is most commonly a manifestation of bacterial pneumonia, particularly streptococcal pneumonia.

Case 2

A 63-year-old male patient presented with nonproductive cough, and a chest radiograph demonstrated a right middle lobe opacity with mild volume loss (**Fig. 6A**). The patient was thought to have CAP based on the radiographic findings; however, 3 weeks after antibiotic treatment, the opacity was unchanged. The degree of middle lobe volume loss was less pronounced than is usually seen in nonobstructive middle lobe atelectasis, that is, middle lobe syndrome.[22] Chest CT was performed (**Fig. 6B**) and demonstrated a patent right middle lobe bronchus and air bronchograms, making postobstructive pneumonitis unlikely. The patient was subsequently referred

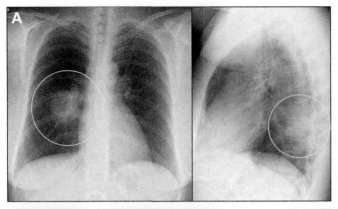

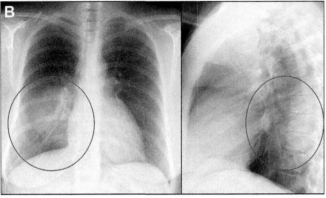

Fig. 5. Case 1. A 50-year-old woman with cough and fever. (*A*) Initial posteroanterior (PA) and lateral chest radiographs reveal mass in the superior segment of the right lower lobe (*yellow circle*). (*B*) Subsequent radiograph 3 days later demonstrates marked enlargement of the opacity.

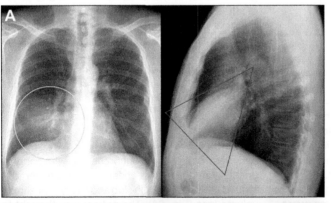

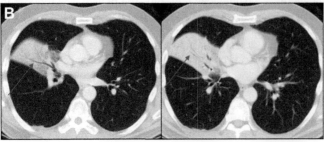

Fig. 6. Case 2. A 63-year-old male with nonproductive cough. (*A*) Initial diagnostic PA and lateral chest radiographs reveal right middle lobar opacity and mild volume loss (*yellow circle* and *blue triangle*). (*B*) Subsequent chest CT demonstrates consolidative opacities in the right middle lobe with patent right middle lobe bronchi and air bronchograms (*red arrows*).

for bronchoscopy for definitive diagnosis. Bronchioloalveolar lavage and biopsy were performed and yielded an atypical lymphoid infiltrate.

Diagnosis: Extranodal marginal B-cell lymphoma of mucosa-associated lymphoid tissue.

Current ATS guidelines do not call for routine radiographic follow-up for suspected infection, and current British Thoracic Society guidelines call for follow-up imaging only in patients with persistent symptoms at 6 weeks or those at high risk for malignancy. A survey of the Society of Thoracic Radiology membership indicated that thoracic radiology subspecialists were most influenced by the age of the patient and the appearance of the abnormality in deciding whether to recommend follow-up.[23] In addition, follow-up imaging or further investigation should be recommended when the clinical presentation is atypical. Any nonresolving area of pulmonary consolidation suggests a diagnosis other than CAP, and one of the major concerns is malignancy. "Air-space" opacities on radiographs may result from malignancy with postobstructive pneumonitis or from infiltrative neoplasms, such as adenocarcinoma with lepidic growth and lymphoproliferative disorders. Other possible causes of a nonresolving pulmonary opacity include postobstructive pneumonitis from benign processes including benign neoplasms and aspirated foreign bodies, atypical infections (such as mycobacterial infections, blastomycosis, or cryptococcosis), lipoid pneumonia, and inflammatory processes including organizing pneumonia and vasculitis. In all cases, detection depends on correlating with clinical presentation so that follow-up imaging or more careful immediate investigation is performed.

Case 3

A 72-year-old man who was visiting the United States from his home in Nigeria presented with fever, nausea, and vomiting. A chest radiograph was performed, which showed a masslike area of consolidation with cavitation in the anterior segment of the left upper lobe (Fig. 7). An initial diagnosis of pneumonia was made, possibly related to aspiration, given the history of vomiting; however, there was no report of acute cough or sputum production.

The differential diagnosis for cavitary disease does include a wide array of bacterial infections including multiple streptococcal species and *K pneumoniae*[24] sometimes in the form of a cavitary mass or abscess. Additional differential diagnoses include noninfectious diseases such as granulomatosis with polyangiitis and malignancy. The finding of cavitation in the mid and upper lung zones should also raise the possibility of tuberculosis; this is particularly true in any patient who, as in this case, has risk factors such as time spent in an endemic region, and in a patient without acute respiratory symptoms.

Diagnosis: Postprimary Tuberculosis

Tuberculosis is not a common disease in the United States. However, in 2019 it remained the leading cause of infectious disease death among adults worldwide, with the World Health Organization estimating that there were 10 million new cases that year.[25] Tuberculosis is most prevalent in Southeast Asia and Africa, and the 20 countries with the highest disease burden, predominantly in Asia and Africa, accounted for 84% of cases in 2019 (see articles by Teo and colleagues and Ryzdak and colleagues in this issue). In patients without travel history outside the United States, residence in communal living facilities, such as homeless shelters, nursing homes, and prisons, is also a risk factor for tuberculosis.

Approximately 90% of patients with an initial tuberculosis infection have an immune response that sequesters the disease such that it never becomes symptomatic, resulting in "latent" tuberculosis. Almost 5% of patients will have an initial uncontained infection, or "primary tuberculosis," and another 5% will initially contain the infection but will later develop active "postprimary tuberculosis."[26] These patients classically develop cavitary disease in the apical and posterior segments of the upper lobes and the superior segments of the lower lobes, possibly because of high oxygen tension and poor lymphatic drainage in those regions. However, the absence of cavitation should not cause a radiologist to exclude tuberculosis. Cavitation is only seen in roughly 20% to 45% of radiographs of patients with active postprimary tuberculosis.[26] In an appropriate clinical setting, any upper lobe opacities should suggest the possibility of tuberculosis. CT increases the sensitivity for the detection of cavitation, identifying smaller and more subtle cavities, but cavitation is still not seen in all patients with active postprimary disease.

In the United States, nontuberculous mycobacterial infection is substantially more common than tuberculosis. Nontuberculous mycobacterial infection has a variety of radiographic presentations, including the "classic" presentation, described as a mimic of tuberculosis, presenting with apical, frequently cavitary, opacities.[26] This manifestation of nontuberculous mycobacterial infection is usually seen in older patients,

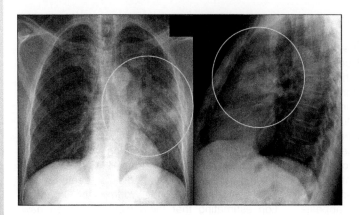

Fig. 7. Case 3. A 72-year-old Nigerian man visiting the United States, with fever, nausea, and vomiting. PA and lateral chest radiographs reveal masslike consolidation with cavitation in the left upper lobe (*yellow circles*).

predominantly those with chronic obstructive pulmonary disease and should be considered in a patient from the United States with radiographic findings like those illustrated in this case.

Case 4

A 19-year-old male presented with symptoms of cough and fever. A chest radiograph (**Fig. 8**) demonstrates opacities in the right mid and lower lung zones with minimal blunting of the right costophrenic angle suggesting a small pleural effusion. These findings in isolation would be consistent with CAP with parapneumonic effusion; however, additional findings include a right paratracheal opacity and enlargement of the right hilum, suggesting lymphadenopathy (see **Fig. 8**, arrows). Radiographically evident lymphadenopathy in the setting of lung opacities should lead to

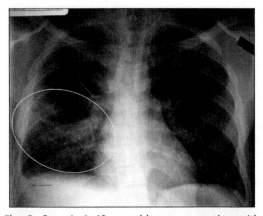

Fig. 8. Case 4. A 19-year-old man presenting with cough and fever. Chest radiograph demonstrates right mid to lower lung heterogeneous opacities (*yellow oval*) with a small right pleural effusion (*blue arrow*). Additional right paratracheal opacities and right hilar enlargement (*red arrows*) are evident.

investigation for diseases other than bacterial pneumonia, including malignancy and primary tuberculosis.

Diagnosis: Primary Tuberculosis

Hilar and mediastinal lymph nodes may be enlarged in the setting of infection, but studies in *S pneumoniae* infection and in bacterial empyema demonstrate only mild lymph node enlargement at CT in this setting,[27–29] in keeping with conventional wisdom that lymph nodes that are sufficiently enlarged that they are evident on radiographs are rare in conventional bacterial pneumonia. The differential diagnosis for radiographically evident lymphadenopathy in the setting of acute infection includes infection by atypical pathogens, including fungal infections. Another potential consideration is acute infection in the setting of an underlying disease, such as neoplasm or sarcoidosis. Neoplasm is also a differential consideration for pulmonary opacities with lymphadenopathy, particularly lymphoma in a young patient such as this one, and also lung carcinoma.

Tuberculosis initially infects the lungs by inhalation of droplet particles, which do not have a strong predilection for specific pulmonary zones but may cause lower lung infection because they are relatively heavy. Primary tuberculosis generally causes nonspecific radiographic opacities that usually are not cavitary and enlargement of ipsilateral hilar and mediastinal lymph nodes, which at CT have low attenuation centrally due to caseation necrosis. These findings usually heal over time as a result of host immune response, frequently although not always leaving calcified nodules and/or calcifications in hilar and mediastinal lymph nodes.

In approximately 5% of patients, the primary infection is not contained; these patients are considered to have progressive primary

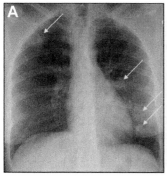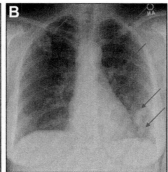

Fig. 9. Case 5. Young woman with fever. (*A*) Initial chest radiograph depicts bilateral nodular opacities (*yellow arrows*) suggesting multifocal community-acquired pneumonia. (*B*) Subsequent chest radiograph 5 days later shows increasing size and number of nodular opacities (*blue arrows*) with more definite cavitation of the right upper lobar nodule (*red arrow*).

tuberculosis. Primary tuberculosis has historically been a disease of children, but in the developed world because tuberculosis is less prevalent, it is now the pattern seen in approximately 23% to 34% of cases of tuberculosis in adults.[26]

Case 5

A young woman presented to the emergency department with fever. Clinically, the patient had an acute onset of infectious symptoms, and a radiograph was performed (**Fig. 9**A), which demonstrated bilateral pulmonary opacities. A diagnosis of pulmonary infection was suggested, and the patient was discharged from the emergency department with a prescription for oral antibiotics.

Closer review of the radiograph reveals that the opacities represent scattered bilateral pulmonary nodules, measuring between a centimeter and approximately 3 cm in diameter. Potential causes of multiple pulmonary nodules include metastases; sarcoidosis; vasculitides, particularly granulomatosis with polyangiitis; rheumatoid arthritis; and a few infections. Fungal infections may present with multiple pulmonary nodules; those that are most likely to present this way would be coccidioidomycosis or paracoccidioidomycosis in patients with appropriate travel history or opportunistic fungi such as aspergillosis in immunocompromised patients. In an immunocompetent patient, a common infectious cause of multiple nodules is hematogenous spread of bacterial infection, or septic emboli.

Diagnosis: Pulmonary Septic Emboli

This patient returned to the emergency department 5 days later, and, as demonstrated in **Fig. 9**B, the nodules had increased in size and number with a more evident area of cavitation in the nodule at the right lung apex. These findings are consistent with evolution of pulmonary septic emboli. The patient was found to be bacteremic and required intravenous antibiotics as well as echocardiography to exclude endocarditis.

Septic embolism is commonly thought of as occurring in patients with a history of intravenous drug abuse but has also been described in patients with septic thrombophlebitis, classically in the internal jugular vein (Lemierre syndrome); indwelling catheters and other hardware; and other infections, including periodontal infections, pyomyositis, sinusitis and orbital abscess, and abdominal infections.[30] These are severe infections with a reported mortality in some series of approximately 10%. A growing clinical concern is septic emboli from community-acquired infections with methicillin-resistant *S aureus*.

SUMMARY

In conclusion, chest radiography for the investigation of possible CAP remains a common part of radiologic practice. Given this, even in a setting apart from the COVID-19 pandemic, the radiologist can contribute to the care of these patients beyond the simple identification of lobar pneumonia. Radiographs should always be interpreted in light of the clinical setting; subtle findings may correlate with acute interstitial or bronchopneumonia patterns in patients with infectious symptoms, and a masslike presentation that may suggest neoplasm to the untrained observer may also raise the possibility of acute infection. The radiologist should assess for pleural fluid and multilobar involvement, because these may affect clinical decisions about hospital and ICU admission and microbiologic assessment. In contrast, alternative diagnoses should always be considered in patients with a clinical presentation that is discordant from the radiographic finding of apparent pneumonia, at least with follow-up to assess for resolution. When upper lobe cavitation is present, further investigation for tuberculosis should ensue if the onset of symptoms is not acute. Lymphadenopathy evident on a radiograph or multiple pulmonary nodules, particularly when cavitary, should always suggest additional clinical evaluation rather than empirical treatment of CAP. Keeping these principles in mind will allow the radiologist to be a valuable contributor to patient care in the setting of suspected CAP.

CLINICS CARE POINTS

- Chest radiographs in patients with clinical signs and symptoms of pneumonia should be assessed for subtle bronchopneumonia and interstitial patterns of infection and masslike "round pneumonia" in addition to more classic lobar or segmental pneumonia patterns.

- When pneumonia is diagnosed on chest radiographs, reports should always describe pleural fluid and multilobar involvement if present, as these findings may alter management.

- If pneumonia is suspected in patients without classic clinical signs and symptoms of pneumonia, follow-up radiographs should be recommended to confirm the diagnosis based on treatment response and exclude an alternative or underlying process.

- When lymphadenopathy is evident on chest radiographs, atypical infections or neoplasm should be considered as possible diagnoses and, if no immediate further investigation is planned, follow-up radiographs should be obtained.

- If multiple pulmonary nodules are seen in a patient with symptoms of acute respiratory infection, there is a broad differential diagnosis, but septic emboli should be considered.

- Predominantly upper lobe opacities and indolent or subacute presentation should raise the possibility of tuberculosis or nontuberculous mycobacterial infection, particularly when cavitation is present.

DISCLOSURE

None of the authors has a relationship with a commercial company that has a direct financial interest in the subject matter or materials discussed in this article, or with a company making a competing product.

REFERENCES

1. Torres A, Cilloniz C, Niederman MS, et al. Pneumonia. Nat Rev Dis Prim 2021. https://doi.org/10.1038/s41572-021-00259-0.

2. Cao AMY, Choy JP, Mohanakrishnan LN, et al. Chest radiographs for acute lower respiratory tract infections. Cochrane Database Syst Rev 2013;2013(12). https://doi.org/10.1002/14651858.CD009119.pub2.

3. Aagaard E, Maselli J, Gonzales R. Physician practice patterns: chest x-ray ordering for the evaluation of acute cough illness in adults. Med Decis Making 2006;26(6):599–605.

4. Basi SK, Marrie TJ, Huang JQ, et al. Patients admitted to hospital with suspected pneumonia and normal chest radiographs: Epidemiology, microbiology, and outcomes. Am J Med 2004;117(5):305–11.

5. Self WH, Courtney DM, McNaughton CD, et al. High discordance of chest x-ray and computed tomography for detection of pulmonary opacities in ED patients: Implications for diagnosing pneumonia. Am J Emerg Med 2013;31(2):401–5.

6. Claessens Y, Debray M, Tubach F, et al. Early Chest Computed Tomography Scan to Assist Diagnosis and Guide Treatment Decision for Suspected Community-acquired Pneumonia. Am J Respir Crit Care Med 2015;192(8):974–82.

7. Mandell LA, Wunderink RG, Anzueto A, et al. Infectious Diseases Society of America/American Thoracic Society Consensus Guidelines on the management of community-acquired pneumonia in adults. Clin Infect Dis 2007;44(SUPPL. 2).

8. Metlay JP, Waterer GW, Long AC, et al. American thoracic society documents Diagnosis and Treatment of Adults with Community-acquired Pneumonia. Am J Respir Crit Care Med 2019;200(7). https://doi.org/10.1164/rccm.201908-1581ST.

9. Lim W, Baudouin S, George R, et al. BTS guidelines for the management of community acquired pneumonia in adults: update 2009. Thorax 2009;64(Suppl 3). https://doi.org/10.1136/THX.2009.121434.

10. Van Vugt SF, Verheij TJM, De Jong PA, et al. Diagnosing pneumonia in patients with acute cough: Clinical judgment compared to chest radiography. Eur Respir J 2013;42(4):1076–82.

11. Niederman M, Mandell L, Anzueto A, et al. Guidelines for the management of adults with community-acquired pneumonia. Diagnosis, assessment of severity, antimicrobial therapy, and prevention. Am J Respir Crit Care Med 2001;163(7):1730–54.

12. Bartlett J, Dowell S, Mandell L, et al. Practice guidelines for the management of community-acquired pneumonia in adults. Infectious Diseases Society of America. Clin Infect Dis 2000;31(2):347–82.

13. Tang KL, Eurich DT, Minhas-Sandhu JK, et al. Incidence, correlates,and chest radiographic yield of

new lung cancer diagnosis in 3398 patients with pneumonia. Arch Intern Med 2011;171(13):1193–8.

14. Macdonald C, Jayathissa S, Leadbetter M. Is post-pneumonia chest X-ray for lung malignancy useful? Results of an audit of current practice. Intern Med J 2015;45(3):329–34.

15. Fine MJ, Auble TE, Yealy DM, et al. A prediction rule to identify low-risk patients with community-acquired pneumonia. Pneumologie 1997;51(8):834.

16. Hansell DM, McAdams HP. Imaging of diseases of the chest. Mosby, 2010; 2010 [Edinburgh?]

17. Fraser RS, Muller NL, Colman N, et al. Fraser and Paré's diagnosis of diseases of the chest. 4th edition. Philadelphia: Saunders, c1999; 1999.

18. Gharib AM, Stern EJ. Radiology of pneumonia. Med Clin North Am 2001;85(6):1461–91.

19. Boersma WG, Daniels JMA, Löwenberg A, et al. Reliability of radiographic findings and the relation to etiologic agents in community-acquired pneumonia. Respir Med 2006;100(5):926–32.

20. Putman CE, Curtis AM, Simeone JF, et al. Mycoplasma pneumonia. Clinical and roentgenographic patterns. Amerjroentgenol 1975;124(3):417–22.

21. Durning SJ, Sweet JM, Chambers SL. Pulmonary Mass in Tachypneic, Febrile Adult*. Chest 2003; 124(1):372–5.

22. Gudbjartsson T, Gudmundsson G. Middle lobe syndrome: a review of clinicopathological features, diagnosis and treatment. Respiration 2012;84(1):80–6.

23. Humphrey K, Gilman M, Little B, et al. Radiographic follow-up of suspected pneumonia: survey of Society of Thoracic Radiology membership. J Thorac Imaging 2013;28(4):240–3.

24. Gafoor K, Patel S, Girvin F, et al. Cavitary Lung Diseases: A Clinical-Radiologic Algorithmic Approach. Chest 2018;153(6):1443–65.

25. World Health Organization. GLOBAL TUBERCULOSIS REPORT 2020. Published online 2020.

26. Nachiappan A, Rahbar K, Shi X, et al. Pulmonary Tuberculosis: Role of Radiology in Diagnosis and Management. Radiographics 2017;37(1):52–72.

27. Haramati L, Alterman D, White C, et al. Intrathoracic lymphadenopathy in patients with empyema. J Comput Assist Tomogr 1997;21(4):608–11.

28. Stein DL, Haramati LB, Spindola-Franco H, et al. Intrathoracic lymphadenopathy in hospitalized patients with pneumococcal pneumonia. Chest 2005; 127(4):1271–5.

29. Chopra A, Modi A, Chaudhry H, et al. Assessment of Mediastinal Lymph Node Size in Pneumococcal Pneumonia with Bacteremia. Lung 2018;196(1): 43–8.

30. Ye R, Zhao L, Wang C, et al. Clinical characteristics of septic pulmonary embolism in adults: A systematic review. Respir Med 2014;108(1):1–8.

Viral Pneumonias

Jennifer Febbo, MD[a],*, Jonathan Revels, DO[a], Loren Ketai, MD[b]

KEYWORDS

- Viral pneumonia • Tomography x- ray computed • Community-acquired infections
- Immunocompromised hosts

KEY POINTS

- Radiologic findings of influenza usually appear as bronchiolitis, bronchopneumonia, or manifestations of airway-centric infection. H1N1 influenza may have a similar appearance but can also cause an organizing pneumonia pattern.
- The respiratory syncytial virus, parainfluenza virus, and human metapneumovirus have a predilection for airway-centric infection. They usually cause mild symptoms in immunocompetent adults but more likely to cause bronchopneumonia in immunocompromised patients.
- Adenovirus causes nonsegmental consolidation, particularly in the setting of outbreaks of novel serotypes. In the setting of other viral lower respiratory tract infections, lobar consolidation usually suggests bacterial superinfection.
- Cytomegalic virus (CMV) and herpes simplex virus in the respiratory tract of hospitalized patients represent reactivation of latent infection, which is not always pathogenic. When pathogenic, such as in the setting of lung transplants, CMV often causes ground-glass opacities and micronodules.

INTRODUCTION

Viral pneumonia upended the world in 1918 and again in 2020, but it has also been a major source of respiratory illness in the intervening century. More than 200 species of virus are capable of infecting humans and 3 to 4 new human viruses are discovered each year.[1] A handful of these viruses infect the lower respiratory tract, causing significant morbidity and mortality among humans and resulting in over \$6.4 billion in hospital stays.[2] Although many pathogens causing community-acquired pneumonias still go undiagnosed, the development of real-time polymerase chain reactions (PCRs) for numerous respiratory viruses has dramatically increased the documentation of viral pneumonias over the last 2 decades.[3] Recognition of radiologic features that prompt testing for viral pathogens could reduce the use of unnecessary antibiotics, and in selected cases prompt institution of antiviral agents.[4,5]

Most viral pneumonias are community-acquired; however, a few are associated with health care settings. Immunocompromised patients are often infected with these community-acquired viruses, but are at greater risk of severe infection, including with those which are typically indolent. This article will review the imaging of community-acquired and health care–associated viral pneumonia, as well as viral pneumonia in the immunocompromised host. COVID-19 is specifically discussed by Sing and colleagues elsewhere in this issue.

COMMUNITY-ACQUIRED VIRAL PNEUMONIA

The overwhelming majority of viral pneumonias are community acquired. Some of these viruses, such as RSV and parainfluenza, are acquired as children and result in mild, self-limited illness. Among adults with pneumonia in whom a pathogen can be detected, viruses are the primary or coinfecting

[a] University of New Mexico, 2211 Lomas Boulevard NE, Albuquerque, NM 87106, USA; [b] Department of Radiology, MSC 10 5530, 1 University of New Mexico, Albuquerque, NM 87131-0001, USA
* Corresponding author.
E-mail address: jfebbo@salud.unm.edu

Radiol Clin N Am 60 (2022) 383–397
https://doi.org/10.1016/j.rcl.2022.01.010
0033-8389/22/© 2022 Elsevier Inc. All rights reserved.

pathogen in 26% of cases requiring hospitalization.[4] Immunocompetent patients requiring hospitalization are generally elderly and often have underlying conditions such as chronic obstructive pulmonary disease (COPD).[5] The main pathogens comprising community-acquired viral pneumonia are influenza, human metapneumovirus (HMPV), respiratory syncytial virus (RSV), adenovirus, and rhinovirus. Hantavirus pulmonary infections are much less common, but are clinically important because they can cause severe, often fatal, respiratory failure in otherwise healthy, young adults.

INFLUENZA

Before the COIVD-19 pandemic, influenza was the principal cause of severe viral pneumonia in the world. Influenza can be broadly categorized into one of the multiple groups (A, B, C, or D), influenza A is most predominant.[6] In the United States, between the years 2010 and 2018, 4 to 23 million medical visits and 12,000 to 79,000 deaths occurred each year due to influenza.[7] Cases decreased dramatically in 2020 likely due to personal public health measures (eg, mask wearing) and reduced medical office visits instituted to minimize the spread of COVID-19.[8]

Most patients with influenza experience a self-limited upper respiratory infection of the airways, which only occasionally progresses to the lower respiratory tract.[6,9,10] Influenza pneumonia is typically mild, but in pregnant patients,[11] elderly patients, and/or those with chronic underlying disease, such as heart failure or COPD, the pneumonia can be severe and sometimes fatal.[10,12,13]

Influenza is predominantly an airway-centric infection and imaging manifestations often reflect this (Table 1). In severe infections, however, diffuse disease can obscure the underlying airway findings. Radiographs typically demonstrate ill-defined reticulonodular opacities in a central distribution (in contrast to peripheral/subpleural reticular opacities seen in edema), reflecting the airway-centric process. Less commonly, radiographs can also show multifocal consolidation. On computed tomography (CT), features of bronchitis (bronchial wall thickening) and bronchiolitis (tree-in-bud opacities) may be present[6,9] (Fig. 1). When airspace opacities occur, ground-glass opacities and multifocal consolidation are more common than localized consolidation, and often occur in a peribronchial distribution[9] (Figs. 2 and 3). Pleural effusions are rarely seen in the pneumonias caused by influenza as the sole pathogen.[6,9] Secondary infections are common in severe cases of influenza, and are suggested by radiological features such as focal lobar consolidation or worsening opacities following initial improvement.[6,9] In a series of patients accrued before 2009, diffuse airspace disease was only rarely caused by influenza and was more typical of bacterial pneumonia.[9] Acute respiratory distress syndrome (ARDS), however, is seen in other variants of influenza (see below, H1N1).

New strains arise as influenza viruses circulate in swine, birds, and humans, and genetic reassortment occurs between viruses from different animals.[14] One such reassortment resulted in the swine-origin H1N1 pandemic in 2009. This influenza A subtype was classified as H1N1 based on the surface glycoproteins hemagglutinin (H) and neuraminidase (N), which promote propagation of the virus into lower respiratory tract cells.[14] Similar to seasonal influenza infections, most patients experienced an uncomplicated clinical course, but a small percentage of patients developed severe respiratory distress.[15] Although the overall mortality from H1N1 influenza was not increased markedly compared with circulating strains, there was a dramatic shift in mortality toward younger patients, such that 87% of fatalities occurred in patients younger than 65 years.[16]

Although radiographs in swine-origin H1N1 infections are usually normal. Chest radiographs and CTs in swine-origin H1N1 that progresses to pneumonia often include features of consolidation within multiple lobes, with lower lobe predominance.[17] H1N1 can also result in an organizing pneumonia pattern, with peribronchovascular and peripheral/subpleural ground-glass opacities and consolidation[18,19] (Fig. 4). Finally, H1N1 can progress to ARDS (Fig. 5). Compared with ARDS by other types of severe community-acquired pneumonia, H1N1-related ARDS may lead to worse oxygen exchange and increased use of extracorporeal membrane oxygenation.[20]

Some animal-origin influenza viruses can replicate in human cells but have not yet acquired genetic constituents that enable efficient human-to-human transmission. Two such viruses include H5N1 and H7N9 influenza. Together, over 2,000 human infections have been reported with these organisms, accompanied by a high mortality rate.[21] Reports of imaging are limited to very small series. In general consolidation and ground-glass opacities were multifocal at the time at initial imaging and commonly progressed to bilateral disease within several days.[22,23] Pleural effusions were reported to be more frequent in H5N1 than usually seen in human influenza, but remained rare in H7N9 influenza. Occasional pneumatoceles and cavities were also reported with H5N1 pneumonia.[22]

Table 1
Imaging patterns of viral pneumonia by etiology

	Diffuse Ground Glass	Consolidation—Not Bronchocentric	Consolidation—Bronchocentric	Organizing Pneumonia	Tree-In-Bud Micronodules	Micronodules, Not Tree-In-Bud	Linear/Interstitial
Seasonal influenza	+	+	++		++	+	
H1N1	++	+	++	++	+	+	
Adenovirus	+	+++	+		+	+	
HMPV	+		+		+++	+	
RSV	+		+		+++	+	
Parainfluenza	+		++		+++	+	
Hantavirus	+++	++					+++
HSV	++		++			+	+
CMV	+++	++	+		+	++	
VZV	+	+				+++	

Increasing + indicates increasing relative frequency of the associated pattern. The purpose of this table is to indicate general trends; the absence of a + is not to suggest a complete absence of this finding on all imaging.

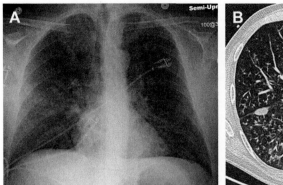
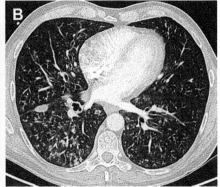

Fig. 1. Influenza B in a 60-year-old man. (*A*) Frontal chest radiograph demonstrates perihilar-predominant bilateral reticulonodular opacities with bronchial wall thickening. (*B*) Axial chest CT shows extensive bilateral centrilobular nodules, including tree-in-bud distribution, and bronchial wall thickening indicating bronchiolitis and bronchitis, airway-centric disease. Incidental focal fluid within the right major fissure.

Testing for influenza can be performed by a variety of means including nasal swab, respiratory aspirate, or respiratory lavage. The rapid influenza detection method can return results in less than 15 minutes, has a high specificity for the detection of influenza (>98%), but the sensitivity ranges between 50% and 70%.[7] Reverse transcription–polymerase chain reaction (RT-PCR) has a higher sensitivity for detection of influenza and it should be performed in cases where there is clinical suspicion for influenza infection but a negative rapid test.[7] Viral cultures may be performed when there is clinical concern for possible drug resistance or a variant influenza that may be related to an emerging pandemic.[7]

Treatment of seasonal influenza with one of four antiviral medications: oseltamivir, peramivir, baloxavir, or zanamivir is recommended within 24 to 48 hours of the onset of symptoms.[23,24] Oseltamivir or zanamivir are used in the treatment of swine-origin H1N1 influenza.[23]

ADENOVIRUS

Adenovirus is spread through fecal-oral route in children and aerosolized droplets among adults. Its overall incidence peaks in summer months; however, epidemics are typically seen in winter or early spring.[25–27] Most adenovirus infections (80%) that occur in children are mild; however, pneumonia can occur in up to 20% of infants.[27]. Among immunocompetent adults, lower respiratory tract infections occur in small epidemic outbreaks within closely confined groups of adults such as within the military. There are numerous serotypes of adenovirus, with serotypes −1 through 7, −21, and −14 responsible for most febrile respiratory illnesses in adults. Serotype 14, one of the newer serotypes to affect North America manifested as a military base outbreak of pneumonia in 2006. Likely abetted by limited humoral immunity in the populace, the serotype rapidly spread to over 15 states by 2007.[27].

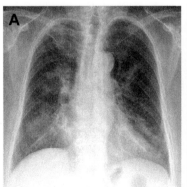
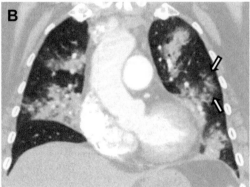

Fig. 2. Influenza A in a 73-year-old woman. (*A*) Frontal chest radiograph shows bilateral centrally distributed hazy opacities. (*B*) Coronal chest CT demonstrates bilateral peribronchovascular consolidation consistent with bronchopneumonia. There are also small acinar nodules in the left upper lobe (*arrows*).

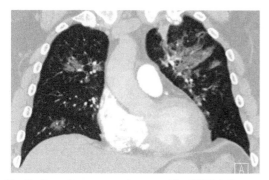

Fig. 3. Bronchopneumonia caused by H3N1 influenza A in a 66-year-old man. Coronal chest CT demonstrates bilateral peribronchovascular ground-glass opacities with interlobular septal thickening.

Chest radiographs of adenovirus pneumonia are similar to nonviral community-acquired pneumonia, and are less likely to produce a dominant airway centric pattern compared with the virus described in the next section. Radiographs may show unilateral or bilateral consolidation, and patchy hazy opacities.[28,29] On chest CT, most patients demonstrate unilateral or bilateral consolidation[9,29,30] (**Fig. 6**). Patchy ground-glass opacities are less common and nodules are infrequent. Although pleural effusions are uncommon on chest radiographs, they have been seen on CT in up to three-fourths of patients.[30] Lymphadenopathy is seen in approximately one-third of patients who undergo CT scanning.

Diagnosis of adenovirus pneumonia can be achieved through PCR, immunohistochemical staining, or culture of bronchoalveolar lavage (BAL) fluid. Outbreaks of adenovirus pneumonia have led to oral immunization against adenovirus by the military; however, immunization is not currently available for civilians. There is no specific antiviral drug approved to target adenovirus. As adenovirus is a DNA virus, some patients with severe pneumonia are treated with cidofovir, an antiviral agent that inhibits DNA polymerase.[27]

HMPV, RSV, AND PARAINFLUENZA

RSV and parainfluenza virus have long been recognized as causing lower respiratory tract infections. HMPV is a relatively newly discovered pathogen, first classified as a paramyxovirus in 2001. More recently, HMPV and RSV have been moved to the family Pneumoviridae. Nevertheless, both share many characteristics with parainfluenza virus, particularly the propensity for airway infection.[6,31,32] These viruses are typically acquired as children; however, reactivation or reinfection can occur in adulthood secondary to waning immunity.[5] HMPV, RSV, and parainfluenza viruses have been detected in 4%, 3%, and 2% of hospitalized adults with community-acquired pneumonia, respectively.[4]

Among immunocompromised hosts, these viruses are important pathogens. Infections occur in 5% to 10% of hematopoietic stem cell transplant (HSCT) and transplant patients in the first 100 days posttransplant, and affect the lower tract in approximately 5% to 50% of these cases.[33,34] RSV, HMPV, and parainfluenza can all result in rapidly fatal pneumonia in immunocompromised patients.[5,6,25,32,35]

HMPV, RSV, and parainfluenza pulmonary infections have a propensity for airway-centric involvement secondary to preferential infection of ciliated respiratory epithelial cells.[31] Airway centric infection manifests as centrilobular nodules with and without tree-in-bud configuration, bronchial wall thickening, and as peribronchiolar

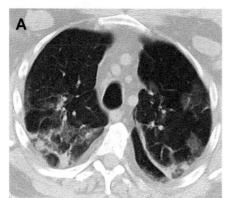
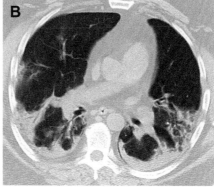

Fig. 4. H1N1 in a 44-year-old man. (A, B) Axial chest CT images show bilateral peribronchovascular and peripheral ground-glass opacities and consolidation in an organizing pneumonia pattern.

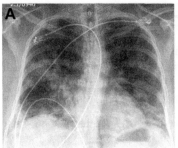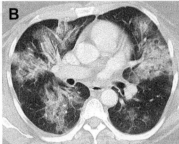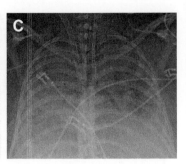

Fig. 5. Forty-three-year-old otherwise healthy woman with H1N1 infection demonstrating progression from bronchopneumonia to ARDS. (A) Initial frontal chest radiograph demonstrates bilateral hazy perihilar and basilar airspace opacities. (B) Axial chest CT on the same day shows bilateral peribronchovascular ground-glass opacities, with areas of interlobular septal thickening. (C) Frontal chest radiograph 11 days later shows near-complete opacification of both lungs and an extracorporeal membrane oxygenation (ECMO) catheter.

ground-glass opacities or consolidation[6,9,31,34,36] (Figs. 7–9). In a retrospective evaluation of 100 (both immunocompetent and immunocompromised) patients diagnosed with HMPV, the most commonly observed radiographic abnormality was bilateral, peribronchovascular airspace opacities.[32] CTs were performed only a minority of the cohort, most commonly demonstrating bilateral, ground-glass opacities. Centrilobular nodules were present in slightly less than half of these patients.[32] Although findings of small airway disease can be obscured in cases of extensive pneumonia in immunocompromised hosts, in a small series of patients with either HSCT or lung transplant, small nodules or tree in bud opacities were still observed on CTs in more than a third of patients.[37]

Most CT findings of RSV and parainfluenza are similar to those seen with HMPV. Both demonstrate tree-in-bud opacities and bronchial wall thickening on CT in most patients.[38] Ground-glass opacities or consolidation are seen in one-fourth to one-third of patients.[9] Parainfluenza may be more likely than RSV to cause patchy basilar multifocal consolidation.[39] Pleural effusions occasionally occur in RSV pneumonia, which differs from parainfluenza and HMPV pneumonia in which associated effusions are rare.[6,9]

Imaging cannot confidently differentiate HMPV, RSV, and parainfluenza pneumonias from other common community-acquired pathogens causing airway centric infections, such as mycoplasma or Hemophilus influenza (Fig. 10). In addition, HMPV can cause nodular consolidation in

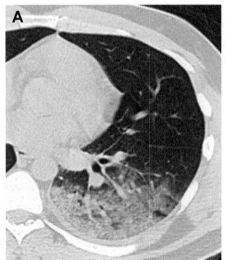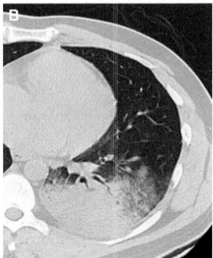

Fig. 6. Adenovirus in an otherwise healthy man in his early 20s. (A, B) Axial chest CT images demonstrate focal left lower lobe mixed consolidation and ground-glass opacities.

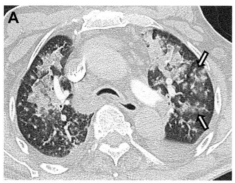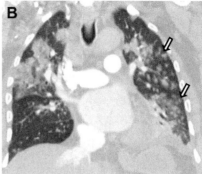

Fig. 7. Human metapneumovirus in a 63-year-old man. (*A*) Axial and (*B*) coronal chest CT images demonstrate bilateral peribronchovascular consolidation and ground-glass opacities indicative of bronchopneumonia. Centrilobular nodules (*arrows*) are also consistent with airway-centric disease. Incidental note of probable tracheomalacia on (*A*).

approximately a third of cases, a feature more often considered to be associated with bacterial pneumonia.[32] Accordingly, specific diagnosis of these airway-centric infections is usually based on RT-PCR or serology. Therapy in symptomatic adults is supportive as there are no current targeted therapies.[5]

RHINOVIRUS

Rhinovirus, a primary respiratory-tract pathogen, which peaks in incidence in summer and fall, is best known for causing, "the common cold," a syndrome of upper respiratory symptoms including rhinorrhea and cough.[40,41] In addition, rhinovirus is increasingly recognized as a cause of community-acquired pneumonia, albeit more frequently among immunocompromised than immunocompetent patients. In the former, it may be more common than the airway-centric viruses (eg, RSV, HMPV) infections described earlier. Coinfections with other viruses or with bacterial pathogens are common in both patient groups.[40,42]

There are relatively few studies depicting the radiologic appearance of rhinovirus pneumonia. A selected series of patients in which BAL was performed, focused predominantly on immunocompromised patients. Imaging demonstrated bilateral opacities in most cases, approximately half of which were predominantly peribronchial.[42] Nodules were also present, but were less common (**Fig. 11**). Mortality from rhinovirus-associated pneumonia and influenza pneumonia were similar in this cohort. In general, however, in the absence of bacterial coinfection, rhinovirus may be less likely to cause severe symptoms than the viruses discussed earlier. This observation and the current lack of an effective antiviral agent targeting rhinovirus render its detection of uncertain clinical importance. Treatment is currently supportive or should be directed at the copathogen.

HANTAVIRUS

Hantavirus is a potential cause for fulminant pneumonia in an otherwise healthy adult with a relevant environmental exposure. It is a zoonotic infection acquired through inhaling aerosolized rodent excreta. "New World" hantaviruses have resulted in several small outbreaks in the western United States, the first in the Four Corners area in

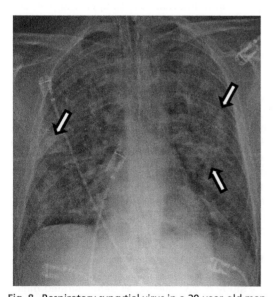

Fig. 8. Respiratory syncytial virus in a 29-year-old man with acute myelogenous leukemia status poststem cell transplant. Frontal chest radiograph demonstrates bilateral reticulonodular opacities and bronchial wall thickening compatible suggesting bronchiolitis and bronchitis. There are more focal airspace opacities in the right mid and lower lung, and left perihilar lung (*arrows*) likely representing associated pneumonia.

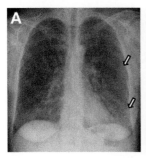 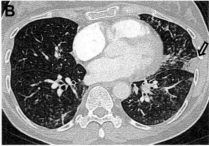 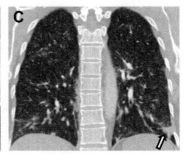

Fig. 9. Parainfluenza in a 61-year-old woman with multiple myeloma on chemotherapy. (*A*) Frontal chest radiograph shows bronchial wall thickening central reticulonodular opacities. There are also patchy airspace opacities in the left mid and lower lung (*arrows*). (*B*) Axial and (*C*) coronal CT images demonstrate bilateral solid and ground-glass centrilobular nodules, as well as localized consolidation in the lingula and left lower lobe (*arrow*).

1993.[43,44] (In contrast to New World hantaviruses, "Old World" viruses in Asia and Europe and most commonly result in hemorrhagic fever with renal syndrome.). In North and South America, New World hantavirus can manifest as cardiovascular and respiratory failure referred to as Hantavirus Pulmonary Syndrome (HPS). In these patients, hantavirus directly infects lung endothelial cells and macrophages, which leads to extensive pulmonary edema and shock.[43]

Radiologically, HPS may mimic cardiogenic pulmonary edema; albeit, with a normal cardiac silhouette. Early findings include Kerley B lines and peribronchial cuffing, all suggesting interstitial edema[45,46] (**Fig. 12**). Most patients rapidly progress to extensive bilateral predominantly perihilar or bibasilar hazy airspace opacities on chest radiographs (**Fig. 13**). Reports of CT findings in

hantavirus are limited to small case series or case reports, and may be skewed toward less severely affected patients who are hemodynamically stable. Available reports have shown bilateral central or basilar-predominant ground-glass opacities with smooth interlobular septal thickening, occasionally with concurrent small ill-defined nodules or focal consolidation.[47,48] The majority of patients have small pleural effusions.

Diagnosis can be confirmed serologically through positive IgM and IgG analysis, or through reverse transcriptase PCR for the viral genome. Hantavirus is associated with a high morbidity rate, 40% worldwide; however, treatment is primarily supportive and no FDA-approved methods are currently available.[43]

HOSPITAL-ASSOCIATED VIRAL PNEUMONIA

Although most viral infections are community-acquired, a few viruses such as Herpes simplex virus (HSV) contribute to morbidity and mortality in immunocompetent adults in the hospital setting. HSV infection can produce bronchopneumonia secondary to reactivation of existing virus within immunocompromised patients (eg, with hematologic malignancies) and in some immunocompetent patients with underlying conditions (eg, burns, major surgeries, diabetes, and prolonged mechanical ventilation.).[49,50]

Because the incidence of HSV infection is low, studies of radiologic findings combine immunocompetent and immunocompromised patients. In one study of 23 patients, all demonstrated multifocal patchy or segmental airspace opacities on radiographs, which were both central and peripheral in the majority.[50] Approximately half of patients had pleural effusions. Chest CT findings of multifocal ground-glass opacities combined with areas of peribronchiolar consolidation and interlobular septal and bronchial wall thickening have

Fig. 10. Haemophilus influenzae pneumonia in a 50-year-old woman with emphysema. Axial chest CT demonstrates numerous centrilobular nodules throughout both lungs, some of which have tree-in-bud morphology, consistent with infectious bronchiolitis imaging appearance is very similar to the previous cases of parainfluenza pneumonia.

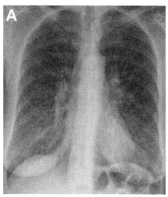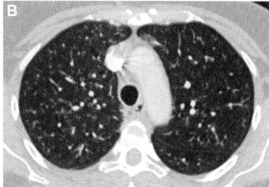

Fig. 11. Fifty-nine-year-old woman with productive cough and positive rhinovirus PCR. (*A*) Frontal chest radiograph shows subtle bilateral micronodules throughout both lungs. (*B*) Axial chest CT confirms bilateral 2-3 mm centrilobular tree-in-bud nodules in the upper lobes.

been reported in most patients.[50,51] Nodules are less common in HSV infection than in varicella, but may be present on CT in 30% of patients (see Brixey and colleagues' article, "Non-Imaging Diagnostic Tests For Pneumonia,"in this issue). These may be centrilobular ground-glass nodules or discrete nodules larger than 5 mm, some of which can manifest a halo sign. Pleural effusions may be seen but lymphadenopathy is uncommon. In critically ill patients, oral and BAL positivity for HSV is nonspecific and by itself is not proof of HSV pneumonia (**Fig. 14**). For example, HSV has been detected in up to 71% of respiratory samples from ARDS patients.[52]

Several other viruses have been implicated in nosocomial infections, but their role remains uncertain. Like HSV, CMV can reactivate after latent infection and has been implicated as another source of ventilator-acquired pneumonia (see below). Controversy exists regarding whether CMV positivity actually worsens clinical outcomes or contributes to lung injury.[53,54] Acanthamoeba polyphaga mimivirus (mimivirus) is an ameba-associated virus, which has recently been isolated within the lower respiratory tract of hospitalized adults and adults in long-term care facilities.[55] However, its status as a true pathogen is controversial, and suspected cases of mimivirus pneumonia are limited to case reports.[56,57]

VIRAL PNEUMONIA IN THE IMMUNOCOMPROMISED PATIENT

Community-acquired viral respiratory infections also commonly affect immunocompromised individuals. Viruses that usually result in limited symptoms in immunocompetent hosts can cause severe pneumonia in those patients. Immunocompromised hosts most at risk for severe viral pneumonia include those following HSCT, or solid organ transplantation.[6] Radiologic studies of community-acquired pneumonia frequently combine both immunocompetent and immunocompromised patients to increase sample size, and therefore in the case of several pathogens, the imaging appearance in both patient groups has been reviewed above. Cytomegalovirus (CMV) is a ubiquitous pathogen whose association with pneumonia is largely confined to immunocompromised adults. Varicella pneumonia is most common in immunocompromised patients but remains a cause of severe pneumonia in immunocompetent adults in countries without universal varicella vaccination.

CYTOMEGALOVIRUS

CMV causes a systemic infection that can present acutely with mononucleosis, pharyngitis, fever,

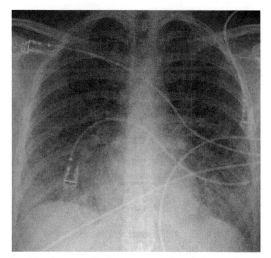

Fig. 12. Linear reticular pattern of early hantavirus in a 26-year-old woman. Frontal chest radiograph demonstrates fine reticular and hazy opacities with lower lung predominance.

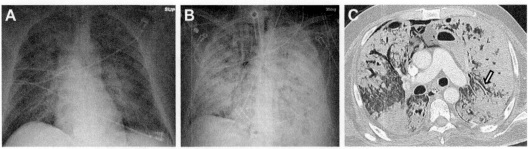

Fig. 13. Progression of hantavirus to ARDS in a 54-year-old man. (*A*) AP chest radiograph demonstrates bilateral perihilar hazy opacities in a "bat wing," pattern as well as Kerley B lines, with normal size of the cardiac silhouette and no pleural effusions. (*B*) AP frontal chest radiograph 3 days later demonstrates extensive bilateral consolidation and hazy opacities which obscure the cardiac silhouette. There is a small right pneumothorax, and lucencies along the right mediastinum and right heart border representing pneumomediastinum. ECMO cannula is in place. (*C*) Chest CT shows extensive bilateral consolidation. Pneumomediastinum and Macklin effect in the left lower lobe suggest barotrauma (*arrow*).

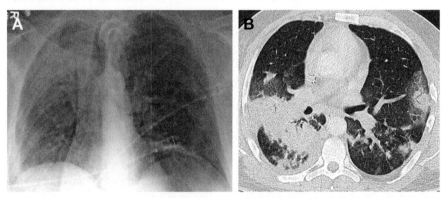

Fig. 14. Forty-four-year-old man with pseudomonas pneumonia. Herpes virus demonstrated on bronchoscopy performed on during after 2 weeks of hospitalization. (*A*) Frontal chest radiograph shows a right upper lung consolidation, more suggestive of bacterial pneumonia. (*B*) Axial chest CT demonstrates extensive consolidation in the superior segment of the right lower lobe, and additional smaller foci of consolidation in the left lower lobe. The multifocal consolidation is most consistent with a bacterial pneumonia. Presence of HSV virus on bronchoscopy may be incidental and not contribute significantly to the patient's pneumonia.

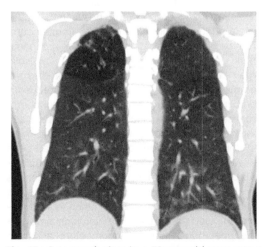

Fig. 15. Cytomegalovirus in a 52-year-old man status postrenal transplant. Coronal chest CT with dominant findings of bilateral lower lobe peribronchovascular ground-glass opacities. There are a few nodules in the right lung apex. (*Courtesy of* B Little, MD, Jacksonville, Florida.).

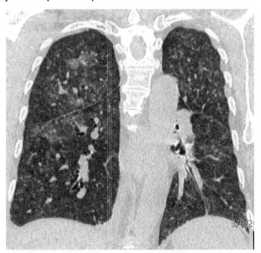

Fig. 16. CMV in a 62-year-old female with a history of orthotopic heart transplant for nonischemic cardiomyopathy. Her CMV prophylaxis was stopped early on posttransplant due to thrombocytopenia/anemia. Coronal chest CT demonstrates diffuse bilateral nodules with mild peribronchovascular ground-glass opacities. (*Courtesy of* F Dako, MD, MPH, Philadelphia, Pennsylvania.).

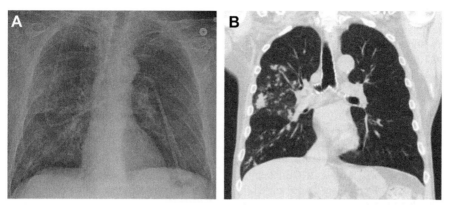

Fig. 17. Varicella pneumonia in a 72-year-old man with multiple myeloma status postautologous transplant complicated. (*A*) Frontal radiograph demonstrates multiple nodules in the right lung. (*B*) Coronal chest CT demonstrates a focal area of nodular consolidation with clustered adjacent centrilobular micronodules. Fewer micronodules are present in the lower lobe. (*Courtesy of* S Moran, MD, Seattle, Washington.).

and lymphadenopathy.[58] The virus commonly establishes chronic, latent infection that can reactivate in immunocompromised hosts such as after HSCT, solid organ transplant (particularly lung transplant), and among those with acquired immunodeficiency syndrome (AIDS). Although it is not specifically a respiratory pathogen, it can cause severe pneumonia in these patients. CMV prophylaxis is very effective in the setting of HSCT, reducing infection from 20% to 70% to 1% to 3%, but is less so in lung transplant recipients (see Michelle Hershman and Scott Simpson's article "Thoracic Infections in Solid Organ Transplants; Radiological Features and Approach to Diagnosis," in this issue).[59]

Because CMV within the lungs usually represents reactivation of a systemic infection rather than inhaled pathogen its manifestations in the lung are pleomorphic and not confined to airway disease. The most common abnormality on chest radiographs is bilateral hazy opacities, which manifest as bilateral ground-glass opacities on chest CT.[60–62] Multiple centrilobular micronodules are also a common finding. In severe cases, multifocal consolidation can predominate or be intermixed with ground-glass opacities (**Figs. 15** and **16**). Interlobular septal thickening and pleural effusions are less common findings. Nodules with halo sign are uncommon and cavitary nodules have been reported but are rare.[60,62,63]

CMV is the most common viral infection among patients living with HIV, but has become much less prevalent following the advent of HAART. In the setting of HIV findings, CMV infection findings are similar to those described earlier. Radiographs commonly demonstrate bilateral hazy opacities

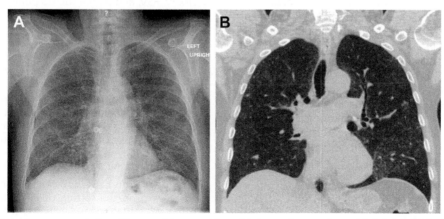

Fig. 18. Varicella pneumonia in a 54-year-old man with multiple myeloma, relapsed following HSCT. (*A*) Frontal chest radiograph shows diffuse bilateral reticular and micronodular opacities. (*B*) Coronal chest CT confirms the diffuse solid and ground-glass micronodules in a random distribution. The distribution suggests a hematogenous component of spread of infection. (*Courtesy of* S Moran, MD, Seattle, Washington.).

seen as ground-glass opacities on CT. Consolidation, discrete masses, and nodules can also occur, and airway abnormalities (bronchiectasis and bronchial wall thickening) can be seen on CT.[64] Pneumocystis jiroveci pneumonia (PJP) can be difficult to distinguish from CMV as both infections are seen in patients with very low CD4 counts and can manifest as diffuse ground-glass opacities. However, CMV infection is associated with micronodules and macronodules more frequently than pneumocystis.[62] Consolidation and the halo sign have also been seen in CMV to a significantly higher degree. The relative likelihood of CMV versus PJP is also highly dependent on viral/and or pneumocystis prophylaxis, respectively.

Diagnosis of CMV pneumonitis is difficult, similar to HSV pulmonary infection (see above, "hospital-associated viral pneumonias"). As with other latent infections, the presence of CMV virus on viral cultures of BAL fluid is not proof of pathogenic CMV infection.[54,64] More definitive diagnosis can be made by BAL cytology or other methods (see Brixey et al.).[64] First-line treatment is with the systemic antiviral intravenous ganciclovir. Foscarnet and cidofovir are antivirals which may be used for resistant infections.[5]

VARICELLA

Varicella, member of the herpes family, can cause severe pneumonia in immunocompromised patients and unvaccinated immunocompetent adults. Most children in the United States are vaccinated against the varicella virus after 12 months of age;[65] however, vaccination is only widespread in predominantly high socioeconomic countries.[66] Individuals who did not receive the vaccination and were not infected as children are at risk of contracting varicella as an adult, and between 5% to 15% of infected adults develop pneumonia.[65] Compared with children, varicella pneumonia in adults is associated with a 4 to 50 fold greater risk of hospitalization and a 174 fold greater risk of death.[66] Severe pneumonia typically develops an average of 3 days after the characteristic varicella rash and can rapidly progress to acute respiratory distress syndrome.[67] Mortality of intubated patients reaches 50%.[65]

Chest radiographs demonstrate ill-defined nodules measuring less than 1 cm, which may coalesce. Occasional findings include consolidation, hilar lymphadenopathy, or pleural effusions.[6,67] Chest CT in immunocompetent hosts often display 1 to 10 mm centrilobular nodules with and without ground glass halos, as well as randomly-distributed nodules.[68,69] CTs of immunocompetent and immunosuppressed patients with severe pneumonia contain centrilobular nodules in 50%, consolidation and ground-glass opacities in less than half, and effusions in approximately one-third of cases (**Figs. 17** and **18**).[68] Randomly distributed 2 to 3 mm calcified nodules are typical of healed infection.[6]

First-line therapy of varicella is the antiviral acyclovir, administered intravenously. In the setting of typical skin rash and exposure history, therapy is often initiated before the diagnosis is confirmed with PCR.[5]

SUMMARY

Viral pneumonia is prevalent among both immunocompetent and immunocompromised hosts, typically causing more severe disease in the latter. Several viral pneumonias, such as influenza, HMPV, RSV, and parainfluenza demonstrate similar airway-centric distribution, the likelihood of a specific organism often dependent on seasonal epidemics. Other viral pneumonias, such as adenovirus, frequently cause pneumonias with imaging findings indistinguishable from community-acquired bacterial pneumonias. For a few organisms, additional factors are central to the likelihood of infection, for example, environmental exposure for Hantaviruses and vaccination status for Varicella. In organisms that typically cause chronic infections in humans, such as HSV and CMV, the relationship between infection and clinical pneumonia is complex and incompletely understood.

CLINICS CARE POINTS

- HMPV, RSV, and parainfluenza pulmonary infections have a propensity for airway centric involvement with associated imaging findings of bronchiolitis and bronchopneumonia. Since this imaging appearance can be mimicked by bacterial pathogens, diagnosis is usually based on PCR.

- Influenza is also an airway centric infection causing bronchiolitis and bronchopneumonia. Diffuse airspace disease is rare in most seasonal outbreaks but occurs more commonly with infection with novel influenza viruses, such as H1N1 and avian influenza.

- Adenovirus can cause lobar type consolidation, which in the setting of infection with other virus pathogens (including influenza) suggests bacterial co-infection.

- Both HSV and CMV infections represent systemic reactivation of a latent infection rather than an acute primary pulmonary infection and positive respiratory cultures are not proof of pneumonia. Among immunocompromised hosts (patients living with advanced AIDS), CMV most commonly presents with ground glass opacities and centrilobular micronodules.

• Varicella and Hantavirus can cause severe pneumonia in otherwise healthy adults, one in the absence of prior vaccination or childhood infection, the other following specific environmental exposure. Imaging is dominated by micronodules in the setting of varicella, and linear interstitial opacities in the setting of Hantavirus Pulmonary Syndrome (HPS).

DISCLOSURE

The authors have nothing to disclose.

REFERENCES

1. Woolhouse M, Scott F, Hudson Z, et al. Human viruses: discovery and emergence. Philos Trans R Soc Lond B Biol Sci 2012;367(1604):2864–71.
2. Liang L, Moore B, Soni A, Healthcare cost and utilization project: statistical brief #261Agency for Healthcare Research and Quality: Rockville, MD. National Inpatient Hospital Costs: The Most Expensive Conditions by Payer. 2017. Accessed. https:// www.hcup-us.ahrq.gov/reports/statbriefs/sb261-Most-Expensive-Hospital-Conditions-2017.pdf. [Accessed 1 June 2021]. Available at.
3. Tiveljung-Lindell A, Rotzén-Ostlund M, Gupta S, et al. Development and implementation of a molecular diagnostic platform for daily rapid detection of 15 respiratory viruses. J Med Virol 2009;81(1): 167–75.
4. Jain S, Self WH, Wunderink RG, et al, CDC EPIC Study Team. Community-acquired pneumonia requiring hospitalization among U.S. Adults. N Engl J Med 2015;373(5):415–27.
5. Dandachi D, Rodriguez-Barradas MC. Viral pneumonia: etiologies and treatment. J Investig Med 2018;66(6):957–65.
6. Koo HJ, Lim S, Choe J, et al. Radiographic and CT features of viral pneumonia. Radiographics 2018; 38(3):719–39.
7. Chow EJ, Doyle JD, Uyeki TM. Influenza virus-related critical illness: prevention, diagnosis, treatment. Crit Care 2019;23(1):214.
8. Olsen SJ, Azziz-Baumgartner E, Budd AP, et al. Decreased influenza activity during the COVID-19 pandemic — United States, Australia, Chile, and South Africa, 2020. MMWR Morbidity Mortality Wkly Rep 2020;69(37):1305–9.
9. Miller WT, Mickus TJ, Barbosa E, et al. CT of viral lower respiratory tract infections in adults: comparison among viral organisms and between viral and bacterial infections. AJR Am J Roentgenol 2011; 197(5):1088–95.
10. Oikonomou A, Müller NL, Nantel S. Radiographic and high-resolution CT findings of influenza virus pneumonia in patients with hematologic malignancies. Am J Roentgenology 2003;181(2):507–11.
11. ACOG Committee Opinion No. 753: Assessment and Treatment of Pregnant Women With Suspected or Confirmed Influenza. Obstet Gynecol 2018; 132(4):e169–73.
12. Oliveira EC, Marik PE, Colice G. Influenza pneumonia. Chest 2001;119(6):1717–23.
13. McElhaney JE, Verschoor CP, Andrew MK, et al. The immune response to influenza in older humans: beyond immune senescence. Immun Ageing 2020; 17(1).
14. Cheng VC, To KK, Tse H, et al. Two years after pandemic influenza A/2009/H1N1: what have we learned? Clin Microbiol Rev 2012;25(2):223–63.
15. Ajlan AM, Quiney B, Nicolaou S, et al. Swine-origin influenza A (H1N1) viral infection: radiographic and CT findings. Am J Roentgenology 2009;193(6):1494–9.
16. Shrestha SS, Swerdlow DL, Borse RH, et al. Estimating the burden of 2009 pandemic influenza A (H1N1) in the United States (April 2009-April 2010). Clin Infect Dis 2010;52(Supplement 1): S75–82.
17. Abbo L, Quartin A, Morris MI, et al. Pulmonary imaging of pandemic influenza H1N1 infection: relationship between clinical presentation and disease burden on chest radiography and CT. Br J Radiol 2010;83(992):645–51.
18. Cornejo R, Llanos O, Fernández C, et al. Organizing pneumonia in patients with severe respiratory failure due to novel A (H1N1) influenza. BMJ Case Rep 2010;2010. bcr0220102708.
19. Torrego A, Pajares V, Mola A, et al. Influenza A (H1N1) organiZing pneumonia. BMJ Case Rep 2010;2010. bcr12.2009.2531.
20. Töpfer L, Menk M, Weber-Carstens S, et al. Influenza A (H1N1) vs non-H1N1 ARDS: analysis of clinical course. J Crit Care 2014;29(3):340–6.
21. Li YT, Linster M, Mendenhall IH, et al. Avian influenza viruses in humans: lessons from past outbreaks. Br Med Bull 2019;132(1):81–95.
22. Qureshi NR, Hien TT, Farrar J, et al. The radiologic manifestations of H5N1 avian influenza. J Thorac Imaging 2006;21(4):259–64.
23. Rewar S, Mirdha D, Rewar P. Treatment and prevention of pandemic H1N1 influenza. Ann Glob Health 2016;81(5):645.
24. Gaitonde DY, Moore FC, Morgan MK. Influenza: diagnosis and treatment. Am Fam Physician 2019; 100(12):751–8.

25. Lee N, Qureshi ST. Other viral pneumonias: coronavirus, respiratory syncytial virus, adenovirus, hantavirus. Crit Care Clin 2013;29(4):1045–68.

26. Stefanidis K, Konstantelou E, Yusuf GT, et al. Radiological, epidemiological and clinical patterns of pulmonary viral infections. Eur J Radiol 2021;136:109548.

27. Lynch JP 3rd, Kajon AE. Adenovirus: epidemiology, global spread of novel serotypes, and advances in treatment and prevention. Semin Respir Crit Care Med 2016;37(4):586–602.

28. Cha MJ, Chung MJ, Lee KS, et al. Clinical features and radiological findings of adenovirus pneumonia associated with progression to acute respiratory distress syndrome: a single center study in 19 adult patients. Korean J Radiol 2016;17(6):940–9.

29. Tan D, Fu Y, Xu J, et al. Severe adenovirus community-acquired pneumonia in immunocompetent adults: chest radiographic and CT findings. J Thorac Dis 2016;8(5):848–54.

30. Jiang J, Wan R, Pan P, et al. Comparison of clinical, laboratory and radiological characteristics between COVID-19 and adenovirus pneumonia: a retrospective study. Infect Drug Resist 2020;13:3401–8.

31. Marinari LA, Danny MA, Simpson SA, et al. Lower respiratory tract infection with human metapneumovirus: chest CT imaging features and comparison with other viruses. Eur J Radiol 2020;128:108988.

32. Keske Ş, Gümüş T, Köymen T, et al. Human metapneumovirus infection: diagnostic impact of radiologic imaging. J Med Virol 2019;91(6):958–62.

33. Gabutti G, De Motoli F, Sandri F, et al. Viral respiratory infections in hematological patients. Infect Dis Ther 2020;9(3):495–510.

34. Pochon C, Voigt S. Respiratory virus infections in hematopoietic cell transplant recipients. Front Microbiol 2019;9:3294.

35. El Chaer F, Shah DP, Kmeid J, et al. Burden of human metapneumovirus infections in patients with cancer: risk factors and outcomes. Cancer 2017;123(12):2329–37.

36. Godet C, Le Goff J, Beby-Defaux A, et al. Human metapneumovirus pneumonia in patients with hematological malignancies. J Clin Virol 2014;61(4):593–6.

37. Shahda S, Carlos WG, Kiel PJ, et al. The human metapneumovirus: a case series and review of the literature. Transpl Infect Dis 2011;13(3):324–8.

38. Herbst T, Van Deerlin VM, Miller WT Jr. The CT appearance of lower respiratory infection due to parainfluenza virus in adults. AJR Am J Roentgenol 2013;201(3):550–4.

39. Kim MC, Kim MY, Lee HJ, et al. CT findings in viral lower respiratory tract infections caused by parainfluenza virus, influenza virus and respiratory syncytial virus. Medicine (Baltimore) 2016;95(26):e4003.

40. To KKW, Yip CCY, Yuen KY. Rhinovirus - From bench to bedside. J Formos Med Assoc 2017;116(7):496–504.

41. Moriyama M, Hugentobler WJ, Iwasaki A. Seasonality of respiratory viral infections. Annu Rev Virol 2020;7(1):83–101.

42. Choi SH, Huh JW, Hong SB, et al. Clinical characteristics and outcomes of severe rhinovirus-associated pneumonia identified by bronchoscopic bronchoalveolar lavage in adults: comparison with severe influenza virus-associated pneumonia. J Clin Virol 2015;62:41–7.

43. Munir N, Jahangeer M, Hussain S, et al. Hantavirus diseases pathophysiology, their diagnostic strategies and therapeutic approaches: a review. Clin Exp Pharmacol Physiol 2020;48:20–34.

44. Centers for Disease Control. "Hantavirus: Outbreaks." Reviewed Jan 17, 2018. Available at: https://www.cdc.gov/hantavirus/outbreaks/index.html. Accessed May 25, 2021.

45. Ketai LH, Williamson MR, Telepak RJ, et al. Hantavirus pulmonary syndrome: radiographic findings in 16 patients. Radiology 1994;191(3):665–8.

46. Boroja M, Barrie JR, Raymond GS. Radiographic findings in 20 patients with Hantavirus pulmonary syndrome correlated with clinical outcome. AJR Am J Roentgenol 2002;178(1):159–63.

47. de Lacerda Barbosa D, Zanetti G, Marchiori E. Hantavirus Pulmonary Syndrome: High-resolution Computed Tomography Findings. Arch Bronconeumol 2017;53(1):35–6.

48. Gasparetto EL, Davaus T, Escuissato DL, et al. Hantavirus pulmonary syndrome: high-resolution CT findings in one patient. Br J Radiol 2007;80(949):e21–3.

49. Aquino SL, Dunagan DP, Chiles C, et al. Herpes simplex virus 1 pneumonia: patterns on CT scans and conventional chest radiographs. J Comput Assist Tomogr 1998;22(5):795–800.

50. Chong S, Kim TS, Cho EY. Herpes simplex virus pneumonia: high-resolution CT findings. Br J Radiol 2010;83(991):585–9.

51. Hammer MM, Gosangi B, Hatabu H. Human herpesvirus alpha subfamily (Herpes Simplex and Varicella Zoster) viral pneumonias: CT findings. J Thorac Imaging 2018;33(6):384–9.

52. Luyt CE, Combes A, Deback C, et al. Herpes simplex virus lung infection in patients undergoing prolonged mechanical ventilation. Am J Respir Crit Care Med 2007;175:935–42.

53. Papazian L, Fraisse A, Garbe L, et al. Cytomegalovirus. An unexpected cause of ventilator-associated pneumonia. Anesthesiology 1996;84(2):280–7.

54. Coisel Y, Bousbia S, Forel JM, et al. Cytomegalovirus and herpes simplex virus effect on the prognosis of mechanically ventilated patients suspected to have

ventilator-associated pneumonia. PLoS One 2012; 7(12):e51340.

55. La Scola B, Marrie TJ, Auffray JP, et al. Mimivirus in pneumonia patients. Emerg Infect Dis 2005;11(3): 449–52.

56. Sakhaee F, Vaziri F, Bahramali G, et al. Pulmonary infection related to mimivirus in patient with primary ciliary dyskinesia. Emerg Infect Dis 2020;26(10): 2524–6.

57. Saadi H, Reteno DG, Colson P, et al. Shan virus: a new mimivirus isolated from the stool of a Tunisian patient with pneumonia. Intervirology 2013;56(6): 424–9.

58. de Melo Silva J, Pinheiro-Silva R, Dhyani A, et al. Cytomegalovirus and epstein-barr infections: prevalence and impact on patients with hematological diseases. Biomed Res Int 2020;2020: 1627824.

59. Clausen ES, Zaffiri L. Infection prophylaxis and management of viral infection. Ann Transl Med 2020; 8(6):415.

60. Franquet T, Lee KS, Müller NL. Thin-section CT findings in 32 immunocompromised patients with cytomegalovirus pneumonia who do not have AIDS. AJR Am J Roentgenol 2003;181(4):1059–63.

61. Moon JH, Kim EA, Lee KS, et al. Cytomegalovirus pneumonia: high-resolution CT findings in ten non-AIDS immunocompromised patients. Korean J Radiol 2000;1(2):73–8.

62. Du CJ, Liu JY, Chen H, et al. Differences and similarities of high-resolution computed tomography features between pneumocystis pneumonia and cytomegalovirus pneumonia in AIDS patients. Infect Dis Poverty 2020;9:149.

63. Najjar M, Siddiqui AK, Rossoff L, et al. Cavitary lung masses in SLE patients: an unusual manifestation of CMV infection. Eur Respir J 2004;24(1):182–4.

64. McGuinness G, Scholes JV, Garay SM, et al. Cytomegalovirus pneumonitis: spectrum of parenchymal CT findings with pathologic correlation in 21 AIDS patients. Radiology 1994;192(2):451–9.

65. Denny JT, Rocke ZM, McRae VA, et al. Varicella pneumonia: case report and review of a potentially lethal complication of a common disease. J Investig Med High Impact Case Rep 2018;6. 2324709618770230.

66. Wutzler P, Bonanni P, Burgess M, et al. Varicella vaccination - the global experience. Expert Rev Vaccines 2017;16(8):833–43.

67. Mirouse A, Vignon P, Piron P, et al. Severe varicella-zoster virus pneumonia: a multicenter cohort study. Crit Care 2017;21(1):137.

68. Gasparetto EL, Warszawiak D, Tazoniero P, et al. Varicella pneumonia in immunocompetent adults: report of two cases, with emphasis on high-resolution computed tomography findings. Braz J Infect Dis 2005;9(3):262–5.

69. Kim JS, Ryu W, Lee SI, et al. High resolution CT findings of varicella-zoster pneumonia. Am J Roentgenology 1999;172(1):113–6.

Nontuberculous Mycobacterial Infections

Faisal Jamal, MBBS, Mark M. Hammer, MD*

KEYWORDS

- Nontuberculous mycobacteria • *Mycobacterium avium* complex • Bronchiectasis

KEY POINTS

- Pulmonary manifestations of NTM are mostly seen in elderly population with or without underlying lung disease. MAC is the most common agent.
- The most common imaging pattern is bronchiectatic disease in elderly females without prior lung disease, with imaging findings of bronchiectasis and nodules most commonly involving the midlung zones.
- The second most commonly seen pattern is cavitary disease in elderly males with preexisting underlying lung disease, with similar radiological findings as pulmonary tuberculosis.
- Diagnostic criteria include both imaging and recurrent isolation of mycobacterium from the sputum or one isolation from bronchial wash in a symptomatic patient.

INTRODUCTION

Mycobacterial species other than *Mycobacterium tuberculosis* and *Mycobacterium leprae* constitute nontuberculous mycobacteria (NTM), also termed atypical mycobacteria. NTM infections are increasing worldwide likely due to increase in immunocompromised patients, improved diagnostic techniques, and increased life expectancy, particularly in elderly women.[1–3] NTM are ubiquitous organisms commonly found in a variety of environmental sources. Pulmonary manifestations account for 80% to 90% of disease caused by NTM.[4,5] These infections can happen in those with or without preexisting lung diseases such as chronic obstructive pulmonary disease (COPD), bronchiectasis, cystic fibrosis, pneumoconiosis, and prior tuberculosis.[6,7] Depending on the scenario, patients may present acutely or with chronic manifestations, such as chronic cough. Imaging plays a key role in the diagnosis and monitoring of NTM infection.

Epidemiology and Sources of Infection

NTM are ubiquitous free-living organisms and are found abundantly in the natural environment. They have been isolated from tap and surface water resources, soil, animals, and food and milk products.[8,9] Humans are therefore constantly exposed to these organisms, and infection occurs mostly from aerosolized droplets from these environmental sources. Human to human transmission is rare although postulated in some cystic fibrosis lung transplant centers.[2,10] In immunocompromised patients, like patients with HIV/AIDS, infections commonly occur through the gastrointestinal route.[8] These organisms then gain access through lymphovascular invasion of the gastrointestinal tract leading to disseminated infection.[6,11]

Runyon in 1959 classified mycobacteria according to their rate of growth, pigmentation in response to light, and colony morphology. They are classified as *Mycobacterium tuberculosis* complex (TB), rapidly growing NTM, and slowly growing NTM. Slowly growing mycobacteria are divided into 3 groups: photochromogens, scotochromogens, and nonchromogens based on pigmentation with light exposure.[6,9]

Mycobacterium avium complex (MAC), also sometimes called *Mycobacterium avium intracellulare*, is the most common species causing human infections in the United States. It is followed

Department of Radiology, Brigham and Women's Hospital, 75 Francis Street, Boston, MA 02115, USA
* Corresponding author.
E-mail address: mmhammer@bwh.harvard.edu

Radiol Clin N Am 60 (2022) 399–408
https://doi.org/10.1016/j.rcl.2022.01.012

by *Mycobacterium fortuitum* and *Mycobacterium kansasii*, and all 3 of these are slowly growing NTM. Rapid growing *Mycobacterium abscessus* is increasing in prevalence particularly due to its involvement in cystic fibrosis patients.[2,5,12] The prevalence of NTM has been increasing worldwide and is 2 to 3 times more common than tuberculosis in the Western world.[13] MAC is commonly seen in the United States and East Asia, and *M kansasii*, *Mycobacterium xenopi*, and *Mycobacterium malmoense* are more prevalent in Europe.[13]

MAC most commonly causes pulmonary disease, both cavitary and noncavitary forms. Hypersensitivity pneumonitis and solitary pulmonary nodules are less commonly seen. Disseminated infections occur in severely immunocompromised patients such as those with AIDS. *M kansasii* is the second most common respiratory isolate after MAC in the United States.[14] It causes a cavitary pattern of pulmonary disease resembling tuberculosis in COPD patients and disseminated infection in immunocompromised patients such as those with AIDS. However, unlike other NTM, *M kansasii* is not found in soil or natural water supplies but has been frequently recovered from tap water in endemic areas. Rapidly growing *M abscessus* typically causes pulmonary disease in patients with bronchiectasis, similar to the bronchiectatic type typically caused by MAC. The rapid growing *M fortuitum* typically causes skin and soft tissue as well as catheter-related infections mostly by direct inoculation; and *Mycobacterium chelonae* causes disseminated infection in immunocompromised patients as well as rare infection in patients with esophageal dysmotility.[12,13]

Diagnostic Criteria

Making the diagnosis of NTM is sometimes difficult because these organisms frequently colonize the airways in patients with preexisting lung disease, such as those with COPD or bronchiectasis. Moreover, cultures can also be falsely negative in infected patients, particularly in those without cavities.[15] As a result, the American Thoracic Society requires clinical and radiologic criteria, in addition to microbiological results, for appropriate diagnosis (**Box 1**).

Clinical symptoms are nonspecific and include dry or productive cough, shortness of breath, fatigue, malaise, and hemoptysis. Fever and weight loss are less commonly seen. As infection can coexist with preexisting pulmonary disease, symptoms and physical examination may be masked by the underlying pulmonary condition. Thus, it may be difficult to attribute any symptoms to the mycobacterial infection; following patients

over time may be necessary to correlate the course of the infection with clinical symptoms.

Microbiological evaluation and drug susceptibility testing are essential for the accurate diagnosis and identification of NTM species and their appropriate management.[5,16]

Sputum testing

Smear and culture of at least 3 separate expectorated morning sputum specimens are recommended. Sputum sent for culture must be decontaminated first for elimination of common bacteria and fungi. In addition, in patients with suspected tuberculosis, sputum nucleic acid amplification tests should be performed for exclusion of that diagnosis. At least 2 positive sputum cultures are needed for the diagnosis of NTM infection.

Bronchial lavage and biopsy

In case of negative sputum testing, additional testing such as bronchoscopy with bronchoalveolar lavage (BAL) or transbronchial biopsy can be performed. At least one positive BAL culture is adequate. Alternatively, lung or transbronchial biopsy with mycobacterial histopathological features and culture is diagnostic. For either sputum or BAL samples, nucleic acid probes are also commercially available that are highly accurate and can identify MAC and *M kansasii* within a day.[17,18]

Clinical Syndromes and Imaging Findings

Cavitary type (classical)

This form typically occurs in white, middle-aged to elderly males with preexisting lung diseases such as COPD or prior granulomatous disease (including tuberculosis and sarcoidosis). It is clinically and radiologically similar in appearance to postprimary, or reactivation, tuberculosis.[6,19,20] Patients commonly develop cough with sputum, fatigue, and weight loss, which can simulate relapse of prior tuberculosis. MAC is the frequent culprit; however, *M kansasii* and *M abscessus* can also cause similar patterns of disease.[20] Cough and dyspnea are common symptoms, which are difficult to distinguish from the underlying disease such as COPD. Fever and hemoptysis are less common compared with tuberculosis.[2]

In patients with pre-existing bronchiectasis, such as from treated tuberculosis, MAC can develop in prior areas of lung involvement. It is characterized by upper lobe cavitary lesions (**Fig. 1A, B**) as well as centrilobular and tree in bud nodules (**Fig. 1B, C**). Peribronchial consolidation, architectural distortion, and scarring can also occur, as seen in tuberculosis. Computed tomography (CT) will better characterize the cavities and show associated volume loss and traction bronchiectasis. Spread of infection through bronchi is common and may involve the contralateral lung; it is characterized on CT by tree-in-bud nodules.[6,15,20] Reportedly, NTM infections are more indolent with smaller cavities compared with TB, but this distinction is not helpful clinically.[15] Lymphadenopathy and pleural effusions are relatively uncommon.[15,20,21]

Nodular-bronchiectatic type (non-classic)

This is the most frequently seen type in the United States and Canada. It commonly develops in nonsmoking middle-aged to elderly white women without underlying lung disease and is sometimes referred to as the Lady Windermere syndrome.[22] MAC and *M kansasii* are the most common culprits; however, *M chelonae* and *M abscessus* can also cause this type of infection. The clinical presentation is indolent, with many years of chronic progressive cough with or without sputum, and recurrent respiratory infections.[22] Fever, dyspnea, and other constitutional symptoms such as weight loss may also occur.[2] This syndrome is associated with bronchiectasis, although it is not clear if bronchiectasis is the predisposing factor leading to the infection or is the result of the infection, likely both may occur.[20] Notably, cystic fibrosis transmembrane conductance regulator (CFTR) gene mutations are seen at increased prevalence in patients with this form of NTM, even in patients without clinically apparent cystic fibrosis, and this may be a predisposing factor to developing NTM infection.[23] Sputum cultures are less sensitive for the diagnosis as compared with the cavitary form, and thus more invasive approaches such as BAL may be required.

Chest x-ray may show atelectasis and scarring, most commonly affecting the right middle lobe and lingula (Fig. 2). CT shows bronchiolitis (centrilobular and tree in bud nodules) and bronchiectasis with predilection for the midlung zones, particularly

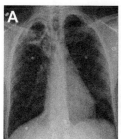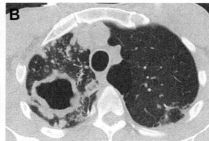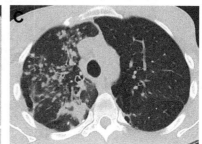

Fig. 1. 72-year-old man with *M kansasii*. (*A*) Chest radiograph shows cavitary consolidation in right upper lung with adjacent nodular opacities. (*B*) and (*C*), Axial chest CT shows cavity in right apical segment with adjacent centrilobular and tree in bud nodules. Note the underlying paraseptal emphysema.

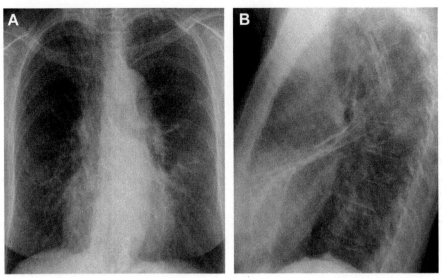

Fig. 2. 69-year-old woman with MAC. (*A*) Frontal and (*B*) lateral chest radiographs show areas of atelectasis and scarring in the right middle lobe and the lingula with bronchiectasis.

the right middle lobe and lingula (**Fig. 3**). Cavities and consolidation are uncommonly seen in this form as compared with the cavitary form of NTM[22,24] (**Fig. 4**). Bronchiectatic airways may also contain foci of mucous plugging and are associated with air trapping (mosaic attenuation). Lymphadenopathy is rare. Atelectasis and scarring are commonly seen in the regions of bronchiectasis, again particularly in the right middle lobe and lingula.[20,25,26] In addition, bronchiectatic NTM is associated with scoliosis and pectus excavatum.[27]

The imaging differential diagnosis for bronchiectatic NTM includes allergic bronchopulmonary aspergillosis (ABPA), which also presents with bronchiectasis. However, ABPA does not commonly demonstrate mid-lung predominance, and is more likely to manifest an upper lobe predilection. The presence of high-attenuation mucus in dilated airways is characteristic of ABPA, though

not always present. Patients will have a history of asthma or cystic fibrosis; diagnostic testing will show elevated total and aspergillus-specific IgE levels.[28] Other causes of bronchiectasis (eg, cystic fibrosis, ciliary dyskinesia, or chronic aspiration) tend to involve the upper or lower lung zones predominantly, rather than the mid-lung zones as with NTM.

Hypersensitivity pneumonitis

This entity, also known as hot tub lung, represents an immune reaction to inhalation of MAC, typically related to repeated exposure from hot tubs by aerosolization.[29] It is subacute in presentation and characterized by fever, cough, and dyspnea. Hot tub lung is similar in appearance and presentation to other forms of hypersensitivity pneumonitis, best characterized on CT by centrilobular or confluent ground glass with areas of air trapping. Patients

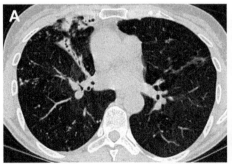
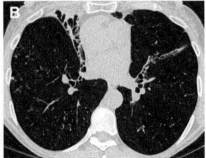

Fig. 3. 67-year-old woman with MAC. Axial CT images (*A*, *B*) show bronchiectasis in the right middle lobe and lingula with tree-in-bud nodules in the middle and lower lobes. Also, note mosaic attenuation indicative of air trapping.

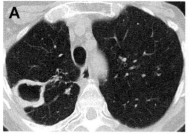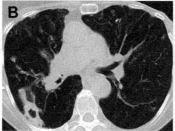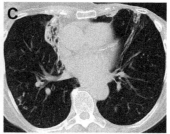

Fig. 4. 76-year-old woman with MAC, predominantly the nodular-bronchiectatic form. Axial chest CT images show midlung-predominant bronchiectasis (*B, C*) as well as several cavities in the right upper and lower lobes (*A, B*).

may develop fibrosis with long-term exposure.[13,30] Lung biopsies will show features of hypersensitivity pneumonitis such as cellular bronchiolitis and non-necrotizing granulomas, and cultures are often positive for MAC. The treatment is avoiding the exposure, as well as use of steroids.[2,13,30,31]

Solitary pulmonary nodules

MAC pulmonary infection can present as solitary (or multiple) pulmonary nodules, occasionally resembling lung cancer.[32] The patients are typically asymptomatic.[20]

On CT, the nodules may display calcification and therefore be confidently diagnosed as benign. However, they are often noncalcified, causing a diagnostic dilemma (**Fig. 5**). Several clues may help make the correct diagnosis preoperatively. These include a tubular or branching morphology, indicating bronchiectasis with endobronchial mucus. The presence of multiple clustered nodules is also very helpful in suggesting this diagnosis. The nodules may also be cavitary (**Fig. 6**).[6,20]

Disseminated in Immunocompromised Patients

Patients with HIV

NTM may cause disseminated disease in patients with HIV/AIDS. MAC is the most common agent involved, and this entity is typically seen in patients with CD4 count less than 100 cells/mm³.[21] Dissemination occurs by hematogenous spread from the gastrointestinal tract, which is often the initial site of infection.

Patients typically present with systemic symptoms like fever, weight loss, abdominal pain, and diarrhea. Hepatosplenomegaly and lymphadenopathy are commonly found on physical examination. Blood culture or lymph node biopsy is needed for diagnosis.

CT imaging typically shows disseminated lymphadenopathy, particularly in the mediastinum and abdomen[33] (**Fig. 7**). Disseminated infection can also involve other organs such as the liver and bone marrow leading to microabscesses and osteomyelitis.[34] Lung involvement may present as miliary nodules or, rarely, consolidation. Pleural effusions are uncommon.[20] In these severely immunocompromised patients, disseminated MAC may occur simultaneously with other opportunistic infections (eg, *Candida, Pneumocystis, Cytomegalovirus*) or Kaposi sarcoma[20] (**Fig. 8**).

In addition to MAC, *M xenopi* also causes disseminated disease in patients with HIV/AIDS, whereas *M kansasii* causes localized infection to the lungs, which can manifest as consolidation, often with lymphadenopathy and pleural effusions.

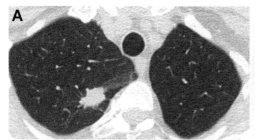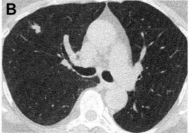

Fig. 5. 67-year-old woman with a history of breast cancer status postlumpectomy and radiotherapy presenting with chronic cough with sputum. Axial CT chest shows (*A*) right apical nodule (*B*) additional right upper lobe nodule. Subsequent FDG PET-CT showed FDG avidity in both nodules (not shown). She underwent VATS with 2 wedge resections. Pathology showed necrotizing granulomas with AFB stain suspicious for Mycobacteria. A culture of the tissue was negative and a BAL culture showed no growth. An induced sputum sample obtained was smear-positive and recovered *Mycobacterium mucogenicum*.

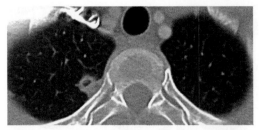

Fig. 6. 41-year-old woman with a history of colon cancer and Lynch syndrome. Axial chest CT shows a solitary cavitary nodule in the right upper lobe. Surgical resection revealed necrotizing granuloma and acid-fast bacilli, presumed NTM.

Other immunocompromised patients such as those with solid organ transplants, hematologic malignancies, or those on immunosuppressive drugs (particularly TNF-alpha inhibitors) can also develop disseminated NTM, usually with MAC and *M kansasii*, but this occurs much less commonly than in patients with HIV/AIDS.[20,33] As discussed earlier, NTM may be isolated from blood cultures in disseminated disease. Clinical and radiological manifestations are similar to those seen in patients with HIV. Localized abscess may also be seen throughout the body in disseminated infection[20] (**Fig. 9**).

The differential diagnosis of disseminated NTM in immunocompromised patients includes other disseminated infections (TB, bacterial, and fungal), although mycobacteria are more commonly associated with necrotic lymphadenopathy than other agents. Disseminated malignancy, including Kaposi sarcoma and lymphoma, may also lead to diffuse lymphadenopathy.

Immune reconstitution inflammatory syndrome

Immune reconstitution inflammatory syndrome (IRIS) may develop in patients with HIV and MAC infection after beginning antiretroviral therapy. IRIS represents a response of the now healthier immune system to a pre-existing infection. IRIS has been associated with a variety of preexisting pathogens, such as tuberculosis, MAC, cryptococcus, cytomegalovirus, and *Pneumocystis jirovecii*. Fever, shortness of breath, night sweats, and weight loss are common symptoms and mimic worsening of the infection itself.[35] Patients with AIDS with low pretreatment CD4 count (<100 cells/μL) are at particular risk.[36,37] The diagnosis is made on clinical grounds and based on positive virological and immunologic response to antiretroviral therapy,[38] although occasionally repeat biopsy may be pursued. The treatment for IRIS is to continue both antiretroviral and antimicrobial therapies. Steroids may be needed in those patients who develop severe symptoms.[39]

Radiological findings mimic worsening of the infection in the setting of improving immunologic function. The most common finding consists of intrathoracic lymphadenopathy, which may be necrotic. Consolidation and tree in bud nodules, as well as pleural and pericardial effusions, may also occur though less commonly.[20]

MonoMAC syndrome

Monocytopenia and mycobacterial infection (MonoMAC syndrome) is a clinical phenotype of germline GATA2 mutations, resulting in loss of function of a gene controlling many aspects of hematopoiesis and lymphatic formation.[40] Patients present with peripheral cytopenias and are at risk of transformation to acute leukemia. Bone marrow biopsy will show a hypocellular bone marrow; the diagnosis is then made via gene sequencing.[40] Severe and recurrent NTM infections, as well as opportunistic fungal (most commonly Histoplasma) and disseminated human papillomavirus infections, are commonly seen.[40,41] Imaging patterns are similar to other disseminated NTM infections including lymphadenopathy and nodular opacities in the lungs (**Fig. 10**).

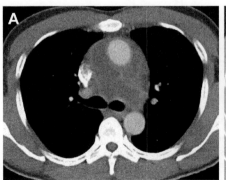
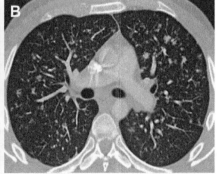

Fig. 7. 43-year-old man with HIV/AIDS. Axial CT images show (*A*) extensive necrotic mediastinal lymphadenopathy and (*B*) diffusely scattered nodules in both lungs.

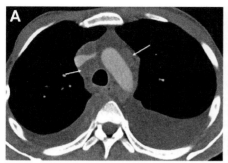
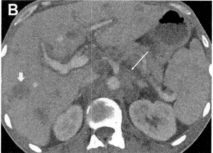

Fig. 8. 37-year-old man with AIDS and CD4 count of 14/μL, diagnosed with cutaneous and lymph node Kaposi sarcoma as well as disseminated MAC infection. CT images show (A) mediastinal and abdominal lymphadenopathy (white arrows), biopsy-proven MAC, as well as (B) multiple hepatic lesions, likely Kaposi sarcoma (broad white arrow).

Patients with Esophageal Dysmotility

Rapidly growing mycobacterial species such as M fortuitum and M chelonae have been isolated in infections in patients with esophageal dysfunction, such as from achalasia, hiatal hernia, stroke, and prior esophagectomy. Chronic aspiration is most likely the mechanism of infection and may be complicated by lipoid pneumonia.[20,42] Chest radiograph and CT show unilateral or bilateral patchy nodular or consolidative opacities resembling aspiration.[6] Lung abscesses due to recurrent aspiration have also been described.[43,44] Treatment of esophageal disorders is important for prevention and recovery in these patients.[42]

Management

The need for and goals of treatment for NTM depend on multiple factors, including the clinical syndrome and patient immune status. Here we will briefly review considerations for the most common agent, MAC. Note that patients must first meet the clinical, radiographic, and microbiologic criteria for NTM infection (see Box 1).

The mainstay of therapy for MAI is prolonged, multiagent therapy as detailed below. Because these agents are sometimes difficult to tolerate, a risk-benefit analysis must be considered for each patient. For patients with noncavitary nodular bronchiectatic disease, close observation with serial sputum cultures and CT imaging is an initial option. More than half of patients with nodular bronchiectatic disease eventually progress with time and require treatment; however, some untreated patients may clear MAC from their sputum spontaneously.[45]

For patients with cavitary disease or positive sputum culture, treatment should be considered.[46,47] The goal of therapy is achieving 12 months of negative culture[16] and imaging stability. In patients with macrolide-sensitive noncavitary MAC infection, at least 3-drug combination therapy is advised, usually a combination of a macrolide (azithromycin or clarithromycin), rifampin, and ethambutol.[16,48] For patients with severe (cavitary) and life-threatening infections, a parenteral aminoglycoside such as amikacin should be used for an initial 8 to 12 weeks of therapy or even longer. For those who have mild disease and cannot tolerate 3 drugs, a 2-drug regimen (azithromycin or clarithromycin and ethambutol) can be considered.[49]

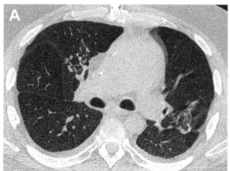
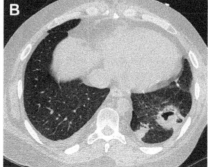

Fig. 9. 57-year-old man status postcardiac transplant, with M kansasii infection. Axial chest CT images show tree-in-bud nodules in the right upper lobe and a left lower lobe cavity, representing a lung abscess.

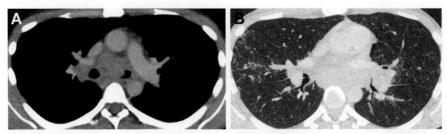

Fig. 10. 33-year-old man with MonoMAC syndrome (GATA2 mutation). (*A*) CT shows extensive mediastinal and hilar lymphadenopathy and (*B*) tree-in-bud nodules in the right middle lobe (*arrow*).

In patients with macrolide-resistant infection, ethambutol is still used as an immunomodulator, and a combination of rifamycin or rifabutin, ethambutol, clofazimine, and a parenteral aminoglycoside are used. For *M kansasii* infection, the preferred regiment is combination therapy with isoniazid, rifampin, and ethambutol.[5,50]

Surgical resection by lobectomy for localized disease or pneumonectomy for extensive cavitary disease is considered in some patients who fail medical therapy.[44,51,52] One study showed that only 16% of patients were culture-positive after surgery compared with 44% before surgery.[53]

SUMMARY

NTM infections are on the rise worldwide, particularly in the Western world. They cause a wide range of pulmonary and systemic manifestations described by various clinical and radiological types. The two most common types are as follows: classical cavitary type, seen with preexisting lung disease, and the nonclassical bronchiectatic type, seen in elderly women without preexisting lung disease. Disseminated infections by the hematogenous route are common in immunocompromised patients including those with HIV.

CLINICS CARE POINTS

- Bronchiectatic NTM presents with bronchiectasis and tree-in-bud nodules in the mid-lung zones.
- Cavitary NTM disease is most common in elderly males with pre-existing lung disease and simulates tuberculosis.
- Disseminated NTM infections occur in severely immunocompromised patients, particularly those with HIV/AIDS.

DISCLOSURE

The authors have nothing to disclose.

REFERENCES

1. Stout JE. Evaluation and management of patients with pulmonary nontuberculous mycobacterial infections. Expert Rev Anti Infect Ther 2006;4(6):981–93.
2. Weiss CH, Glassroth J. Pulmonary disease caused by nontuberculous mycobacteria. Expert Rev Respir Med 2012;6(6):597–612.
3. Jones D, Havlir DV. Nontuberculous mycobacteria in the HIV infected patient. Clin Chest Med 2002;23(3):665–74.
4. Wassilew N, Hoffmann H, Andrejak C, et al. Pulmonary disease caused by non-tuberculous mycobacteria. Respiration 2016;91(5):386–402.
5. Griffith DE, Aksamit T, Brown-Elliott BA, et al. An official ATS/IDSA statement: diagnosis, treatment, and prevention of nontuberculous mycobacterial diseases. Am J Respir Crit Care Med 2007;175(4):367–416.
6. Miller WT Jr. Spectrum of pulmonary nontuberculous mycobacterial infection. Radiology 1994;191(2):343–50.
7. Chapman JS. The atypical mycobacteria. Am Rev Respir Dis 1982;125(3 Pt 2):1l9–24.
8. Goslee S, Wolinsky E. Water as a source of potentially pathogenic mycobacteria. Am Rev Respir Dis 1976;113(3):287–92.
9. Gruft H, Falkinham JO 3rd, Parker BC. Recent experience in the epidemiology of disease caused by atypical mycobacteria. Rev Infect Dis 1981;3(5):990–6.
10. Aitken ML, Limaye A, Pottinger P, et al. Respiratory outbreak of Mycobacterium abscessus subspecies massiliense in a lung transplant and cystic fibrosis center. Am J Respir Crit Care Med 2012;185:231–2.
11. O'Brien RJ. The epidemiology of nontuberculous mycobacterial disease. Clin Chest Med 1989;10(3):407–18.
12. Falkinham JO 3rd. Environmental sources of nontuberculous mycobacteria. Clin Chest Med 2015;36(1):35–41.
13. Marras TK, Wallace RJ Jr, Koth LL, et al. Hypersensitivity pneumonitis reaction to Mycobacterium

avium in household water. Chest 2005;127(2): 664–71.

14. Prevots DR, Shaw PA, Strickland D, et al. Nontuberculous mycobacterial lung disease prevalence at four integrated health care delivery systems. Am J Respir Crit Care Med 2010;182(7):970–6.

15. Erasmus JJ, McAdams HP, Farrell MA, et al. Pulmonary nontuberculous mycobacterial infection: radiologic manifestations. Radiographics 1999;19(6): 1487–505.

16. Daley CL, Iaccarino JM, Lange C, et al. Treatment of nontuberculous mycobacterial pulmonary disease: an official ATS/ERS/ESCMID/IDSA clinical practice guideline. Clin Infect Dis 2020;71(4):e1–36.

17. Goto M, Okuzumi K, Oka S, et al. Identification of mycobacteria by the acridinium-ester labeled DNA probes for M. tuberculosis and M. avium-intracellulare complex in culture and its clinical application. Kansenshogaku Zasshi 1992;66(1):81–6.

18. Body BA, Warren NG, Spicer A, et al. Use of Gen-Probe and Bactec for rapid isolation and identification of mycobacteria. Correlation of probe results with growth index. Am J Clin Pathol 1990;93(3): 415–20.

19. Ahn CH, McLarty JW, Ahn SS, et al. Diagnostic criteria for pulmonary disease caused by Mycobacterium kansasii and Mycobacterium intracellulare. Am Rev Respir Dis 1982;125(4):388–91.

20. Martinez S, McAdams HP, Batchu CS. The many faces of pulmonary nontuberculous mycobacterial infection. AJR Am J Roentgenol 2007;189(1): 177–86.

21. Kilby JM, Gilligan PH, Yankaskas JR, et al. Nontuberculous mycobacteria in adult patients with cystic fibrosis. Chest 1992;102(1):70–5.

22. Reich JM, Johnson RE. Mycobacterium avium complex pulmonary disease. Incidence, presentation, and response to therapy in a community setting. Am Rev Respir Dis 1991;143(6):1381–5.

23. Jang MA, Kim SY, Jeong BH, et al. Association of CFTR gene variants with nontuberculous mycobacterial lung disease in a Korean population with a low prevalence of cystic fibrosis. J Hum Genet 2013;58(5):298–303.

24. Koh WJ, Lee KS, Kwon OJ, et al. Bilateral bronchiectasis and bronchiolitis at thin-section CT: diagnostic implications in nontuberculous mycobacterial pulmonary infection. Radiology 2005;235(1):282–8.

25. Wittram C, Weisbrod GL. Mycobacterium avium complex lung disease in immunocompetent patients: radiography-CT correlation. Br J Radiol 2002;75(892):340–4.

26. Hollings NP, Wells AU, Wilson R, et al. Comparative appearances of non-tuberculous mycobacteria species: a CT study. Eur Radiol 2002;12(9):2211–7.

27. Kartalija M, Ovrutsky AR, Bryan CL, et al. Patients with nontuberculous mycobacterial lung disease exhibit unique body and immune phenotypes. Am J Respir Crit Care Med 2013;187(2):197–205.

28. Jeong YJ, Kim KI, Seo IJ, et al. Eosinophilic lung diseases: a clinical, radiologic, and pathologic overview. Radiographics 2007;27(3):617–37 [discussion: 637-9].

29. Cappelluti E, Fraire AE, Schaefer OP. A case of "hot tub lung" due to Mycobacterium avium complex in an immunocompetent host. Arch Intern Med 2003; 163(7):845–8.

30. Pham RV, Vydareny KH, Gal AA. High-resolution computed tomography appearance of pulmonary Mycobacterium avium complex infection after exposure to hot tub: case of hot-tub lung. J Thorac Imaging 2003;18(1):48–52.

31. Embil J, Warren P, Yakrus M, et al. Pulmonary illness associated with exposure to Mycobacterium-avium complex in hot tub water. Hypersensitivity pneumonitis or infection? Chest 1997;111(3):813–6.

32. Lim J, Lyu J, Choi CM, et al. Non-tuberculous mycobacterial diseases presenting as solitary pulmonary nodules. Int J Tuberc Lung Dis 2010;14(12):1635–40.

33. Aronchick JM, Miller WT Jr. Disseminated nontuberculous mycobacterial infections in immunosuppressed patients. Semin Roentgenol 1993;28(2): 150–7.

34. Nalaboff KM, Rozenshtein A, Kaplan HM. Imaging of mycobacterium avium-intracellulare infection in AIDS patients on highly active antiretroviral therapy: reversal syndrome. AJR Am J Roentgenol 2000;175(2):387–90. https://doi.org/10.2214/ajr.175.2.1750387.

35. Goebel FD. Immune reconstitution inflammatory syndrome (IRIS)–another new disease entity following treatment initiation of HIV infection. Infection 2005; 33(1):43–5.

36. Ratnam I, Chiu C, Kandala NB, et al. Incidence and risk factors for immune reconstitution inflammatory syndrome in an ethnically diverse HIV type 1-infected cohort. Clin Infect Dis 2006;42(3):418–27. https://doi.org/10.1086/499356.

37. Manabe YC, Campbell JD, Sydnor E, et al. Immune reconstitution inflammatory syndrome: risk factors and treatment implications. J Acquir Immune Defic Syndr 2007;46(4):456–62.

38. Breton G, Duval X, Estellat C, et al. Determinants of immune reconstitution inflammatory syndrome in HIV type 1-infected patients with tuberculosis after initiation of antiretroviral therapy. Clin Infect Dis 2004;39(11):1709–12.

39. Meintjes G, Stek C, Blumenthal L, et al. Prednisone for the prevention of paradoxical tuberculosis-associated IRIS. N Engl J Med 2018;379(20): 1915–25.

40. Camargo JF, Lobo SA, Hsu AP, et al. MonoMAC syndrome in a patient with a GATA2 mutation: case report and review of the literature. Clin Infect Dis 2013;57(5):697–9.

41. Vinh DC, Patel SY, Uzel G, et al. Autosomal dominant and sporadic monocytopenia with susceptibility to mycobacteria, fungi, papillomaviruses, and myelodysplasia. Blood 2010;115(8):1519–29.

42. Hadjiliadis D, Adlakha A, Prakash UB. Rapidly growing mycobacterial lung infection in association with esophageal disorders. Mayo Clin Proc 1999; 74(1):45–51.

43. Banerjee R, Hall R, Hughes GR. Pulmonary Mycobacterium fortuitum infection in association with achalasia of the oesophagus. Case report and review of the literature. Br J Dis Chest 1970;64(2): 112–8.

44. Shiraishi Y, Nakajima Y, Katsuragi N, et al. Pneumonectomy for nontuberculous mycobacterial infections. Ann Thorac Surg 2004;78(2):399–403.

45. Kwon BS, Lee JH, Koh Y, et al. The natural history of non-cavitary nodular bronchiectatic Mycobacterium avium complex lung disease. Respir Med 2019; 150:45–50.

46. Pan SW, Shu CC, Feng JY, et al. Microbiological persistence in patients with mycobacterium avium complex lung disease: the predictors and the impact on radiographic progression. Clin Infect Dis 2017;65(6):927–34.

47. Hwang JA, Kim S, Jo KW, et al. Natural history of Mycobacterium avium complex lung disease in untreated patients with stable course. Eur Respir J 2017;49(3):1600537.

48. van Ingen J. Diagnosis of nontuberculous mycobacterial infections. Semin Respir Crit Care Med 2013; 34(1):103–9.

49. Haworth CS, Banks J, Capstick T, et al. British Thoracic Society guidelines for the management of non-tuberculous mycobacterial pulmonary disease (NTM-PD). Thorax 2017;72(Suppl 2):ii1–64.

50. Nachiappan AC, Rahbar K, Shi X, et al. Pulmonary Tuberculosis: Role of Radiology in Diagnosis and Management. Radiographics 2017;37(1):52–72.

51. Shiraishi Y, Fukushima K, Komatsu H, et al. Early pulmonary resection for localized Mycobacterium avium complex disease. Ann Thorac Surg 1998; 66(1):183–6.

52. Nelson KG, Griffith DE, Brown BA, et al. Results of operation in Mycobacterium avium-intracellulare lung disease. Ann Thorac Surg 1998;66(2):325–30.

53. Yu JA, Pomerantz M, Bishop A, et al. Lady Windermere revisited: treatment with thoracoscopic lobectomy/segmentectomy for right middle lobe and lingular bronchiectasis associated with nontuberculous mycobacterial disease. Eur J Cardiothorac Surg 2011;40(3):671–5.

North American Endemic Fungal Infections

Jeffrey P. Kanne, MD

KEYWORDS

- Fungus • Infection • Histoplasmosis • Blastomycosis • Coccidioidomycosis

KEY POINTS

- Endemic fungal infection is a common cause of community-acquired pneumonia, although many infections may be asymptomatic.
- The diagnosis of fungal pneumonia is often delayed because of the clinical and radiographic overlap with common community-acquired bacterial infections and lack of clinical suspicion.
- Chronic cavitary fungal infection can mimic neoplasia and mycobacterial infection.
- Disseminated endemic fungal infection most commonly affects patients who are immunosuppressed or who have a high inoculum of organisms.
- Histoplasmosis is the most common cause of fibrosing mediastinitis, a rare immunologic response to *H capsulatum*.

INTRODUCTION

Endemic fungal infections in North America consist of histoplasmosis, blastomycosis, and coccidioidomycosis. The incidence and prevalence vary greatly depending on geography, with histoplasmosis being the most widespread. Most cases of blastomycosis occur in the Upper Midwest, and coccidioidomycosis is limited to parts of the western United States. Because many infections are subclinical, the true incidence of these infections is unknown. Furthermore, compulsory reporting of cases to local or state public health authorities varies.[1] When symptomatic, the endemic fungal infections primarily cause an acute respiratory illness similar to bacterial and viral pneumonias.

Radiography and selective use of computed tomography (CT) are usually adequate for evaluation of patients with endemic fungal pneumonia. MR imaging may be used to evaluate extrathoracic disease including bone and joint and central nervous system (CNS) involvement. PET/CT might have a limited role in highly selective cases to identify disseminated disease, although it is not commonly used. Although imaging findings often overlap with those of other community-acquired pneumonias, the radiologist can be the first to suggest the diagnosis of endemic fungal infection by considering the imaging findings in the context of local prevalence, risk factors for fungal disease, and temporal evolution of disease.

This article reviews the clinical and imaging manifestations of histoplasmosis, blastomycosis, and coccidioidomycosis with figures highlighting the different radiologic manifestations of disease. Although *Cryptococcus gattii* is an emerging cause of fungal infection in parts of the United States, discussion of this infection is beyond the scope of this article.

HISTOPLASMOSIS

Histoplasmosis is caused by inhalation of spores of the dimorphic fungus *Histoplasma capsulatum* (Fig. 1). Histoplasmosis is the most common endemic mycosis in North America and is the leading cause of hospitalization and death among these infections, with the growing number of immunocompromised patients contributing to the increase.[2,3]

Department of Radiology, University of Wisconsin School of Medicine and Public Health, 600 Highland Avenue MC 3252, Madison, WI 53792-3252, USA
E-mail address: JKanne@uwhealth.org

Radiol Clin N Am 60 (2022) 409–427
https://doi.org/10.1016/j.rcl.2022.01.007

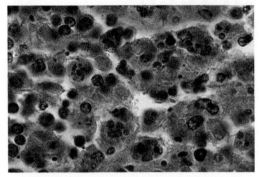

Fig. 1. *Histoplasma capsulatum.* High-power photomicrograph (H&E stain) shows intracellular *H capsulatum.* (*Courtesy of* J Torrealba, MD, Dallas, TX.)

Mycology

H capsulatum primarily lives in soil contaminated by bird and bat guano.[4] Two variants of *H capsulatum* exist: widespread *H capsulatum* var. *capsulatum* and *H capsulatum* var. *duboisii*, which is found exclusively in Africa, primarily in Central and Western Africa and Madagascar.[5]

Epidemiology

Histoplasmosis was first described in 1906 in a worker at the Panama Canal[6] and is now recognized as endemic in regions on all continents except Antarctica (**Fig. 2**).[4,7] Human immunodeficiency virus (HIV) infection and increased use of immunosuppressive therapies have led to a better understanding of the true global nature of the disease.[4,7] Traditionally, the Mississippi and Ohio River Valleys in the United States and parts of Central and South America are considered the main

endemic regions.[4,8] However, highly endemic areas have also been identified in parts of Central and South America, Sub-Saharan Africa (especially Nigeria), parts of Southeast Asia, Northern and Northeastern India, and Eastern Australia.[1] Most cases of histoplasmosis in Europe are acquired from travel elsewhere, although *H capsulatum* has been identified in the soil of the Po River Valley in Italy.[1,9]

Pathogenesis

The respiratory tract is the portal of entry for *H capsulatum.* Inhaled conidia or mycelial fragments transform into yeast form both inside and outside phagocytes within the alveoli.[10] Phagocytes allow viable organisms to spread to lymph nodes and other organs, playing a role in the pathogenesis of histoplasmosis. In most cases, host immune response clears the infection, and infection remains subclinical.[11] Immunocompromised patients and patients inhaling a large inoculum are at risk for disseminated infection.[12]

Diagnosis

Although *H capsulatum* can be identified on light microscopy, either in phagocytic cells or, less commonly, in extracellular tissue, the organisms can be difficult to distinguish from other pathogens and can be easily overlooked if few. Culture is more useful in patients with disseminated chronic histoplasmosis, leading to a diagnosis in 50% to 85% of patients. Blood and bone marrow reportedly have the highest yield.[13] However, slow growth in culture is impractical for rapid diagnosis.[4] Galactomannan urine and serum antigen testing gives positive result in 80% to 95% of

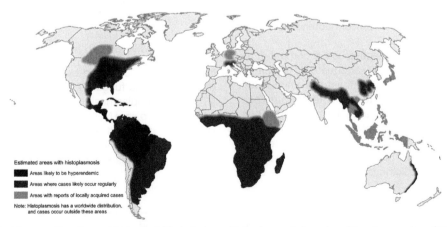

Fig. 2. World map estimating regions most likely to have histoplasmosis based on literature review. (*From* Ashraf N, Kubat RC, Poplin V, et al. Re-drawing the maps for endemic mycoses. Mycopathologia 2020;185(5):843–65. Used under a Creative Commons Attribution 4.0 International License. http://creativecommons.org/licenses/by/4.0/.)

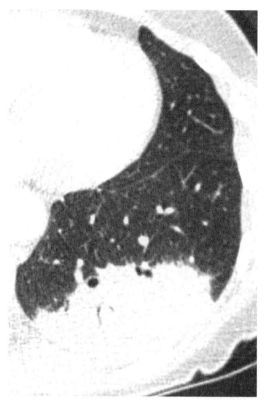

Fig. 3. A 56-year-old female was on adalimumab with acute histoplasmosis. Unenhanced CT image shows dense consolidation in the left lower lobe.

patients with acute pulmonary histoplasmosis or progressive disseminated histoplasmosis. There is cross-reactivity in patients with blastomycosis and other fungal infections including coccidioidomycosis.[13,14] Antibodies to *H capsulatum* develop 4 to 8 weeks after initial infection and can be detected by immunodiffusion, complement fixation, and enzyme immunoassay. Some antibodies

can persist for years after infection, whereas others wane after a few months. As with antigen testing, cross-reaction can occur in patients with blastomycosis or coccidioidomycosis.[4,15,16] Although polymerase chain reaction (PCR) testing is commercially available for histoplasmosis, its role in diagnosis remains unclear.[17–19]

Clinical Disease

Acute pulmonary histoplasmosis

Approximately 90% of patients infected with *H capsulatum* are asymptomatic.[4] Symptomatic infections are associated with higher inoculums, immunosuppression, extremes of age, and more virulent strains of the organism.[20–22] Symptomatic acute pulmonary histoplasmosis typically occurs after a 14-day median incubation period and is characterized by cough, shortness of breath, fever, and chills,[4] similar to other forms of community-acquired pneumonia.[23] Chest pain and rheumatologic symptoms such as arthralgia, arthritis, and erythema nodosum occur in a small number of patients.[24] Most patients recover within 1 to 2 weeks. Patients with severe infection can develop acute respiratory distress syndrome (ARDS) or progress to disseminated disease.[4] The liver, spleen, skin, and bone marrow are the most common sites of disseminated disease.

On chest imaging, symptomatic acute pulmonary histoplasmosis is typically characterized by bilateral lung consolidation with hilar and mediastinal lymph node enlargement, similar to other severe community-acquired pneumonias (**Fig. 3**).[4] However, pleural effusion is uncommon. Hepatosplenomegaly may be apparent on chest CT. Lung nodules, lymphadenopathy, or both can be incidentally detected in asymptomatic patients with acute infection (**Fig. 4**). Immunocompromised patients or patients with a large inoculum can have a

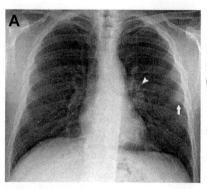
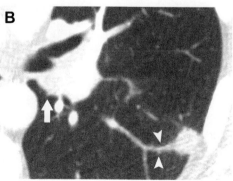

Fig. 4. A 52-year-old male had asymptomatic acute histoplasmosis. (*A*) Posteroanterior radiograph shows left hilar lymph node enlargement (*arrowhead*) and a well-defined left lung nodule (*arrow*). (*B*) Unenhanced CT image shows a well-defined large left lower lobe nodule with subtle perilymphatic nodules along the draining vein (*arrowheads*) and left hilar lymph node enlargement (*arrow*).

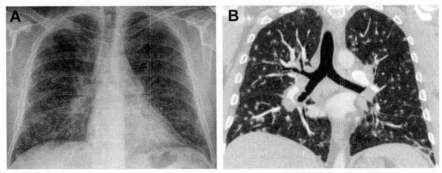

Fig. 5. A 50-year-old male had disseminated histoplasmosis. (*A*) PA radiograph shows diffuse small lung nodules. (*B*) Coronal reformatted maximum intensity projection from contrast-enhanced CT shows the random distribution of small nodules indicating hematogenous spread.

miliary pattern of randomly distributed tiny nodules on imaging (**Fig. 5**).

Subacute pulmonary histoplasmosis

Symptomatic, subacute infections are characterized by milder but prolonged symptoms and result from a lower inoculum of *H capsulatum*. Chest imaging findings include mediastinal and hilar lymphadenopathy (**Fig. 6**). Lung findings may be absent or limited, most often a dominant nodule with nearby perilymphatic nodules and less often a small focus of consolidation.[25] Nodules consist of necrotizing or nonnecrotizing granulomata. Organisms can be identified with special staining of biopsy specimens, but because they are typically not viable, they do not grow in culture. Nodules

can persist indefinitely, and some can calcify or cavitate.[4,12]

Chronic pulmonary histoplasmosis

Chronic infection with *H capsulatum* can mimic chronic pulmonary tuberculosis and typically affects older males with structural lung disease, particularly emphysema.[20] Patients develop productive cough, shortness of breath, chest pain, weight loss, and night sweats, which wax and wane and recur with acute exacerbations. Chronic histoplasmosis is characterized by cavities, scar, and pleural thickening, most commonly affecting the upper lobes (**Fig. 7**). Background emphysema or other structural lung disease is common. Consolidation around preexisting bullae can mimic

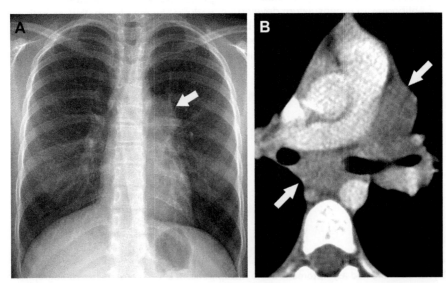

Fig. 6. A 11-year-old female with subacute histoplasmosis. (*A*) PA radiograph shows left hilar and mediastinal lymph node enlargement (*arrow*). (*B*) Contrast-enhanced CT image shows enlarged subcarinal and subaortic homogeneous lymph nodes (*arrows*).

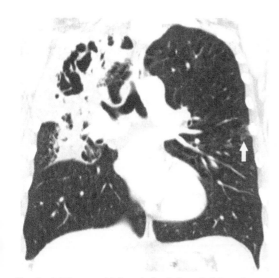

Fig. 7. A 54-year-old female had chronic histoplasmosis. Coronal reformatted unenhanced CT image shows a large, complex, and thick-walled right upper lobe cavity with adjacent consolidation. Small bronchiolocentric nodules (*arrow*), reflecting airway spread of inflammatory debris, are in the left lung.

cavities. Lymphadenopathy is not common, but calcified lymph nodes are often present. Progressive scar and volume loss ensue. The imaging findings can mimic those of tuberculosis and chronic necrotizing aspergillosis.[4,20]

Mediastinal lymphadenitis

Mediastinal lymphadenitis occurs in acute and subacute histoplasmosis. As with many cases of acute histoplasmosis, symptoms are uncommon but occur more often in children because of mass effect on their relatively smaller and more pliable airways. Patients can also develop signs and symptoms of venous congestion from mediastinal vein compression or dysphagia from esophageal compression.[26] On CT, enlarged lymph nodes are homogeneous (**Fig. 8**).[27] Urine antigen testing often obviates tissue sampling.

Mediastinal granuloma

Mediastinal granuloma is an uncommon manifestation of histoplasmosis, which can occur during acute infection or develop later. This manifestation is characterized by a confluent, heterogeneous lymph node mass often involving the paratracheal and subcarinal lymph nodes (**Fig. 9**),[28–30] contrasting to the homogeneous lymph nodes of mediastinal lymphadenitis. Scattered or peripheral

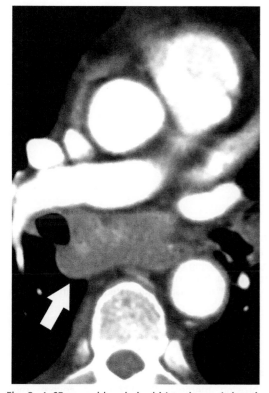

Fig. 8. A 65-year-old male had histoplasmosis lymphadenitis. Contrast-enhanced CT image shows a large, heterogeneously enhancing subcarinal lymph node (*arrow*). Granulomatous inflammation and *H capsulatum* were identified on transbronchial biopsy.

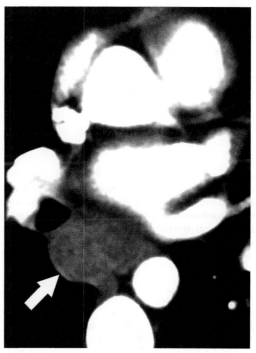

Fig. 9. A 34-year-old female had histoplasmosis mediastinal granuloma. Contrast-enhanced CT image shows enlarged subcarinal lymph node (*arrow*) containing small low-attenuation foci reflecting necrosis.

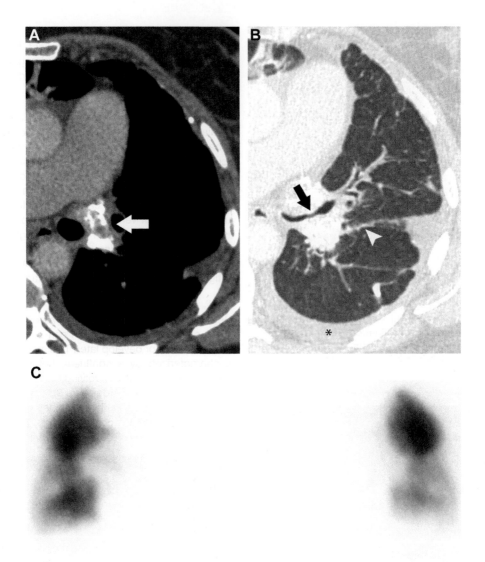

Anterior 1275K   Posterior 956K

Fig. 10. A 46-year-old female had fibrosing mediastinitis. (*A*) Contrast-enhanced CT image (soft tissue window settings) shows a partially calcified left hilar and mediastinal mass (*arrow*) occluding the left pulmonary artery. (*B*) Contrast-enhanced CT image (lung window settings) shows narrowing of the left upper lobe bronchus (*arrow*), fissural thickening (*arrowhead*) reflecting subpleural edema from central venolymphatic obstruction, and small left pleural effusion (*astrisk*). (*C*) Planar image from ^{99m}Tc99 macroaggregated albumin perfusion scan shows no perfusion to the left lung.

calcifications are sometimes apparent on CT. Many patients are asymptomatic, but symptoms can arise from local mass effect.[4] Rare complications include adhesions and fistulae. Delayed symptoms can arise from superinfection or flares of immune response.

Fibrosing mediastinitis

Fibrosing mediastinitis (FM) is a severe, rare immune-mediated complication most commonly resulting from previous histoplasmosis characterized by formation of a solid, fibrotic mediastinal or hilar mass, which can slowly invade and narrow

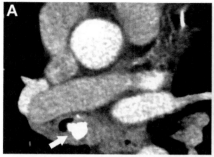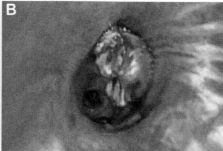

Fig. 11. A 64-year-old male had hemoptysis resulting from a broncholith. (*A*) Contrast-enhanced CT images show a large calcification (*arrow*) in an enlarged subcarinal lymph node protruding into the lumen of the bronchus intermedius. (*B*) Bronchoscopic image after partial debulking shows calcific endoluminal mass.

adjacent structures.[29,31] The exact mechanism leading to FM is unclear, but an abnormal immune response to residual antigens of *H capsulatum* is postulated. Hemoptysis is the most common manifestation typically from venous congestion or bronchial artery hypertrophy. More severe complications include complications include superior vena cava syndrome, pulmonary venous infarction, or autoamputation of the lung.[12]

CT findings of FM include a partially calcified, confluent mediastinal mass invading and narrowing or occluding adjacent structures (**Fig. 10**). Usually, the mass affects one side of the mediastinum.[12] Occasionally, the fibrotic process is limited to the hilum.

The diagnosis of FM is usually established by clinical and imaging findings, because biopsy results are not specific and invasive procedures can be high risk. Antigen testing is usually negative, and organisms typically do not grow in culture. Serum antibodies only indicate past infection.[12]

Broncholith

Calcified mediastinal or hilar lymph nodes and occasionally more peripheral peribronchial lymph nodes can erode into the adjacent airways causing hemopytsis and airway obstruction (**Fig. 11**).[32] Patients sometimes expectorate small pieces of calcium (lithoptysis). Other complications include obstructive bacterial infection or rarely bronchoesophageal fistula.[33]

Histoplasmoma

A histoplasmoma is a slowly growing nodule with a fibrous capsule and necrotic center.[34] Most are well circumscribed, and some may develop peripheral or target-like patterns of calcification (**Fig. 12**). Histoplasmomas are reported to occur more often in the lower lobes.[34,35] Growth may prompt evaluation for malignancy. Biopsy may

show *H capsulatum*, but organisms rarely grow on culture.

Treatment

Because most cases of acute histoplasmosis resolve spontaneously in immunocompetent patients, treatment is not recommended. However, treatment with antifungal agents is recommended for patients with moderate to severe acute disease and for immunocompromised patients. Chronic pulmonary histoplasmosis and progressive disseminated histoplasmosis are always treated. Surgery is an option for symptomatic patients with mediastinal granuloma to reduce mass effect and repair fistulae. Treatment of FM should be limited to preserving patency of blood vessels and airways because of high mortality rates resulting from exuberant collateral vessels and distorted tissue planes.[12]

BLASTOMYCOSIS
Mycology

Blastomycosis is caused by dimorphic fungi of the genus *Blastomyces*. Until recently, *Blastomyces dermatitidis* (**Fig. 13**) was the sole species in the genus. In 2011, *Blastomyces gilchristii*, a separate but phenotypically identical species, was identified and has been linked to outbreaks in northern Wisconsin and northwest Ontario, where it is the dominant species.[36–38] *B dermatitidis* and *B gilchristii* cause identical clinical syndromes, thus speciation is rarely performed in medical laboratories, and both will herein be referred to collectively as *B dermatitidis*. Other species in the *Blastomyces* genus cause atypical forms of blastomycosis.

Epidemiology

Defining the full geographic distribution of *B dermatitidis* is hampered by the latency between

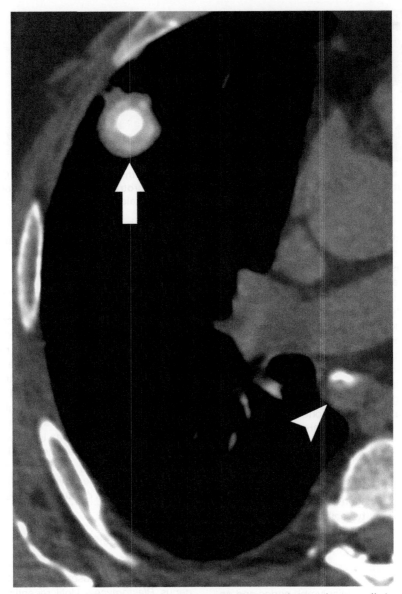

Fig. 12. A 61-year-old male had histoplasmoma. Unenhanced CT image shows a large, well-circumscribed right upper lobe nodule (*arrow*) with dense central calcification and a fainter peripheral ring of calcification and soft tissue. A partially calcified mediastinal lymph node (*arrow*) is also present.

exposure and symptoms, lack of skin testing or other reliable markers of exposure, and the difficulty in isolating the fungus in the environment. However, most infections occur in North America with traditional endemic areas including the Great Lakes basin and the St Lawrence, Mississippi, and Ohio River basins (**Fig. 14**).[1,39] The reported incidence of blastomycosis is 0.5 to 100 cases per 100,000 persons per year with central and northern Wisconsin[40] and northwestern Ontario[41]

considered hyperendemic regions. In addition to isolated cases, outbreaks of blastomycosis have been linked to construction, excavation, and outdoor recreational activities. B dermatitidis grows in moist, acidic, and sandy soils often near bodies of water.[42] *Blastomyces helicus* was described in 2015 and primarily affects immunocompromised patients in North America outside of traditional endemic areas; it has been linked to prairie dog dens in the western United States.[43] *Blastomyces*

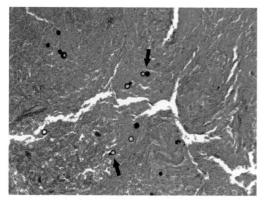

Fig. 13. *B dermatitidis*. Photomicrograph (high-powered methenamine silver stain) shows broad-based budding yeast bodies of *B dermatitidis* (*arrows*). (*From* Johnson EM, Martin MD, Sharma R, et al. Blastomycosis: the great pretender. J Thorac Imaging 2020;37(1)W5–W11.)

percursus and *Blastomyces emzantsi* have been linked to infections in patients in Israel and Africa, including South Africa.[44]

Pathogenesis

Inhalation of the mold form of *B dermatitidis* is the primary portal of entry into the body.[45] Cutaneous inoculation is rare.[46] At body temperatures, the organism begins replicating in yeast form within pulmonary macrophages.[47] Innate and adaptive immunity are primarily responsible for clearing the infection.[48] Dissemination is typically through hematogenous routes. The typical incubation period is 4 to 6 weeks, although symptomatic disease can occur years or even decades after infection, presumably from reactivation or latent infection.[49,50] Both relapse of incompletely treated infection and reinfection can occur.

Diagnosis

The diagnosis of blastomycosis is often delayed because of similarities to more common community-acquired infections. Fewer than 5% of patients are estimated to be correctly diagnosed with blastomycosis at presentation.[50] Definitive diagnosis requires identification of *B dermatitidis* in culture from sputum, bronchoalveolar lavage fluid, or tissue. A commercially available DNA probe assay assists in rapid confirmation. Because of its unique morphologic appearance, *B dermatitidis* is easily identified on light microscopy of tissue or fluid specimens, allowing for initiation of therapy pending culture confirmation.[51] Serum and urine antigen testing can also help establish a provisional diagnosis of blastomycosis with sensitivity up to 90%. However, cross-reactivity with *H capsulatum* precludes distinguishing these 2 infections. At present, antibody testing has not been proved to be useful for diagnosis blastomycosis, although a new enzyme immunoassay has potential.[49]

Clinical Disease

Acute pulmonary blastomycosis
Acute pulmonary blastomycosis occurs in 70% to 90% of patients with blastomycosis, reflecting the respiratory tract as the primary portal of entry.[52,53] More than 50% of patients have subclinical disease, and most cases are self-limited. In contrast

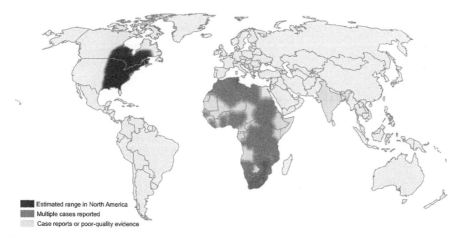

Estimated range in North America
Multiple cases reported
Case reports or poor-quality evidence

Fig. 14. World map estimating regions most likely to have blastomycosis based on literature review. Note this map is specific to *B. dermatitidis* complex. Other species are not included. (*From* Ashraf N, Kubat RC, Poplin V, et al. Re-drawing the maps for endemic mycoses. Mycopathologia 2020;185(5):843–65. Used under a Creative Commons Attribution 4.0 International License. http://creativecommons.org/licenses/by/4.0/.)

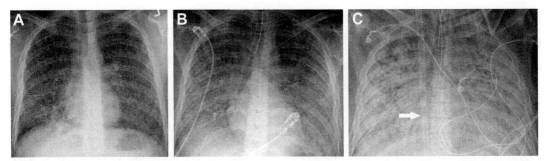

Fig. 15. A 21-year-old male developed fatal acute respiratory distress syndrome. (*A*) Initial bedside anteroposterior (AP) chest radiograph shows diffuse tiny lung nodules. (*B*) AP bedside chest radiograph 1 day later shows nodules coalescing and new endotracheal tube (*C*). AP bedside chest radiograph 2 weeks after presentation shows confluent diffuse lung opacities. Extracorporeal membrane oxygenation support (*arrow*) was required.

to histoplasmosis, blastomycosis more commonly causes symptomatic disease including in immunocompetent patients. Immunocompromised patients are more likely to develop severe infection, disseminated infection, and ARDS.[54] Signs and symptoms of acute pulmonary blastomycosis are indistinguishable from acute community-acquired pneumonias and include cough, fever, chills, malaise, and chest pain.[54,55] Acute infection can progress to ARDS in 7% to 15% of patients, with delay in diagnosis being a significant cause (**Fig. 15**).[50] The reported mortality rate for blastomycosis-associated ARDS is approximately 50%, with reported ranges of 40% to 89%[56]

The most common radiographic finding of acute pulmonary blastomycosis is lung consolidation,

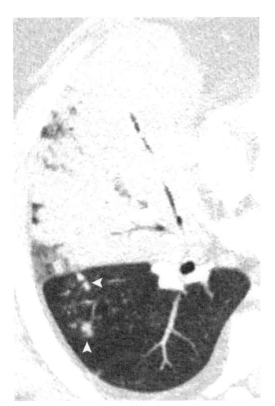

Fig. 16. A 30-year-old male had acute blastomycosis. Contrast-enhanced CT image shows dense middle lobe consolidation. Small nodules are in the right lower lobe (*arrowheads*).

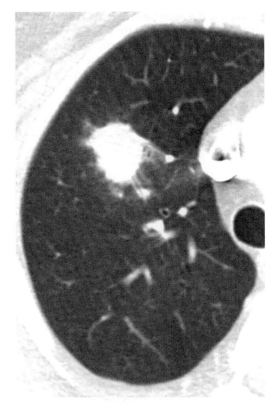

Fig. 17. A 63-year-old female had acute blastomycosis. Contrast-enhanced CT image shows an irregular nodule in the right upper lobe.

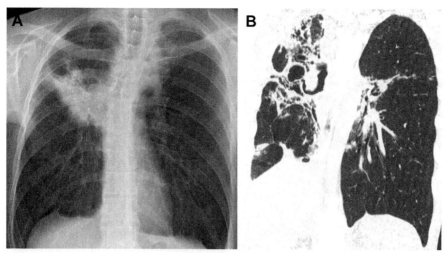

Fig. 18. A 37-year-old male had acute blastomycosis progressing to chronic infection. (*A*) PA chest radiograph at presentation shows right perihilar and left apical lung consolidation. (*B*) Coronal reformatted CT image 2 years later shows extensive scarring primarily in the right lung with bronchiectasis and a complex cavity.

which can be patchy or confluent, similar to acute bacterial infection (**Fig. 16**).[57] On CT, small satellite nodules may be apparent, and pleural effusion, which occurs in fewer than 20% of patients, is usually small. In contrast to histoplasmosis and bacterial infection, lymphadenopathy is often mild and occurs in only approximately 13% of patients. Pleural effusion is even more uncommon occurring in only 2% of patients. These findings and failure to respond to standard community-acquired pneumonia therapy should raise the question of blastomycosis in endemic areas.[57] Other patients with blastomycosis may have a dominant mass or nodule mimicking lung carcinoma (**Fig. 17**).[57] Diffuse lung disease is reported in 5% of patients with acute pulmonary blastomycosis and can have a miliary pattern of random nodules or diffuse consolidation.[56,57]

Chronic pulmonary blastomycosis

Patients with chronic pulmonary blastomycosis can present with ongoing systemic signs and symptoms such as fatigue, weight loss, intermittent fever, and night sweats, similar to chronic histoplasmosis and tuberculosis as well as lymphoma.[50,52] Symptom duration ranges from months to years. Imaging findings range from masslike consolidation to cavitary lesions indistinguishable from chronic histoplasmosis and tuberculosis (**Fig. 18**).[57,58]

Disseminated blastomycosis

Between 20% and 40% of patients with symptomatic blastomycosis develop disseminated disease, most commonly affecting the skin, bone, CNS, and genitourinary (GU) tract.[52,53,59,60] Disseminated disease is more common in

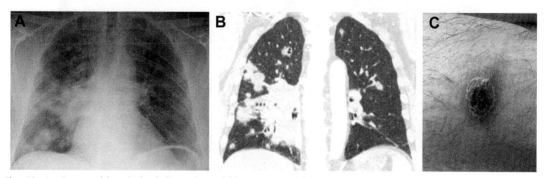

Fig. 19. A 49-year-old male had disseminated blastomycosis. (*A*) PA radiograph shows consolidation in the mid right lung and scattered bilateral lung nodule. (*B*) Coronal reformat shows dense right lower lobe consolidation and scattered bilateral, irregular lung nodules. (*C*) Photograph shows typical pustular skin lesion with a crusted-over central plaque.

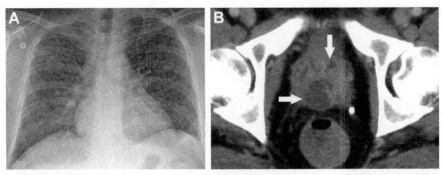

Fig. 20. A 47-year-old male had disseminated blastomycosis and prostatitis. (*A*) Bedside AP chest radiograph shows diffuse tiny lung nodules. (*B*) Contrast-enhanced pelvic CT image shows multiple low-attenuation foci in the prostate gland (*arrows*).

immunocompromised patients. Skin involvement is the most common extrapulmonary site of blastomycosis, affecting 40% to 80% of patients with disseminated disease (**Fig. 19**).[61] Bone or joint involvement occurs in 5% to 20% of patients with disseminated blastomycosis, most commonly causing osteomyelitis.[52,53] Direct extension can cause soft tissue abscess, septic arthritis, and sinus tracts. GU tract involvement occurs in fewer than 10% of patients with disseminated disease. Prostatitis (**Fig. 20**) is most common in males,[62] and tubo-ovarian abscess is most common in females.[50] CNS involvement occurs in 5% to 10% of immunocompetent patients

with blastomycosis (**Fig. 21**). Subacute meningitis is the most common manifestation with brain abscesses much less common.[63]

Treatment
Treatment of blastomycosis depends on the immune status of the patient and the severity of the infection. In contrast to histoplasmosis and coccidioidomycosis, all symptomatic patients with blastomycosis should be treated with antifungal medication to prevent progression or recurrence of disease. Milder infections are typically treated with oral triazole agents, whereas severe infections require initial therapy with amphotericin B.[64]

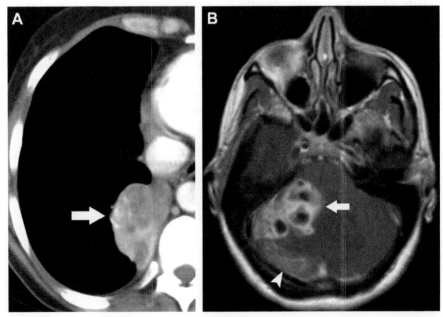

Fig. 21. A 44-year-old female mushroom hunter had disseminated blastomycosis. (*A*) Contrast-enhanced chest CT image shows a large, heterogeneous right lower lobe mass (*arrow*). (*B*) Contrast-enhanced T1-weighted brain MR image shows multiple peripherally enhancing cerebellar masses (*arrow*) and leptomeningeal enhancement (*arrowhead*).

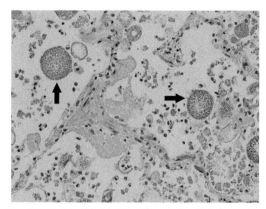

Fig. 22. *C immitis*. Photomicrograph of lung parenchyma shows multiple large thick-walled spherules with abundant basophilic endospores (*arrows*). There is an associated acute inflammation with necrotic debris in this case of *Coccidioides*-related acute pneumonia (hematoxylin-eosin, original magnification ×200). (*Courtesy of* J Torrealba, MD, Dallas, TX.)

Coccidioidomycosis

Mycology

Coccidioidomycosis is caused by the dimorphic fungi *Coccidioides immitis* (**Fig. 22**) and *Coccidioides posadasii*, which are phenotypically identical and cause identical clinical disease.[65] *Coccidioides* species are robust organisms, able to tolerate extremes of temperature and salinity of up to 8%. While in the soil, *Coccidioides* lives in mycelial form obtaining nutrients from dead or decaying organic matter.[66]

Epidemiology

Documentation of clinic cases, skin testing, and soil testing since the latter half of the 1900s have helped define the geographic range of *Coccidioides*. Endemic areas in the United States include Arizona, California, New Mexico, Nevada, Utah, Washington, and Texas with most cases occurring in Arizona and California (**Fig. 23**).[1] *Coccidioides* is also endemic in parts of Central and South America including northern Mexico, Argentina, Brazil, Bolivia, and Paraguay.[1,67] Incidence in the United States has increased since 2014, primarily because of increasing cases in California. *C immitis* is primarily found in California, eastern Washington, and Baja California in Mexico, whereas *C posadasii* is primarily found in other regions. The strongest risk factor for developing coccidioidomycosis is living or working in an endemic region, although even short-term travel to an endemic region is sufficient exposure.[1,68]

Pathogenesis

Although the exact infective dose of *Coccidioides* is unknown, the consensus is that it is quite small requiring just a few anthroconidia.[1,66] Most inhaled organisms can evade phagocytosis. The anthroconidia change into spherules in the terminal bronchiole, furthering their ability to be cleared by macrophages and neutrophils. Ultimately, adaptive host immunity, particularly T lymphocytes, leads to control of infection. Immunocompromised patients including those with HIV infection, pregnant (especially third trimester) or immediately postpartum women, and others with T-cell dysfunction are at increased risk of severe and disseminated disease. In addition, patients of Filipino, African, Native American, and Latino descent are at higher risk of more severe and disseminated disease, presumably because of genetic

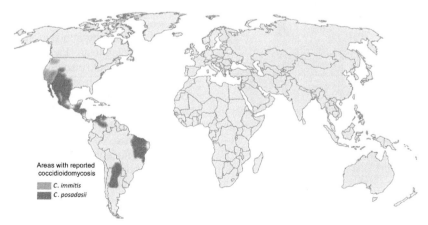

Fig. 23. World map estimating regions with coccidioidomycosis based on literature review. (*From* Ashraf N, Kubat RC, Poplin V, et al. Re-drawing the maps for endemic mycoses. Mycopathologia 2020;185(5):843–65. Used under a Creative Commons Attribution 4.0 International License. http://creativecommons.org/licenses/by/4.0/.)

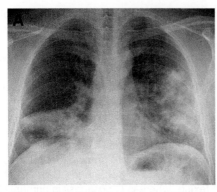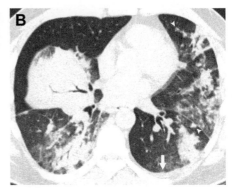

Fig. 24. A 40-year-old male had acute coccidioidomycosis following golfing trip in Arizona. (*A*) PA radiograph shows bilateral lung consolidation. (*B*) Unenhanced CT image shows bilateral dense lung consolidation with adjacent small nodules (*arrowheads*). A small left pleural effusion is present (*arrow*).

susceptibility, although the true mechanism has yet to be elucidated.[1,66,68]

Diagnosis

The diagnosis of coccidioidomycosis is confirmed by culture, identifying *Coccidioides* in tissue specimens or body fluids, or PCR. PCR and culture are

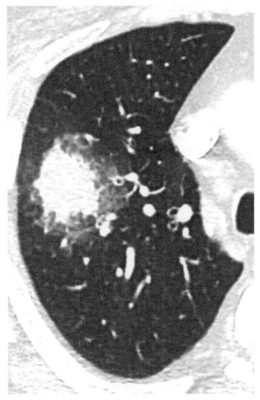

Fig. 25. A 76-year-old male had acute coccidioidomycosis. Contrast-enhanced CT image shows a large right upper lobe mass with surrounding halo of ground-glass opacity.

reported to have a sensitivity of 75% and specificity of 99%.[69] More commonly, the diagnosis is confirmed by a variety of serologic tests including enzyme immunoassay, complement fixation, and immunodiffusion. These tests rely on host ability to produce antibodies against *Coccidioides*, and serologic testing in immunocompromised patients may be limited. Furthermore, unlike with many other infections, serum IgG levels may wane over time resulting in false-negative complement fixation test results.[70] Knowledge of the type and timing of the test and the clinical context, such as timing from onset of symptoms and empirical antifungal therapy, is key to their interpretations.[66]

Clinical Disease

Primary pulmonary coccidioidomycosis

Up to 60% of patients with coccidioidomycosis have subclinical disease.[66,71] As with other endemic mycoses, most symptomatic acute infections are mild and indistinguishable from other forms of community-acquired pneumonia. Failure to respond to standard antibiotics for presumed bacterial community-acquired pneumonia is one clue to the diagnosis. Living in or travel to an endemic area should also raise suspicion. Patients may report a recent maculopapular rash, erythema nodosum, or erythema multiforme-like rash, which have been associated with a good prognosis because they are manifestations of robust host immune response.[66] More severe disease is characterized by diffuse pneumonia and primarily affects immunosuppressed patients or those at greater risk. As with blastomycosis, progression to ARDS is associated with increased mortality.[72]

Lung consolidation is the primary radiologic manifestation of acute pulmonary coccidioidomycosis (**Figs. 24** and **25**).[73] Mediastinal lymphadenopathy and pleural effusion can occur, the latter

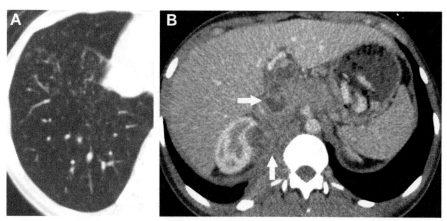

Fig. 26. A 21-year-old female had disseminated coccidioidomycosis. (*A*) Contrast-enhanced CT image shows numerous tiny right lung nodules. (*B*) Contrast-enhanced CT image shows retroperitoneal lymphadenopathy with necrosis (*arrows*).

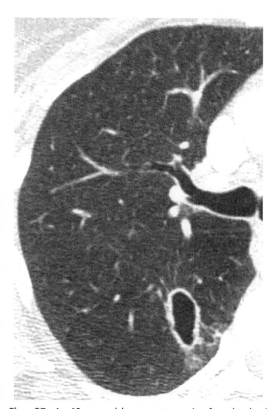

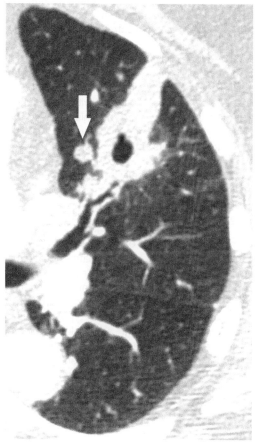

Fig. 27. A 49-year-old asymptomatic female had chronic cavity from coccidioidomycosis. Unenhanced CT image shows a thin-walled cavity in the right lower lobe with a small amount of adjacent ground-glass opacity.

Fig. 28. An 89-year-old male had chronic coccidioido-mycosis. Unenhanced CT image shows a thick-walled left upper lobe cavity with small satellite nodules (*arrow*).

occurs in only up to 15% of patients.[74] Patients with diffuse pneumonia have bilateral lung consolidation and lymphadenopathy.

Disseminated disease

Hematogenous or lymphangitic spread of infection can lead to disseminated coccidioidomycosis (**Fig. 26**). The CNS, skin, bone, and joints are most affected. CNS involvement is most severe, most commonly manifesting as meningitis.[75]

Chronic pulmonary coccidioidomycosis

Approximately 5% of patients, even those with asymptomatic disease, have residual lung nodules or cavities, which may be detected incidentally on chest imaging. Nodules can mimic malignancy but can be managed in accordance with current guidelines in patients in endemic areas. Residual nodules from coccidioidomycosis do not require treatment.[72]

Cavities, like nodules, do not require treatment if asymptomatic. However, cavities can rupture or become superinfected with bacteria or other fungi such as *Aspergillus* species.[72] Patients can also develop pleurisy or intermittent hemoptysis. Cavities typically have thin, small walls, sometimes with mural calcifications, but appearances vary (**Fig. 27**). Not all cavities resolve with therapy.[72,76]

Chronic fibrocavitary disease is an uncommon manifestation of coccidioidomycosis and is characterized by single or multiple cavities and patchy lung consolidation (**Fig. 28**). This disease can mimic chronic pulmonary tuberculosis or histoplasmosis. Patients may present with weight loss, fever, and fatigue. Prolonged antifungal therapy is required. Medically refractory cases may require surgical resection.[66,76,77]

Treatment

Asymptomatic patients or those with mild clinical manifestations do not require treatment, because the infection is typically self-limited, and to date, no data support treatment preventing dissemination. For patients with moderate signs and symptoms, oral triazole therapy is typically given. Amphotericin B along with a triazole is reserved for severe, disseminated disease. Patients with impaired cellular immunity are often given suppressive therapy, usually with fluconazole, after standard therapy is completed to prevent relapse.[66,72]

SUMMARY

Histoplasmosis, blastomycosis, and coccidioidomycosis are common causes of community-acquired pneumonia in their respective endemic geographic regions. Most infected patients have subclinical disease, and those with symptomatic infection typically have mild disease. Imaging findings of acute infection mimic those of bacterial and viral community-acquired pneumonia, whereas imaging findings of chronic disease, often associated with cavities, can mimic mycobacterial disease or aspergillosis. A detailed understanding of the epidemiology, clinical manifestations, thoracic and extrathoracic imaging findings, and available laboratory tests can help the radiologist first suggest the diagnosis of endemic fungal infection or identify complications such as superinfection, reactivation of infection, or chronic disease.

CLINICS CARE POINTS

- Most endemic fungal infections are subclinical or mild.

- Immunocompromised patients and patients with a large innoculum are at higher risk for disseminated disease, which can be life threatening.

- Imaging findings can help suggest the diagnosis of endemic fungal infection, identify complications, and assess response to therapy.

- Knowledge of exposures and travel can help the radiologist consider endemic fungal infection as a cause for a patient's illness.

DISCLOSURE

The author has nothing to disclose.

REFERENCES

1. Ashraf N, Kubat RC, Poplin V, et al. Re-drawing the maps for endemic mycoses. Mycopathologia 2020; 185(5):843–65.

2. Chu JH, Feudtner C, Heydon K, et al. Hospitalizations for endemic mycoses: a population-based national study. Clin Infect Dis 2006;42(6):822–5.

3. Benedict K, Derado G, Mody RK. Histoplasmosis-associated hospitalizations in the United States, 2001-2012. Open Forum Infect Dis 2016;3(1): ofv219.

4. Wheat LJ, Azar MM, Bahr NC, et al. Histoplasmosis. Infect Dis Clin North Am 2016;30(1):207–27.

5. Pakasa N, Biber A, Nsiangana S, et al. African Histoplasmosis in HIV-negative patients, kimpese,

democratic Republic of the Congo. Emerg Infect Dis 2018;24(11):2068–70.

6. Darling ST. A Protozoön general infection producing pseudotubercles in the lungs and focal necroses in the liver, spleen and lymph nodes. JAMA 1906; 46(17):1283–5.

7. Bahr NC, Antinori S, Wheat LJ, et al. Histoplasmosis infections worldwide: thinking outside of the Ohio River valley. Curr Trop Med Rep 2015;2(2):70–80.

8. Wheat LJ, Freifeld AG, Kleiman MB, et al. Clinical practice guidelines for the management of patients with histoplasmosis: 2007 update by the Infectious Diseases Society of America. Clin Infect Dis 2007; 45(7):807–25.

9. Sotgiu G, Mazzoni A, Mantovani A, et al. Histoplasma capsulatum: occurrence in soil from the emilia-romagna region of Italy. Science 1965; 147(3658):624.

10. Horwath MC, Fecher RA, Deepe GS. Histoplasma capsulatum, lung infection and immunity. Future Microbiol 2015;10(6):967–75.

11. Knox KS, Hage CA. Histoplasmosis. Proc Am Thorac Soc 2010;7(3):169–72.

12. Azar MM, Loyd JL, Relich RF, et al. Current concepts in the epidemiology, diagnosis, and management of Histoplasmosis syndromes. Semin Respir Crit Care Med 2020;41(1):13–30. https://doi.org/10.1055/s-0039-1698429.

13. Hage CA, Ribes JA, Wengenack NL, et al. A multicenter evaluation of tests for diagnosis of histoplasmosis. Clin Infect Dis 2011;53(5):448–54.

14. Durkin M, Connolly P, Kuberski T, et al. Diagnosis of coccidioidomycosis with use of the Coccidioides antigen enzyme immunoassay. Clin Infect Dis 2008; 47(8):e69–73.

15. Wheat J, French ML, Kohler RB, et al. The diagnostic laboratory tests for histoplasmosis: analysis of experience in a large urban outbreak. Ann Intern Med 1982;97(5):680 5.

16. Wheat LJ. Histoplasmosis in Indianapolis. Clin Infect Dis 1992;14(Suppl 1):S91–9.

17. Babady NE, Buckwalter SP, Hall L, et al. Detection of Blastomyces dermatitidis and Histoplasma capsulatum from culture isolates and clinical specimens by use of real-time PCR. J Clin Microbiol 2011;49(9): 3204–8.

18. Tang YW, Li H, Durkin MM, et al. Urine polymerase chain reaction is not as sensitive as urine antigen for the diagnosis of disseminated histoplasmosis. Diagn Microbiol Infect Dis 2006;54(4):283–7.

19. Wheat LJ. Improvements in diagnosis of histoplasmosis. Expert Opin Biol Ther 2006;6(11):1207–21.

20. Wheat LJ, Wass J, Norton J, et al. Cavitary histoplasmosis occurring during two large urban outbreaks. Analysis of clinical, epidemiologic, roentgenographic, and laboratory features. Medicine (Baltimore) 1984;63(4):201–9. https://doi.org/10.1097/00005792-198407000-00002.

21. Medoff G, Maresca B, Lambowitz AM, et al. Correlation between pathogenicity and temperature sensitivity in different strains of Histoplasma capsulatum. J Clin Invest 1986;78(6):1638–47.

22. Sepúlveda VE, Williams CL, Goldman WE. Comparison of phylogenetically distinct Histoplasma strains reveals evolutionarily divergent virulence strategies. mBio 2014;5(4):e01376-14.

23. Hage CA, Knox KS, Wheat LJ. Endemic mycoses: overlooked causes of community acquired pneumonia. Respir Med 2012;106(6):769–76.

24. Rosenthal J, Brandt KD, Wheat LJ, et al. Rheumatologic manifestations of histoplasmosis in the recent Indianapolis epidemic. Arthritis Rheum 1983;26(9): 1065–70.

25. Wheat LJ. Histoplasmosis: a review for clinicians from non-endemic areas. Mycoses 2006;49(4): 274–82.

26. Goodwin RA, Alcorn GL. Histoplasmosis with symptomatic lymphadenopathy. Chest 1980;77(2):213–5.

27. Nin CS, de Souza VV, do Amaral RH, et al. Thoracic lymphadenopathy in benign diseases: a state of the art review. Respir Med 2016;112:10–7.

28. Felson B, Klatte EC. Complications of the arrested primary histoplasmic complex. JAMA 1976; 236(10):1157–61.

29. Goodwin RA, Loyd JE, Des Prez RM. Histoplasmosis in normal hosts. Medicine (Baltimore) 1981;60(4): 231–66.

30. Loyd JE, Tillman BF, Atkinson JB, et al. Mediastinal fibrosis complicating histoplasmosis. Medicine (Baltimore) 1988;67(5):295–310.

31. Goodwin RA, Nickell JA, Des Prez RM. Mediastinal fibrosis complicating healed primary histoplasmosis and tuberculosis. Medicine (Baltimore) 1972;51(3): 227–46.

32. Arrigoni MG, Bernatz PE, Donoghue FE. Broncholithiasis. J Thorac Cardiovasc Surg 1971;62(2):231–7.

33. Ford MAP, Mueller PS, Morgenthaler TI. Bronchoesophageal fistula due to broncholithiasis: a case series. Respir Med 2005;99(7):830–5.

34. Goodwin RA, Snell JD. The enlarging histoplasmoma. Concept of a tumor-like phenomenon encompassing the tuberculoma and coccidioidoma. Am Rev Respir Dis 1969;100(1):1–12.

35. Guimarães MD, Marchiori E, Meirelles GS, et al. Fungal infection mimicking pulmonary malignancy: clinical and radiological characteristics. Lung 2013;191(6):655–62.

36. Meece JK, Anderson JL, Fisher MC, et al. Population genetic structure of clinical and environmental isolates of Blastomyces dermatitidis, based on 27 polymorphic microsatellite markers. Appl Environ Microbiol 2011;77(15):5123–31.

37. Brown EM, McTaggart LR, Zhang SX, et al. Phylogenetic analysis reveals a cryptic species Blastomyces gilchristii, sp. nov. within the human pathogenic fungus Blastomyces dermatitidis. PLoS One 2013;8(3): e59237.

38. McTaggart LR, Brown EM, Richardson SE. Phylogeographic Analysis of Blastomyces dermatitidis and Blastomyces gilchristii reveals an Association with North American freshwater Drainage basins. PLoS One 2016;11(7):e0159396.

39. Seitz AE, Younes N, Steiner CA, et al. Incidence and trends of blastomycosis-associated hospitalizations in the United States. PLoS One 2014;9(8): e105466.

40. Baumgardner DJ, Buggy BP, Mattson BJ, et al. Epidemiology of blastomycosis in a region of high endemicity in north central Wisconsin. Clin Infect Dis 1992;15(4):629–35.

41. Dwight PJ, Naus M, Sarsfield P, et al. An outbreak of human blastomycosis: the epidemiology of blastomycosis in the Kenora catchment region of Ontario, Canada. Can Commun Dis Rep 2000; 26(10):82–91.

42. Restrepo A, Baumgardner DJ, Bagagli E, et al. Clues to the presence of pathogenic fungi in certain environments. Med Mycol 2000;38(Suppl 1):67–77.

43. Friedman DZP, Schwartz IS. Emerging fungal infections: new patients, new patterns, and new pathogens. J Fungi (Basel) 2019;5(3):67.

44. Maphanga TG, Birkhead M, Muñoz JF, et al. Human Blastomycosis in South Africa Caused by Blastomyces percursus and Blastomyces emzantsi sp. nov., 1967 to 2014. J Clin Microbiol 2020;58(3):e01661-19.

45. Schwarz J, Baum GL. Blastomycosis. Am J Clin Pathol 1951;21(11):999–1029.

46. Gray NA, Baddour LM. Cutaneous inoculation blastomycosis. Clin Infect Dis 2002;34(10):E44–9.

47. Gauthier G, Klein BS. Insights into fungal morphogenesis and immune evasion: fungal conidia, when situated in mammalian lungs, may switch from mold to pathogenic yeasts or spore-forming spherules. Microbe Wash DC 2008;3(9):416–23.

48. Smith JA, Gauthier G. New Developments in Blastomycosis. Semin Respir Crit Care Med 2015;36(5): 715–28.

49. Schwartz IS, Kauffman CA. Blastomycosis Semin Respir Crit Care Med 2020;41(1):31–41.

50. McBride JA, Gauthier GM, Klein BS. Clinical Manifestations and Treatment of Blastomycosis. Clin Chest Med 2017;38(3):435–49.

51. Patel AJ, Gattuso P, Reddy VB. Diagnosis of blastomycosis in surgical pathology and cytopathology: correlation with microbiologic culture. Am J Surg Pathol 2010;34(2):256–61.

52. Lemos LB, Baliga M, Guo M. Blastomycosis: The great pretender can also be an opportunist. Initial clinical diagnosis and underlying diseases in 123 patients. Ann Diagn Pathol 2002;6(3):194–203.

53. Kralt D, Light B, Cheang M, et al. Clinical characteristics and outcomes in patients with pulmonary blastomycosis. Mycopathologia 2009;167(3):115–24.

54. McBride JA, Sterkel AK, Matkovic E, et al. Clinical Manifestations and Outcomes in Immunocompetent and Immunocompromised Patients With Blastomycosis. Clin Infect Dis 2021;72(9):1594–602.

55. Bariola JR, Vyas KS. Pulmonary blastomycosis. Semin Respir Crit Care Med 2011;32(6):745–53.

56. Mazi PB, Rauseo AM, Spec A. Blastomycosis. Infect Dis Clin North Am 2021;35(2):515–30.

57. Johnson EM, Martin MD, Sharma R, et al. Blastomycosis: the great pretender. J Thorac Imaging 2022; 37(1):W5–11. https://doi.org/10.1097/RTI.0000000000000562.

58. Patel RG, Patel B, Petrini MF, et al. Clinical presentation, radiographic findings, and diagnostic methods of pulmonary blastomycosis: a review of 100 consecutive cases. South Med J 1999;92(3): 289–95.

59. Azar MM, Assi R, Relich RF, et al. Blastomycosis in Indiana: Clinical and Epidemiologic Patterns of Disease Gleaned from a Multicenter Retrospective Study. Chest 2015;148(5):1276–84. https://doi.org/10.1378/chest.15-0289.

60. Kaplan W, Clifford MK, Blastomycosis I. A Review of 198 Collected Cases In Veterans Administration Hospitals. Am Rev Respir Dis 1964;89:659–72.

61. Smith JA, Riddell J, Kauffman CA. Cutaneous manifestations of endemic mycoses. Curr Infect Dis Rep 2013;15(5):440–9.

62. Rolnick D, Baumrucker GO. Genitourinary blastomycosis; case report and review of literature. J Urol 1958;79(2):315–23.

63. Bariola JR, Perry P, Pappas PG, et al. Blastomycosis of the central nervous system: a multicenter review of diagnosis and treatment in the modern era. Clin Infect Dis 2010;50(6):797–804.

64. Chapman SW, Dismukes WE, Proia LA, et al. Clinical practice guidelines for the management of blastomycosis: 2008 update by the infectious diseases society of America. Clin Infect Dis 2008;46(12): 1801–12.

65. Stockamp NW, Thompson GR. Coccidioidomycosis. Infect Dis Clin North Am 2016;30(1):229–46.

66. Kimes KE, Kasule SN, Blair JE. Pulmonary coccidioidomycosis. Semin Respir Crit Care Med 2020;41(1): 42–52.

67. Laniado-Laborín R, Arathoon EG, Canteros C, et al. Coccidioidomycosis in Latin America. Med Mycol 2019;57(Supplement_1):S46–55.

68. Diaz JH. Travel-related risk factors for coccidioidomycosis. J Trav Med 2018;25(1):tay027.

69. Vucicevic D, Blair JE, Binnicker MJ, et al. The utility of Coccidioides polymerase chain reaction testing in

the clinical setting. Mycopathologia 2010;170(5): 345–51.

70. Grys TE, Brighton A, Chang YH, et al. Comparison of two FDA-cleared EIA assays for the detection of Coccidioides antibodies against a composite clinical standard. Med Mycol 2018;57(5):595–600.

71. Smith CE, Beard RR. Varieties of coccidioidal infection in relation to the epidemiology and control of the diseases. Am J Public Health Nations Health 1946; 36(12):1394–402.

72. Bays DJ, Thompson GR. Coccidioidomycosis. Infect Dis Clin North Am 2021;35(2):453–69.

73. Malo J, Luraschi-Monjagatta C, Wolk DM, et al. Update on the diagnosis of pulmonary coccidioidomycosis. Ann Am Thorac Soc 2014;11(2):243–53.

74. Merchant M, Romero AO, Libke RD, et al. Pleural effusion in hospitalized patients with Coccidioidomycosis. Respir Med 2008;102(4):537–40.

75. Bays DJ, Thompson GR, Reef S, et al. Natural History of Disseminated Coccidioidomycosis: Examination of the VA-Armed Forces Database. Clin Infect Dis 2020;73(11):e3814–9.

76. Jude CM, Nayak NB, Patel MK, et al. Pulmonary coccidioidomycosis: pictorial review of chest radiographic and CT findings. Radiographics 2014; 34(4):912–25.

77. Ampel NM. The treatment of Coccidioidomycosis. Rev Inst Med Trop Sao Paulo 2015;57(Suppl 19): 51–6.

Endemic Thoracic Infections in Latin America and the Caribbean

Carlos S. Restrepo, MD[a],*, Jorge Carrillo, MD[b,1], Rolando Reyna, MD[c,2], Fortunato Suarez, MD[d], Sebastian Rossini, MD[e], Daniel Andres Vargas Zapata, MD[f,3]

KEYWORDS

- Chagas disease • Malaria • Amebiasis • Echinococcosis • Cysticercosis • Schistosomiasis
- Paragonimiasis • Ascariasis

KEY POINTS

- Chronic Chagas cardiomyopathy is the most common and serious complication of Chagas disease, and the most common cause of mortality.
- Acute lung injury and adult respiratory distress syndrome are the most severe pulmonary manifestations of malaria.
- Pleuropulmonary amebiasis occur when a subcapsular amebic liver abscess ruptures though the diaphragm into the thoracic cavity.
- After the liver, the lung is the second most commonly affected organ in echinococcosis.
- Pulmonary arterial hypertension is a common complication of schistosomiasis.
- Strongyloides hyperinfection syndrome is typically seen in immunosuppressed patients.
- Imaging findings in acute paracoccidioidomycosis resembles those of primary tuberculosis infection with the combination of airspace disease and lymphadenopathy.

INTRODUCTION

Socioeconomic inequality, poor hygiene, poor sanitation, and lack of access to safe drinking water pose significant public health challenges in Latin America and the Caribbean (LAC) region, where infectious diseases continue to cause significant morbidity, disability, and mortality. Major regional health challenges include limited access to health services, lack of resources, and poor distribution of the existing ones. Diarrheal diseases, along with acute respiratory infections, remain a significant cause of infant and child mortality. Parasitic diseases in particular, which affect more than 1.5 billion people worldwide, are closely associated with income inequality and deficient sanitation. Many of these conditions, which still have significant impact in LAC, are part of the Neglected Infectious Disease (NID) initiative by the World Health Organization (WHO). Ten percent of the global burden of NID occur in LAC, where 17% of the population in rural areas do not have access to safe drinking water, and 37% lack access to sanitation facilities.[1] Developing countries,

[a] Cardiothoracic Imaging, Department of Radiology, The University of Texas Health Science Center at San Antonio; [b] Universidad Nacional de Colombia, Bogotá, Colombia; [c] Hospital Santo Tomás, Panama; [d] Instituto Nacional de Enfermedádes Respiratórias Ismael Cosio Villegas, Código postal 14080, 4502 Calzada de Tlalpan, Ciudad de México, Mexico; [e] Instituto Radiológico Mar del Plata, Calle Mendoza 3267, Mar del Plata, Buenos Aires, 7600 Argentina; [f] The University of Texas Health Science Center at San Antonio

[1] Present address: Diagonal 57 # 1-60 Este Apartamento 303 Torre B, Barrio El Castillo, Bogotá, Colombia.
[2] Present address: PO Box 0819-01586, Ciudad de Panamá, Panamá
[3] Present address: 7714 Louis Pasteur Dr., San Antonio TX 78229.
* Corresponding author. 3323 Ivory Creek, San Antonio, TX 78258.
E-mail address: restrepoc@UTHSCSA.edu

Radiol Clin N Am 60 (2022) 429–443
https://doi.org/10.1016/j.rcl.2022.01.001
0033-8389/22/© 2022 Elsevier Inc. All rights reserved.

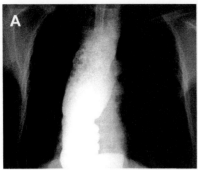 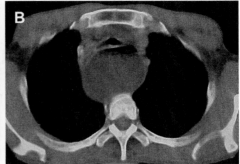

Fig. 1. Chagas megaesophagus. (A) Frontal radiograph after oral barium administration demonstrates dilated entire esophagus in a 54-year-old man with Chagas disease. (B) Noncontrast CT of the chest reveals an abnormally dilated esophagus with retained fluid content.

including those in LAC, bear 98% of the global burden of infectious parasitic diseases.[2] In this article, the thoracic imaging manifestations of several communicable diseases, including 9 parasitic infection and 1 fungal infection that have significant impact in the LAC region will be reviewed.

PROTOZOA
Chagas Disease (American Trypanosomiasis)

Chagas disease is caused by infection with *Trypanosoma cruzi*, a flagellated protozoan that circulates among hematophagous insect vectors and more than 100 species of mammals, including people. It is considered by some to be the most important parasitic disease in the Western Hemisphere, with a disease burden 7.5 times as great as that of malaria. The disease is endemic in 21 countries, from the southern United States to southern Argentina and Chile, where an estimated 6 million people are currently infected, with 28,000 new cases and 12,000 deaths every year.[3,4] The highest prevalence country is Bolivia, follow by Argentina and El Salvador. Even though vector-borne transmission occurs only in the Americas, because of increasing migration, the disease is increasingly being found in non-endemic areas including Europe and Asia, and has become a global health problem. In the United States 300,000 people live with the infection, with up to 45,000 individuals having undiagnosed Chagas cardiomyopathy.[5] Among Latin America-born patients with newly diagnosed nonischemic cardiomyopathies in Los Angeles and New York, 19% and 13% respectively, had Chagas disease.[6,7]

T cruzi penetrates in the host's cells and multiplies (amastigote form), creating pseudocysts that break, giving rise to an inflammatory reaction with scar formation and fibrosis. The pseudocyst rupture releases new amastigotes that circulate and invade new cells, in a cycle of progressive reinfection that predominantly affects the heart, followed by the esophagus and colon through a mechanism that includes inflammation and denervation.[8]

It is estimated that 30% to 50% of infected people who survive the acute phase progress to chronic Chagas' cardiomyopathy, a highly arrhythmogenic condition, also associated with dilated heart and congestive heart failure, which may develop thromboembolic complications such as stroke and systemic embolism.[9]

Chagas gastrointestinal (GI) involvement is less common (14%), and predominantly affects the esophagus and colon, resulting in visceral dilation from intramural neuronal damage with megaesophagus and megacolon (Fig. 1). This complication has significant regional geographic variation, and predominantly presents below the equatorial line, in the southernmost part of South America.[8]

Chronic Chagas cardiomyopathy (CCC) is the most common and serious complication of Chagas disease, and the most common cause of mortality in affected patients. CCC develops after several years or even decades of the indeterminate form of the disease, which is typically asymptomatic. The typical morphologic pattern is a dilated cardiomyopathy, with predominant fibrosis in the apical and posterior wall of the left ventricle, and electric conduction abnormalities with end result of abnormal myocardial contraction. Impaired left ventricular (LV) function with a reduced ejection fraction (<30%), segmental or global LV wall motion abnormalities, LV aneurysm, increased LV diastolic dimension, and cardiomegaly are important independent predictors of mortality.[10]

Contrast-enhanced cardiac magnetic resonance (CMR), in addition to precisely evaluating cardiac morphology and function, may also demonstrate myocardial scar of fibrosis when present. In a substantial number of patients, this

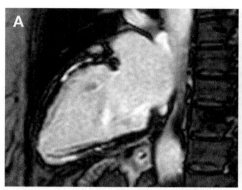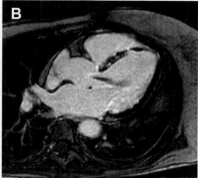

Fig. 2. Chagas cardiomyopathy. (*A*) Cardiac magnetic resonance vertical long axis image after contrast injection shows multiple areas of delayed gadolinium enhancement in a nonvascular distribution in the anterior and inferior wall of the left ventricle. (*B*) Four-chamber view in a different patient. Patchy areas of delayed enhancement are seen in the interventricular septum and apical left ventricle.

allows for risk stratification and robust prognostic evaluation. The prevalence of delayed enhancement in CCC (25%-90%) varies depending on the severity of the disease, with higher prevalence in patients with ventricular tachycardia and LV dysfunction Prevalence also tends to be higher in males.[11,12]

In CCC patients, CMR wall motion abnormalities and delayed enhancement are more commonly seen in the inferolateral and apical segments, with delayed enhancement distribution that may be transmural (36%-50%), subendocardial (27%), subepicardial (12%-23%), or midwall (14%-35%), not infrequently mimicking ischemic and nonischemic cardiomyopathies (**Fig. 2**).[11,12] CMR is particularly indicated in patients with severe ventricular arrhythmias in order to quantify the extent of myocardial fibrosis and the risk of sudden death. This information may influence the decision to place an implantable defibrillator.[13]

MALARIA

Human malaria results from the protozoal infection by 1 of the 5 *Plasmodium* species, transmitted by the *Anopheles* mosquito. More than 80% of malaria cases in South America come from the Amazon rain forest (Venezuela [30%], Brazil [24%], Peru [19%] and Colombia [10%]), where the disease is endemic, with more than half of the cases caused by *Plasmodium vivax*. The incidence of *Plasmodium falciparum* malaria, the second most common type in the region, has decreased in recent years, except in parts of the Pacific coast in Colombia, where *P falciparum* is still the dominant type.[14] According to the WHO, there were 229 million cases of malaria in 2019, with an estimated 409,000 deaths, most in the Sub-Saharan Africa and India (96%).[15]

Malaria infection begins when an infected female *Anopheles* mosquito bites a person, injecting saliva infected with *Plasmodium* sporozoites into the bloodstream, which passes quickly into the human liver, where the sporozoites multiply. The parasites, in the form of merozoites, are released from the liver cells, travel through the right side of the heart, and reach the lungs. In the bloodstream, the merozoites invade erythrocytes and multiply, invading more red cells. This cycle is repeated, causing recurrent fever each time parasites break free and invade more blood cells. Some of the merozoites in these cells develop into sexual forms (male and female gametocytes) that circulate in the blood stream. When a mosquito bites an infected person, it ingests the gametocytes that mate in the gut of the mosquito to form sporozoites. Human infection continues when the mosquito bites another person, injecting saliva with the parasite, beginning a new cycle.

Symptoms and severity of malaria vary depending on which of the 4 parasite species is the cause (or combination thereof, since a patient may contract more than 1 type of malaria at a time), with an incubation period of 10 to 15 days (but may last as long as few months), after which time, malaise, episodic fever, rattling chills, and muscular spasms manifest.

Acute lung injury and adult respiratory distress syndrome (ARDS) are the most severe pulmonary manifestations of malaria. They occur in up to 25% of patients with severe falciparum and vivax malaria, are associated with grave prognosis, and are responsible for up to 40% of malaria deaths. The exact mechanism is not entirely known, but endothelial cell injury and necrosis and altered alveolar capillary permeability are important factors. The histopathology reveals pulmonary edema, intra-alveolar hemorrhage, and hyaline membrane formation.[16] The radiologic manifestations are those of a noncardiogenic pulmonary edema and ARDS with bilateral interstitial and alveolar opacities, which may progress to airspace consolidation associated with variable degree of pleural effusion. Interlobular septal thickening, ground-glass opacities, and small pleural effusion are better appreciated on computed tomography (CT) (**Fig. 3**) (see also article by Ryzdak and colleagues in this issue).[17,18] Differentiation from multilobar pneumonia may be a challenge in these patients with respiratory symptoms, fever, and multifocal pulmonary radiographic abnormalities.[19]

AMEBIASIS

Amebiasis is the parasitic disease caused by the pseudopod forming nonflagellated protozoan *Entamoeba histolytica* (*E histolytica*). It is the third leading cause of death from a parasitic disease worldwide after malaria and schistosomiasis, with an estimated death toll between 40,000 to 100,000 people annually.[20,21]

Amebic colitis, the most common clinical manifestation, is a leading cause of severe diarrhea worldwide and among the leading causes of death in children. Endemic in developing countries, particularly in tropical and subtropical regions, the seroprevalence of *E histolytica* in some rural communities of Latin America with inadequate hygiene is above 40%. In the United States, the incidence of amebiasis is low, with most cases seen in immigrants or returning travelers from endemic regions. Three different types of *Entamoeba* that can cause asymptomatic infestation have been described: *E dispar, E moshkovskii,* and *E bangladeshi',* are morphologically identical to *E hystolytica,* and can potentially infect the intestinal mucosa, but *E histolytica* is the most invasive and responsible of nearly all cases of human amebiasis.[21–23]

E histolytica has cytolytic, phagocytic, and proteolytic capabilities that allow invasion through the mucosa and submucosal tissues and even into the portal circulation. Up to 10% of asymptomatic individuals infected with *E histolytica* develop symptomatic disease during the following year, typically amebic colitis with bloody diarrhea and abdominal pain.[20]

Infection with *E histolytica,* typically from ingestion of quadrinucleated cyst from fecally contaminated food or water (fecal-oral transmission), may be asymptomatic or may cause dysentery or extraintestinal disease, with amebic liver abscess being the most common extraintestinal location. It typically occurs in young men between 20 and 40 years old. Pleuropulmonary amebiasis can occur as a complication when the liver abscess ruptures into the thoracic cavity, which is more likely to occur when the abscess is in a subcapsular location. Not surprisingly, most pleuropulmonary complications of amebic liver abscess occur in the right hemithorax (90%). Imaging manifestations include elevation of the right hemidiaphragm, pleural effusion, parenchymal consolidation in the right lower lobe and/or right middle lobe, and occasionally hydropneumothorax if bronchopleural fistula is present. A different location may result in case of hematogenous or lymphatic spread. Intrapericardial rupture may occur, particularly with left hepatic lobe abscess, but is rare (2%). CT may demonstrate abnormal appearance of the hemidiaphragm with thickening and transdiaphragmatic extension of the abscess, with a characteristic hourglass configuration (**Fig. 4**).[24–26] Amebic liver abscess are commonly unilocular (70%), occasionally with internal septations (30%), and demonstrate rim peripheral enhancement after contrast injection on CT (target sign).[27] Pulmonary amebiasis may rarely result from hematogenous or lymphatic spread from an intestinal infection or from inhalation of dust containing cysts or trophozoites of *E histolytica* (**Fig. 5**).[28]

Pleuropulmonary amebiasis is a serious disease with significant mortality (5%–16%), especially in patients with poor health or malnutrition, in cases with delayed diagnosis, or with inadequate treatment.

CESTODES
Echinococcosis

Recently, a much-needed international consensus on terminology to be used in the field of Echinococcoses has been published with an agreement on 3 names for the disease caused by *Echinococcus spp*: cystic echinococcosis (CE), caused by *E granulosus sensu lato*; alveolar echinococcosis (AE) caused by *E multilocularis*, and neotropical echinococcosis (NE) caused by *E Vogeli* and *E Oligarthra*. Confusing terms like hydatidosis, polycistic echinococcosis, and other, that have been used for centuries are considered to be either confusing or entirely incorrect and should be avoided. Hydatid disease, if used should be only in reference to CE. Because DNA sequencing has identified several subtypes of *E granulosus,* the current recommendation is to add sensu lato (meaning in a wider sense) when in reference to them as a group and sensu stricto when in reference to one subtype in particular.[29]

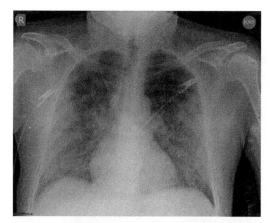

Fig. 3. Acute malaria in a 21-year-old man with plasmodium vivax infection with respiratory distress, thrombocytopenia, and hemoptysis. Chest radiograph demonstrates multifocal ground-glass opacities in the bilateral midlung zones. (Courtesy Tatiana Suarez MD, Medellin, Colombia)

Echinococcosis is a neglected parasitic zoonosis secondary to infection by the larval stage of the cestode (tapeworm) of the genus *Echinococcus*. CE and AE are the most important clinical forms because of their more extensive geographic distribution, with a substantial health and economic burden. CE is found in Africa, Europe, Asia, the Middle East, North America, Central America, and South America. AE has a worldwide distribution, with higher distribution in northern latitudes of Europe, Asia, and North America. NE is endemic and limited to certain areas of Central America and South America.[30] *E granulosus* is endemic in Argentina, Chile, Peru, Uruguay, and southern Brazil, with around 5000 new cases of CE reported annually and 2.9% mortality.[31,32] People are considered to be aberrant intermediate hosts, who become infected by the ingestion of food contaminated with eggs (fecal-oral route), which in the intestine release onchospheres that penetrate the intestinal wall to reach the vasculature and though the circulatory system reach different end organs (especially liver and lungs), where thick-wall multilayer unilocular cysts develop. NE secondary to *Echinococcus vogeli* causes a multicystic disease, whereas *E Oligarthra* produces a unilocular cystic disease.[33]

Initial infection is always asymptomatic. Later, clinical manifestations vary depending on the number and size of the cystic lesions and the location within the affected organ, with most small (<7 cm) encapsulated lesions remaining asymptomatic. Cysts may slowly grow and become symptomatic with abdominal pain and hepatobiliary manifestation caused by mass effect in case of liver lesions and pleuropulmonary manifestation (cough, pain, hemoptysis) in case of pulmonary infection.

The lung is the second most commonly affected organ (20%-30%) after the liver (60%-70%). Other locations (eg, peritoneum, kidney, or brain) are less common. Extrapulmonary intrathoracic disease involving the pleura, mediastinum, heart and great vessels, diaphragm, and chest wall may also occur.[34–36]

A hydatid cyst consists of 3 layers with a variable amount of fluid inside: the pericyst (outermost layer), the exocyst (middle layer), and the endocyst (the innermost layer). In CE, lung involvement typically reveals a single cyst (70%-85%) 1 to 20 cm in diameter, with a predominant lower lobe distribution. Uncomplicated cysts are smooth-wall homogeneous low-density round or oval lesions. Complicated cysts (ruptured or infected) reveal separation between the pericyst and endocyst, creating a variety of imaging signs, including air crescent sign, meniscus sign, inverse crescent sign, air bubble sign, and signet ring sign.

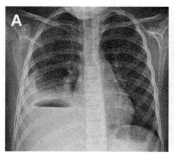
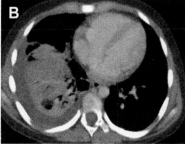
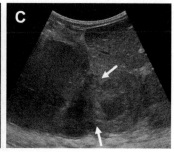

Fig. 4. Pleuropulmonary amebiasis in an 11 year old boy. (*A*) Frontal chest radiograph shows an air fluid level in the right upper quadrant of the abdomen, with a right-side pleural effusion and pulmonary opacity. (*B*) CT shows a consolidative opacity in the right lung surrounded by pleural fluid. (*C*) Right upper quadrant ultrasound, sagittal view reveals the diaphragmatic rupture (*arrows*) with transdiaphragmatic extension of the amebic liver abscess.

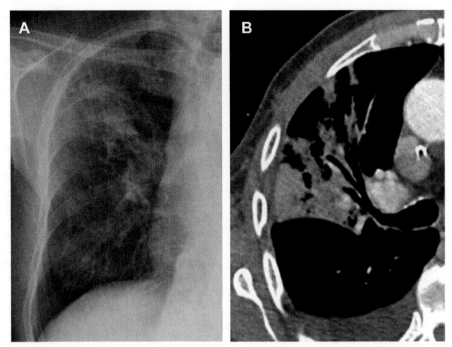

Fig. 5. Pleuropulmonary amebiasis secondary to hematogenous spread. (*A*) Patchy consolidative opacities are appreciated on the chest radiography. (*B*) Contrast-enhanced chest CT soft tissue window demonstrates air-space consolidation and layering right side pleural effusion in a patient with proven amebic pneumonia, and colitis without liver abscess.

Complete rupture is suspected when the cyst is seen connected to a bronchus, also with several imaging signs having been reported, including cumbo sign, whirl sign, and waterlily sign. The air crescent sign or meniscus sign, for example, refers to a thin crescent of air seen between the pericyst and endocyst, whereas the waterlily sign refers to the appearance of a complete collapse of the endocyst, floating in the residual fluid. High-density content and peripheral enhancement suggest superimposed bacterial infection. Larger cysts may present additional abnormalities like atelectasis, bronchiectasis and pleural effusion (**Fig. 6**).[35,37,38]

Cardiac involvement is a rare manifestation of CE (<2%), and occurs through the coronary artery circulation, with LV involvement being the most common location, followed by the right ventricle (60% and 15% respectively). Pericardial disease is seen in less than 10% of the cases.[39] Similar to other organs, the cysts may have variable presentation as single or multiple, with variable wall thickness, rarely becoming solid lesions, difficult to differentiate from a cardiac tumor.[40]

Involvement of the great vessels may occur, either as extrinsic compression from a large mediastinal or pleuropulmonary lesion, or as an infiltrative vascular wall lesion with potential risk for thrombosis, erosion, or rupture (**Fig. 7**).

CYSTICERCOSIS

Cysticercosis, considered by the WHO an NTD, is caused by infection with the larval stage of the pork tapeworm *Taenia solium*, acquired through fecal-oral contamination with eggs from tapeworm carriers. The invasive oncospheres in the eggs cross the small bowel wall, reaching the bloodstream to be carried to the brain, muscles, and other organs where they encyst as cysticerci.[41] Cysticercosis is endemic in Latin America, India, Asia, and Africa in rural and urban areas with poor sanitation and is not uncommonly seen outside of endemic areas in communities with large number of immigrants. Areas of high prevalence are found in Mexico, Bolivia, Ecuador, Peru, Honduras, and Guatemala.[42]

Neurocysticercosis is the most serious clinical form of the disease, manifesting as epilepsy, intracranial hypertension, and hydrocephalus. Nearly 15 million people are estimated to have neurocysticercosis in Latin America and the Caribbean. Pulmonary and heart infection are rare despite the

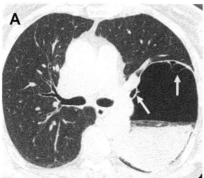
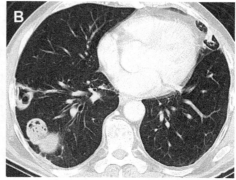

Fig. 6. Pulmonary cystic echinococcosis in 2 different patients. (*A*) CT chest axial image shows a large left side intrapulmonary cyst containing a large air fluid level in a 65-year-old woman. Smaller cysts are visible in the periphery of the dominant cyst's wall (*arrows*). (*B*) CT chest in a 42-year-old man shows multiple air and fluid containing intrapulmonary cysts in the right lower lobe.

high prevalence of cysticercosis in endemic areas, and typically manifest as solitary or multiple nodules in the lung parenchyma, or in the myocardium around 1 cm in diameter. In such cases the possibility of cysticercosis should be considered, in particular if associated with chest wall soft tissue and subcutaneous nodules and brain involvement (**Fig. 8**).[43,44]

TREMATODES
Schistosomiasis

Schistosomiasis or bilharziasis is a parasitic infection caused by trematode parasites of the genus *Schistosoma*, endemic in tropical and subtropical regions. The schistosomes are a group of blood trematodes (fluke worms), with 3 main species infecting people: *Schistosoma haematobium* (Africa, eastern Mediterranean region, and the Arabian peninsula), *S japonicum* (China, the Philippines, and Indonesia), and *Schistosoma mansoni* (Africa, Arabian peninsula, and South America). The females produce hundreds to thousands of eggs per day, with each egg containing a ciliated larva. Infection occurs in fresh water containing larval forms (cercariae). Snails become infected from eggs excreted in human feces or urine. The larvae develop in water snails (intermediate host). The cercariae penetrates the skin of the individual in contact with the water. The parasite migrates in the blood via the lungs to the liver, where they transform into young worms that mature and migrate to the perivesical or mesenteric destination, where they colonize blood vessels for years, producing *Schistosoma* eggs daily, which are eliminated with urine or feces, depending on the species, for the cycle to start again.[45,46] *S mansoni* is found in Latin America primarily in Brazil (90%), Venezuela, Suriname, and the Caribbean, where it is endemic mainly in rural

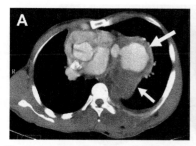
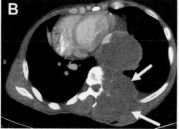
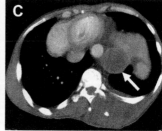

Fig. 7. Cystic echinococcosis with chest wall, mediastinal and aortic involvement. (*A*) Contrast-enhanced chest CT shows an anteriorly displaced aorta adjacent to the heart with a large pseudoaneurysm on the left side of the mid-descending aorta (large *arrow*), and a low-density posterior para-aortic lesion (small *arrow*). (*B*) Axial image at a lower level demonstrates erosive changes on the spine, and posterior chest wall involvement (*arrows*). (*C*) The displaced and compressed aortic lumen is seen adjacent to the lateral wall of the left ventricle. Axial image at the level of the left hemidiaphragm shows the lower aspect of the mediastinal hydatid cyst (*arrow*). (Courtesy Liliana Vega, MD, Mar del Plata, Argentina)

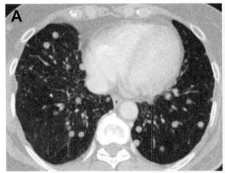
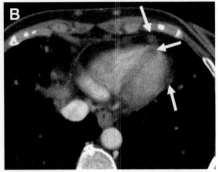

Fig. 8. Chest CT in a female patient with disseminated cysticercosis with pulmonary, cardiac, and soft tissue involvement. (*A*) Lung window axial image shows numerous soft tissue density pulmonary nodules, and subcutaneous nodules in the anterior chest wall. (*B*) Soft tissue window axial image shows additional nodular lesions in the interventricular septum and pericardium (*arrows*). (Courtesy Yashant Aswani, MD.)

areas with poor sanitation. Acute schistosomiasis (Katayama fever) is a systemic hypersensitivity reaction after the primary infection, with patchy pulmonary ground-glass opacities, small pulmonary nodules (2–15 mm) and interlobular septal thickening on imaging examination.[47,48] In chronic infection, the parasites are trapped in tissue, where they induce granulomatous inflammation and fibrosis resulting in 2 main clinical forms: genitourinary and GI schistosomiasis. The fibrotic liver disease derived portal-caval shunting allows ova to leak into the pulmonary capillary bed, resulting in necrotizing and obliterative endarteritis with fibrosis and pulmonary arterial hypertension (PAH), complications seen in as much of 20% of patients with schistosomiasis. In endemic areas with high prevalence of the disease, more than 30% of all cases of PAH are secondary to schistosomiasis.[49,50] Imaging studies may reveal a cardiomegaly with right ventricular enlargement, enlarged pulmonary trunk, and central pulmonary arteries accompanied by a fibrotic liver. No diffuse

parenchymal pulmonary disease (eg, fibrosis, emphysema, or interstitial lung disease) or additional cardiovascular abnormality (eg, intracardiac shunt or chronic thromboembolism) is present to account for PAH. Small pulmonary nodules and small patchy consolidations can also be seen in patients with chronic pulmonary involvement (**Fig. 9**).[51,52]

PARAGONIMIASIS

Paragonimiasis is a foodborne zoonotic disease caused by trematodes of the genus *Paragonimus*. The infection develops after the ingestion of raw or insufficiently cooked meat from freshwater crab, crayfish or from a mammalian host (pigs, wild boar) containing the encysted metacercaria of the flatworm. Of the nearly 50 *Paragonimus* species described, 8 can produce disease in humans, with 3 being responsible for most cases: *Plasmodium westermani* in Asia, *Plasmodium mexicanus* in Central and South America with highest

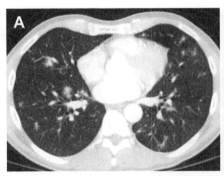
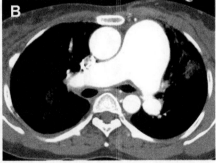

Fig. 9. Acute and chronic schistosomiasis in 2 different patients. (*A*) Acute pulmonary schistosomiasis in a young male. Contrast-enhanced chest CT, lung window axial image reveals small lung nodules with peripheral ground-glass halo scattered in the bilateral lungs. (*B*) Chronic schistosomiasis in a female patient. Contrast-enhanced CT shows pulmonary hypertension with significantly enlarged pulmonary trunk and central pulmonary arteries (*arrows*).

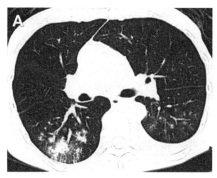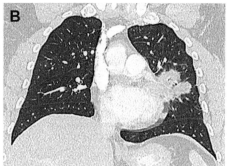

Fig. 10. Acute pulmonary paragonimiasis in 2 different patients. (*A*) Chest CT lung window axial image demonstrates patchy and nodular bibasilar bilateral pulmonary opacities, with interlobular septal thickening in the right lower lobe. (*B*) Coronal reformatted contrast-enhanced chest CT. Lung window image shows patchy rounded opacities in the left upper lobe.

incidence in Ecuador and Peru, and *P. kellicotti* in North America. It is estimated that 1 million people worldwide get infected annually.[53,54]

Paragonimus has a complex life cycle, with 2 intermediate hosts and a definitive mammalian host. After human ingestion, the parasite infective larvae migrate to the peritoneal cavity after penetrating the duodenal wall, ultimately reaching the pleura and lung through the diaphragm. In the lung, the larvae mature into adult flukes, with development of pulmonary cystic cavities.[55] Clinical presentation includes fever, dyspnea, hemoptysis, cough, pleuritic chest pain, and eosinophilic pleural effusion. Abnormalities on imaging examination, which are present in most cases (>90%), vary according to the stage of the disease and geographic distribution. During the transdiaphragmatic and pleural migration, effusion (20%-60%), pneumothorax (5%-17%), and pleural thickening (7%) may occur. Intrapulmonary migration of the worms manifests with airspace consolidation (50%) and linear or bandlike opacities (40%) representing worm migration tracts. Once the parasite ceases migration, lung nodules and thin-walled cysts 1 to 3 cm in diameter appear, some revealing ovoid internal structure from the presence of the worm within. Pulmonary cysts may appear fluid- or air-filled depending on the presence of bronchial communication (**Figs. 10 and 11**).[56–58] Pericardial effusion and omental inflammation are additional findings that have been reported in North American paragonimiasis but are uncommon in Asian paragonimiasis.[59]

NEMATODES
Ascariasis

Ascariasis is the infection produced by the roundworm *Ascaris lumbricoides*, a soil-transmitted helminth with a worldwide distribution in tropical and subtropical areas with poor sanitation and fecal contamination of food and water. Ingested eggs hatch larvae in the intestinal lumen, which are absorbed into the portal circulation reaching the liver initially and later the heart and lung parenchyma through the pulmonary circulation. Larvae are coughed up to the tracheobronchial tree and end swallowed, re-entering the GII tract.[24] Roughly 1 billion people are affected worldwide, with prevalence greater than 20% in several Latin America and Caribbean countries and the highest rates among school-age children.[60,61] Typically during the second week of infection, as the larvae invade the lung, there may be tissue damage and an allergic response. This manifests as respiratory symptoms, which may be associated with eosinophilia in blood with pulmonary radiographic abnormality, also known as Löffler syndrome (in recognition of Dr. Wilhelm Löffler, who described it)[31]

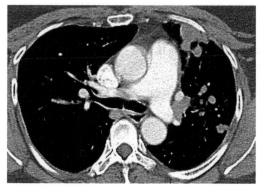

Fig. 11. Chronic pulmonary paragonimiasis in a 44-year-old patient. Contrast-enhanced chest CT axial image shows fluid density cyst scattered throughout the left lung.

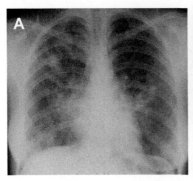 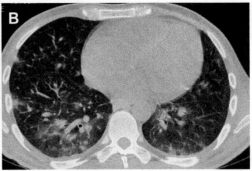

Fig. 12. Pulmonary ascariasis in 2 different patients. (*A*) Frontal chest radiograph shows multifocal patchy ground-glass and nodular bilateral opacities in a parahilar distribution. (*B*) Noncontrast chest CT demonstrates nodular and ground-glass opacities in the bilateral lower lobes.

During this phase, transient patchy nodular or consolidative pulmonary opacities with either unilateral or bilateral distribution may be evident, and typically resolve in about 2 to 4 weeks. Opacities are ground-glass in density, but frank lobar consolidation may occur (**Fig. 12**).[24,25]

In most patients, this stage is asymptomatic; with respiratory manifestation in less than 15% of patients. The severity and magnitude of the pulmonary abnormalities are in part related to the extent of worm burden, but the process is typically transient and self-limited.[62]

STRONGYLOIDIASIS

Strongyloidiasis is a chronic parasitic infection caused by the nematode (roundworm) *Strongyloides stercoralis*, a filariform larva that inhabits the soil and infects people via skin penetration. The parasite is present worldwide in tropical and subtropical regions and remains endemic in the southeastern United States, with between 30 million and 100 million people estimated to be infected worldwide, although estimates as high as 370 million people infected have been reported.[63] Among Latin American countries. the highest prevalence (>20%) is found in Argentina, Ecuador, Venezuela, Peru, and Brazil.[64,65]

After skin penetration, the filariform larvae travel hematogenously to the lungs, reaching the alveolar space, later migrating to the pharynx, where they are swallowed into the proximal small bowel, where they burrow and lay their eggs. In some ways, the life cycle of this parasite is unique. Unlike other soil-transmitted helminths such as hookworm and whipworm, whose eggs do not hatch until they are in the environment, the eggs of *S stercoralis* hatch into larvae in the intestine, allowing permanent cycles of reinfection or autoinfection by which the parasite completes its life cycle within a single host. Most of these larvae will be

excreted in the stool, but some of the larvae may mature into filariform larvae and immediately reinfect the host either by burrowing into the intestinal mucosa and bowel wall, or by penetrating the perianal skin.[63] The infection may be entirely asymptomatic or manifest with minimal nonspecific respiratory symptoms. In immunosuppressed patients (eg, acquired immunodeficiency syndrome [AIDS], corticosteroid therapy, or post-transplant immunosuppression therapy) the parasite may undergo uncontrolled proliferation and dissemination spreading more significantly throughout the lungs, and into to multiple organs (eg, skin, liver, kidneys, lymphatics, and brain), in what is known as hyperinfection syndrome. Affected patients may develop intra-alveolar hemorrhage and adult respiratory distress syndrome.[24,66] Imaging studies may be normal in some patients, but more often will reveal small pulmonary nodules and/or interstitial opacities, or a bronchopneumonia pattern of multifocal patchy alveolar parenchymal opacities that may appear to migrate on follow-up examination. Occasionally a lobar consolidation may occur.[67] On CT, ground-glass opacities and interlobular septal thickening in addition to patchy airspace consolidation are common. In case of hyperinfection syndrome, more extensive multifocal ground-glass and consolidative opacities are seen. These appear disseminated throughout both lungs, commonly associated with interlobular septal thickening, and may be associated with small pulmonary nodules and variable amounts of pleural effusion (**Fig. 13**).[63,68]

FUNGAL INFECTION
Paracoccidioidomycosis

Paracoccidioidomycosis (PCM) is a fungal disease caused by the dimorphic fungus of the genus *Paracoccidioides*, endemic in Latin American countries. Of the 2 species identified, *Plasmodium*

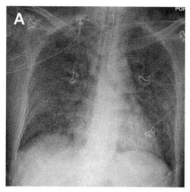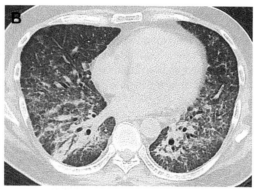

Fig. 13. Strongyloides hyperinfection syndrome in a 47-year-old immunosuppressed man. (*A*) Frontal chest radiograph shows diffuse nodular and ground-glass opacities throughout the bilateral lungs. (*B*) Noncontrast chest CT better demonstrates multifocal interstitial, patchy, and nodular alveolar bilateral pulmonary opacities with interlobular septal thickening.

brasiliensis and *Plasmodium lutzii*, the former is responsible for the majority of clinical human infections.[69]

PCM is the most frequent endemic systemic mycosis in several Latin American countries, with the largest number of cases reported in Brazil, Colombia, Venezuela, and Argentina with smaller endemic areas in Mexico, Ecuador, and Peru. Most cases are in Brazil (80%), with the highest prevalence in midwest and northern parts of the country, where the incidence may be as high as 9.4 cases per 100,000 inhabitants/year. The chronic form of the disease more commonly affects men (75%–95%) between 30 and 60 years old (male:female ratio > 20:1), typically rural workers involved in agricultural activities.[70,71]

Similar to other fungal infections, the lung is the portal of entry for this soil saprophyte. In most cases, the primary pulmonary infection is asymptomatic, with only a small proportion of cases presenting clinical manifestations. A chronic infection

from reactivation of a remote primary infection most commonly affects those with history of smoking (90%) and alcoholism.[71]

The acute form (10%-25%) manifests by fever, hepatosplenomegaly, and generalized lymphadenopathy, rarely with pulmonary disease, different from the chronic form of the disease (75%-90%) that commonly affects the lung parenchyma with pulmonary nodules, airspace consolidation, cavitation and chronic scarring, and fibrosis with bronchiectasis and cicatricial emphysema.[72–74]

In the few individuals with symptomatic acute pulmonary disease, the imaging findings resemble those seen in a primary tuberculosis infection with airspace disease, consolidation, and lymphadenopathy. In the chronic stage of the disease, which is more common, the most frequent CT findings include pulmonary opacities with ground-glass attenuation (60%), nodules (50%), cavitation (40%), parenchymal scarring and fibrosis (30%), and areas of cicatricial emphysema (30%-50%),

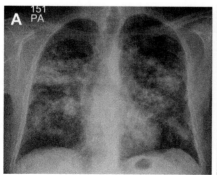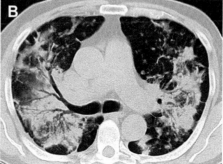

Fig. 14. Paracoccidioidomycosis in a 67-year-old male farmer. (*A*) Frontal chest radiograph shows extensive bilateral ground-glass and consolidative pulmonary opacities. (*B*) Noncontrast chest CT demonstrates air bronchogram within the bilateral areas of air space consolidation and nodular and ground opacities in the bilateral lungs.

often in a predominant peripheral and posterior distribution affecting all lung zones (**Fig. 14**).[75,76] The reverse halo sign (central ground-glass opacity surrounded by denser air–space consolidation in a crescent or ring shape) has also been reported in pulmonary PCM, but is a nonspecific imaging finding that can be seen in several infectious and noninfectious pulmonary pathologies.[77] In the long term, up to 25% of infected patients may develop precapillary pulmonary hypertension, even after declared free of the infection after appropriate antimycotic therapy.[78]

The confirmation of PCM requires the identification of *Paracoccidioides spp* through the examination of fresh sputum or other clinical specimens, such as mucocutaneous lesion, lymph node aspiration, or biopsy.[74]

SUMMARY

Transmissible diarrheal diseases, along with acute respiratory infections, remain a significant cause of morbidity and mortality in developing countries, including Latin America and the Caribbean region where poor sanitation remains a prevalent problem. Contagious and transmissible diseases are particularly affected by societal factors such as education, sociocultural level, income, housing, and access to safe drinking water. Many of the diseases discussed are associated with these deficiencies and disparities, affect the thoracic cavity, and have nonspecific clinical manifestations. Radiologists should be familiar with the epidemiology, pathophysiology, clinical, and imaging manifestations of these entities to contribute to the diagnosis and follow-up of affected patients.

DISCLOSURE

The authors certify that they have no affiliations with or involvement in any organization or entity with any financial interest (such as honoraria; educational grants; participation in speakers' bureaus; membership, employment, consultancies, stock ownership, or other equity interest; and expert testimony or patent-licensing arrangements), or nonfinancial interest (such as personal or professional relationships, affiliations, knowledge, or beliefs) in the subject matter or materials discussed in this article.

REFERENCES

1. Hotez PJ, Bottazzi ME, Franco-Paredes C, et al. The neglected tropical diseases of Latin America and the Caribbean: a review of disease burden and distribution and a roadmap for control and elimination. PLoS Negl Trop Dis 2008;2(9). https://doi.org/10.1371/journal.pntd.0000300.

2. Mueller-Langer F. Neglected infectious diseases: are push and pull incentive mechanisms suitable for promoting drug development research? Health Econ Policy L 2013;8(2). https://doi.org/10.1017/S1744133112000321.

3. Pereiro AC. Guidelines for the diagnosis and treatment of Chagas disease. Lancet 2019;393(10180). https://doi.org/10.1016/S0140-6736(19)30288-0.

4. Pan American Health Organization, World Health Organization. Guidelines for the diagnosis and treatment of Chagas disease.; 2019.

5. Bern C, Montgomery SP. An estimate of the burden of Chagas disease in the United States. Clin Infect Dis 2009;49(5). https://doi.org/10.1086/605091.

6. Traina MI, Sanchez DR, Hernandez S, et al. Prevalence and impact of Chagas disease among Latin American immigrants with nonischemic cardiomyopathy in Los Angeles, California. Circ Heart Fail 2015;8(5). https://doi.org/10.1161/CIRCHEARTFAILURE.115.002229.

7. Kapelusznik L, Varela D, Montgomery SP, et al. Chagas disease in Latin American immigrants with dilated cardiomyopathy in New York City. Clin Infect Dis 2013;57(1). https://doi.org/10.1093/cid/cit199.

8. Coura JR, Borges-Pereira J. Chagas disease: what is known and what should be improved: a systemic review. Revista da Sociedade Brasileira de Medicina Trop 2012;45(3). https://doi.org/10.1590/S0037-86822012000300002.

9. Bern C. Chagas' Disease. N Engl J Med 2015;373(5). https://doi.org/10.1056/NEJMra1410150.

10. Rassi A, Rassi A, Rassi SG. Predictors of mortality in chronic Chagas disease. Circulation 2007;115(9). https://doi.org/10.1161/CIRCULATIONAHA.106.627265.

11. Rochitte CE, Oliveira PF, Andrade JM, et al. Myocardial delayed enhancement by magnetic resonance imaging in patients with Chagas' disease. J Am Coll Cardiol 2005;46(8). https://doi.org/10.1016/j.jacc.2005.06.067.

12. Regueiro A, García-Álvarez A, Sitges M, et al. Myocardial involvement in Chagas disease: Insights from cardiac magnetic resonance. Int J Cardiol 2013;165(1). https://doi.org/10.1016/j.ijcard.2011.07.089.

13. Nunes MCP, Badano LP, Marin-Neto JA, et al. Multimodality imaging evaluation of Chagas disease: an expert consensus of Brazilian Cardiovascular Imaging Department (DIC) and the European Association of Cardiovascular Imaging (EACVI). Eur Heart J - Cardiovasc Imaging 2018;19(4). https://doi.org/10.1093/ehjci/jex154.

14. Recht J, Siqueira AM, Monteiro WM, et al. Malaria in Brazil, Colombia, Peru and Venezuela: current challenges in malaria control and elimination. Malar J

2017;16(1). https://doi.org/10.1186/s12936-017-1925-6.

15. World Health Organization. World Malaria Report 2019.; 2019.

16. Taylor WRJ, Hanson J, Turner GDH, et al. Respiratory manifestations of malaria. Chest 2012;142(2). https://doi.org/10.1378/chest.11-2655.

17. Restrepo CS, Raut AA, Riascos R, et al. Imaging manifestations of tropical parasitic infections. Semin Roentgenol 2007;42(1). https://doi.org/10.1053/j.ro.2006.08.007.

18. Marchiori E, Zanetti G, Hochhegger B, et al. Plasmodium falciparum malaria: another infection of interest to pulmonologists. Jornal Brasileiro de Pneumologia 2013;39(6). https://doi.org/10.1590/S1806-37132013000600015.

19. Elzein F, Mohammed N, Ali N, et al. Pulmonary manifestation of *Plasmodium falciparum* malaria: case reports and review of the literature. Respir Med Case Rep 2017;22. https://doi.org/10.1016/j.rmcr.2017.06.014.

20. Stanley SL. Amoebiasis *The Lancet* 2003;(9362): 361. https://doi.org/10.1016/S0140-6736(03)12830-9.

21. Carrero JC, Reyes-López M, Serrano-Luna J, et al. Intestinal amoebiasis: 160 years of its first detection and still remains as a health problem in developing countries. Int J Med Microbiol 2020;310(1). https://doi.org/10.1016/j.ijmm.2019.151358.

22. Shirley D-AT, Farr L, Watanabe K, et al. A review of the global burden, new diagnostics, and current therapeutics for amebiasis. Open Forum Infect Dis 2018;5(7). https://doi.org/10.1093/ofid/ofy161.

23. Ximénez C, González E, Nieves M, et al. Differential expression of pathogenic genes of Entamoeba histolytica vs E. dispar in a model of infection using human liver tissue explants. PLOS ONE 2017;12(8). https://doi.org/10.1371/journal.pone.0181962.

24. Kunst H, Mack D, Kon OM, et al. Parasitic infections of the lung: a guide for the respiratory physician. Thorax 2011;66(6). https://doi.org/10.1136/thx.2009.132217.

25. Martínez S, Restrepo CS, Carrillo JA, et al. Thoracic manifestations of tropical parasitic infections: a pictorial review. RadioGraphics 2005;25(1). https://doi.org/10.1148/rg.251045043.

26. Fiorentini LF, Bergo P, Meirelles GSP, et al. Pictorial review of thoracic parasitic diseases. Chest 2020; 157(5). https://doi.org/10.1016/j.chest.2019.12.025.

27. Bächler P, Baladron MJ, Menias C, et al. Multimodality imaging of liver infections: differential diagnosis and potential pitfalls. RadioGraphics 2016;36(4). https://doi.org/10.1148/rg.2016150196.

28. Shamsuzzaman SM, Hashiguchi Y. Thoracic amebiasis. Clin Chest Med 2002;23(2). https://doi.org/10.1016/S0272-5231(01)00008-9.

29. Vuitton DA, McManus DP, Rogan MT, et al. International consensus on terminology to be used in the field of echinococcoses. Parasite 2020;27. https://doi.org/10.1051/parasite/2020024.

30. Eckert J, Deplazes P. Biological, epidemiological, and clinical aspects of echinococcosis, a zoonosis of increasing concern. Clin Microbiol Rev 2004; 17(1). https://doi.org/10.1128/CMR.17.1.107-135.2004.

31. Gipson K, Avery R, Shah H, et al. Löffler syndrome on a Louisiana pig farm. Respir Med Case Rep 2016;19. https://doi.org/10.1016/j.rmcr.2016.09.003.

32. PANAFTOSA, Panamerican Health Organization, World Health Organization. Equinococosis: Informe Epidemiológico En La Región de América Del Sur - 2016-2017, n.3. 2019. Available at: https://iris.paho.org/handle/10665.2/50630. Accessed April 23, 2021.

33. D'Alessandro A, Rausch RL. New aspects of neotropical polycystic (*Echinococcus vogeli*) and unicystic (*Echinococcus oligarthrus*) echinococcosis. Clin Microbiol Rev 2008;21(2). https://doi.org/10.1128/CMR.00050-07.

34. Saeedan M bin, Aljohani IM, Alghofaily KA, et al. Thoracic hydatid disease: a radiologic review of unusual cases. World J Clin Cases 2020;8(7). https://doi.org/10.12998/wjcc.v8.i7.1203.

35. Durhan G, Tan AA, Düzgün SA, et al. Radiological manifestations of thoracic hydatid cysts: pulmonary and extrapulmonary findings. Insights into Imaging 2020;11(1). https://doi.org/10.1186/s13244-020-00916-0.

36. Polat P, Kantarci M, Alper F, et al. Hydatid disease from head to toe. RadioGraphics 2003;23(2). https://doi.org/10.1148/rg.232025704.

37. Shehatha J, Alizzi A, Alward M, et al. Thoracic hydatid disease; a review of 763 cases. Heart Lung Circ 2008; 17(6). https://doi.org/10.1016/j.hlc.2008.04.001.

38. Sarkar M, Pathania R, Jhobta A, et al. Cystic pulmonary hydatidosis. Lung India 2016;33(2). https://doi.org/10.4103/0970-2113.177449.

39. Kahlfuß S, Flieger RR, Roepke TK, et al. Diagnosis and treatment of cardiac echinococcosis. Heart 2016;102(17). https://doi.org/10.1136/heartjnl-2016-309350.

40. Dursun M, Terzibasioglu E, Yilmaz R, et al. Cardiac hydatid disease: CT and MRI findings. Am J Roentgenol 2008;190(1). https://doi.org/10.2214/AJR.07.2035.

41. García HH, Gonzalez AE, Evans CA, et al. Taenia solium cysticercosis. The Lancet 2003;362(9383). https://doi.org/10.1016/S0140-6736(03)14117-7.

42. Flisser A, Sarti E, Lightowlers M, et al. Neurocysticercosis: regional status, epidemiology, impact and control measures in the Americas. Acta Tropica 2003;87(1). https://doi.org/10.1016/S0001-706X(03)00054-8.

43. Singh P, Saggar K, Kalia V, et al. Thoracic imaging findings in a case of disseminated cysticercosis. Postgrad Med J 2011;87(1024). https://doi.org/10.1136/pgmj.2010.108555.

44. Bastos AL, Marchiori E, Gasparetto EL, et al. Pulmonary and cardiac cysticercosis: helical CT findings. The Br J Radiol 2007;80(951). https://doi.org/10.1259/bjr/43104295.

45. Colley DG, Bustinduy AL, Secor WE, et al. Human schistosomiasis. Lancet 2014;383(9936). https://doi.org/10.1016/S0140-6736(13)61949-2.

46. Gryseels B, Polman K, Clerinx J, et al. Human schistosomiasis. Lancet 2006;368(9541). https://doi.org/10.1016/S0140-6736(06)69440-3.

47. Nguyen L-Q, Estrella J, Jett EA, et al. Acute schistosomiasis in nonimmune travelers: chest CT findings in 10 patients. Am J Roentgenology 2006;186(5). https://doi.org/10.2214/AJR.05.0213.

48. Al-Jahdali H, Bamefleh H, Elkeir A, et al. Acute pulmonary schistosomiasis. J Glob Infect Dis 2011;3(3). https://doi.org/10.4103/0974-777X.83539.

49. Hovnanian A, Hoette S, Fernandes CJC, et al. Schistosomiasis associated pulmonary hypertension. Int J Clin Pract 2010;64. https://doi.org/10.1111/j.1742-1241.2009.02234.x.

50. Ferreira RCS, Domingues ALC, Bandeira ÂP, et al. Prevalence of pulmonary hypertension in patients with schistosomal liver fibrosis. Ann Trop Med Parasitol 2009;103(2). https://doi.org/10.1179/136485909X398168.

51. Foti G, Gobbi F, Angheben A, et al. Radiographic and HRCT imaging findings of chronic pulmonary schistosomiasis: review of 10 consecutive cases. BJR|caseReps 2019;5(3). https://doi.org/10.1259/bjrcr.20180088.

52. Niemann T, Marti HP, Duhnsen SH, et al. pulmonary schistosomiasis – imaging features. J Radiol Case Rep 2010;4(9). https://doi.org/10.3941/jrcr.v4i9.482.

53. Toledo R, Fried B. In: Digenetic trematodes. Springer; 2019.

54. Yoshida A, Doanh PN, Maruyama H. Paragonimus and paragonimiasis in Asia: An update. Acta Tropica 2019;199. https://doi.org/10.1016/j.actatropica.2019.105074.

55. Vélez ID, Ortega JE, Velásquez LE. Paragonimiasis: a view from Colombia. Clin Chest Med 2002;23(2). https://doi.org/10.1016/S0272-5231(02)00003-5.

56. Im JG, Whang HY, Kim WS, et al. Pleuropulmonary paragonimiasis: radiologic findings in 71 patients. Am J Roentgenology 1992;159(1). https://doi.org/10.2214/ajr.159.1.1609718.

57. Ahn C-S, Shin JW, Kim J-G, et al. Spectrum of pleuropulmonary paragonimiasis: an analysis of 685 cases diagnosed over 22 years. J Infect 2021;82(1). https://doi.org/10.1016/j.jinf.2020.09.037.

58. Strobel M, Maleewong W, Vannavong A, et al. Different chest radiographic findings of pulmonary paragonimiasis in two endemic countries. The Am J Trop Med Hyg 2010;83(4). https://doi.org/10.4269/ajtmh.2010.10-0091.

59. Henry TS, Lane MA, Weil GJ, et al. Chest CT features of North American Paragonimiasis. Am J Roentgenology 2012;198(5). https://doi.org/10.2214/AJR.11.7530.

60. Saboyá MI, Catalá L, Nicholls RS, et al. Update on the mapping of prevalence and intensity of infection for soil-transmitted helminth infections in Latin America and the Caribbean: a call for action. PLoS Negl Trop Dis 2013;7(9). https://doi.org/10.1371/journal.pntd.0002419.

61. Dold C, Holland C v. Ascaris and ascariasis. Microbes Infect 2011;13(7). https://doi.org/10.1016/j.micinf.2010.09.012.

62. Akuthota P, Weller PF. Eosinophilic Pneumonias. Clin Microbiol Rev 2012;25(4). https://doi.org/10.1128/CMR.00025-12.

63. Nabeya D, Haranaga S, Parrott GL, et al. Pulmonary strongyloidiasis: assessment between manifestation and radiological findings in 16 severe strongyloidiasis cases. BMC Infect Dis 2017;17(1). https://doi.org/10.1186/s12879-017-2430-9.

64. Buonfrate D, Mena MA, Angheben A, et al. Prevalence of strongyloidiasis in Latin America: a systematic review of the literature. Epidemiol Infect 2015;143(3). https://doi.org/10.1017/S0950268814001563.

65. Lozada H, Daza JE. Estrongiloidosis pulmonar. Revista chilena de infectología 2016;33(5). https://doi.org/10.4067/S0716-10182016000500016.

66. Vasquez-Rios G, Pineda-Reyes R, Pineda-Reyes J, et al. Strongyloides stercoralis hyperinfection syndrome: a deeper understanding of a neglected disease. J Parasitic Dis 2019;43(2). https://doi.org/10.1007/s12639-019-01090-x.

67. Woodring JH, Halfhill H, Reed JC. Pulmonary strongyloidiasis: clinical and imaging features. Am J Roentgenology 1994;162(3). https://doi.org/10.2214/ajr.162.3.8109492.

68. Bae K, Jeon KN, Ha JY, et al. Pulmonary strongyloidiasis presenting micronodules on chest computed tomography. J Thorac Dis 2018;10(8). https://doi.org/10.21037/jtd.2018.07.32.

69. Turissini DA, Gomez OM, Teixeira MM, et al. Species boundaries in the human pathogen Paracoccidioides. Fungal Genet Biol 2017;106. https://doi.org/10.1016/j.fgb.2017.05.007.

70. Teixeira MM, Theodoro RC, Nino-Vega G, et al. Paracoccidioides species complex: ecology, phylogeny, sexual reproduction, and virulence. PLoS Pathog 2014;10(10). https://doi.org/10.1371/journal.ppat.1004397.

71. vio de Queiroz-Telles F, Peçanha Pietrobom PM, Rosa Júnior M, et al. New insights on pulmonary paracoccidioidomycosis. Semin Respir Crit Care Med 2020;41(01). https://doi.org/10.1055/s-0039-3400544.

72. Martinez R. New trends in paracoccidioidomycosis epidemiology. J Fungi 2017;3(1). https://doi.org/10.3390/jof3010001.

73. Rosa Júnior M, Baldon IV, Amorim AFC, et al. Imaging paracoccidioidomycosis: a pictorial review from head to toe. Eur J Radiol 2018;103. https://doi.org/10.1016/j.ejrad.2018.03.026.

74. Shikanai-Yasuda MA, Mendes RP, Colombo AL, et al. Brazilian guidelines for the clinical management of paracoccidioidomycosis. Revista da Sociedade Brasileira de Medicina Trop 2017;50(5). https://doi.org/10.1590/0037-8682-0230-2017.

75. Souza AS, Gasparetto EL, Davaus T, et al. High-resolution CT findings of 77 patients with untreated pulmonary paracoccidioidomycosis. Am J Roentgenology 2006;187(5). https://doi.org/10.2214/AJR.05.1065.

76. Marchiori E, Valiante PM, Mano CM, et al. Paracoccidioidomycosis: high-resolution computed tomography–pathologic correlation. Eur J Radiol 2011;77(1). https://doi.org/10.1016/j.ejrad.2009.06.017.

77. Marchiori E, Zanetti G, Escuissato DL, et al. Reversed Halo Sign. Chest 2012;141(5). https://doi.org/10.1378/chest.11-1050.

78. Batah SS, Alda MA, Machado-Rugulo JR, et al. Pulmonary paracoccidioidomycosis-induced pulmonary hypertension. Clin Translational Med 2020;10(7). https://doi.org/10.1002/ctm2.213.

Endemic Thoracic Infections in Southeast Asia

Ching Ching Ong, FRCR, Lynette L.S. Teo, FRCR*

KEYWORDS

- Thoracic • Pulmonary • Infections • Imaging • Radiography • CT • Southeast Asia

KEY POINTS

- Many respiratory pathogens that are common worldwide are common in South East Asia (SEA) as well. These pathogens include pneumococcus, Klebsiella, Hemophilus influenza, and influenza virus, the latter however without a discrete seasonal peak seen in temperate climates.
- Tuberculosis is common in SEA, and in that setting, radiography can assist in distinguishing active from latent or inactive disease and assist in identifying abnormal response to treatment that can be associated with drug resistance.
- Melioidosis, a gram-negative bacterial infection, has pleomorphic manifestations and can mimic tuberculosis, although the extent of consolidation tends to be more extensive than in mycobacterial infections.
- Although the epidemiology of fungal infections in general is not well documented in SEA, cryptococcus and aspergillus are both significant pathogens. Aspergillomas and/or chronic pulmonary aspergillosis can be seen in the context of residual parenchymal cavities following tuberculosis.
- Important parasitic diseases in SEA include strongyloidiasis and amebiasis, with clinically important presentations of hyperinfection syndrome and pleuropulmonary disease, respectively.

INTRODUCTION

Respiratory tract infections are leading causes of mortality and morbidity worldwide. Lower respiratory infections are ranked as the fourth leading cause of death in 2019 according to the World Health Organization (WHO).[1]

Southeast Asia (SEA) consists of 11 countries with diverse cultures, ethnicities, religions, and economies: Brunei, Myanmar, Cambodia, Timor-Leste, Indonesia, Laos, Malaysia, the Philippines, Singapore, Thailand, and Vietnam. SEA is home to more than 668 million people, 8.6% of the world's population, with a population density of 154 per km².[2] The region mostly enjoys a hot and humid tropical climate throughout the year, with abundant rainfall.

The epidemiology of respiratory infections is a result of interplay between environmental and socioeconomic factors. Respiratory infections in this region may be due to common pathogens encountered worldwide and certain infections endemic to this region.

Imaging tools in respiratory infections typically include chest radiography (CXR) and computed tomography (CT). According to the American College of Radiology's (ACR) Appropriateness Criteria on acute respiratory illness, CXR is warranted when one or more of the following is present: age greater than or equal to 40 years; dementia; positive results on physical examination; hemoptysis; associated abnormalities (leukocytosis, hypoxemia); or other risk factors, including coronary artery disease, congestive heart failure, or drug-

Department of Diagnostic Imaging, National University Hospital, 1E Kent Ridge Road, Tower block, Level 12, 119228 Singapore
* Corresponding author.
E-mail address: lynette_ls_teo@nuhs.edu.sg

Radiol Clin N Am 60 (2022) 445–459
https://doi.org/10.1016/j.rcl.2022.01.002
0033-8389/22/© 2022 Elsevier Inc. All rights reserved.

induced acute respiratory failure. CXR may also be warranted for any adult with clinical suspicion of pneumonia. Chest CT may be warranted in complicated cases of severe pneumonia and in febrile neutropenic patients with normal or nonspecific CXR findings.[3] Imaging is useful in assessing extent of disease, associated complications, and underlying lung/mediastinal diseases.[4,5]

In this article, the authors discuss selected common respiratory infections and their imaging features encountered in SEA.

IMAGING FINDINGS/PATHOLOGY
Viral

The most common viruses causing community acquired pneumonia (CAP) in adults in the Asia-Pacific region are influenza A and B viruses (5%–15%), and rhinovirus (4%–9%).[6]

Influenza
Influenza viruses are single-stranded ribonucleic acid viruses, members of the Orthomyxoviridae family. They are divided into 3 groups (A, B, and C) according to internal membrane and nucleoprotein antigens.[7] Type A and occasionally type B organisms cause influenza virus pneumonia. Influenza exhibits seasonality, with peak activity in colder months in temperate regions. In tropical countries, influenza activity demonstrates multiple peaks and is identifiable year round.[8,9]

Influenza infections usually involves the upper respiratory tract. Severe complications such as hemorrhagic bronchitis or fulminant pneumonia can occur in individuals with chronic diseases, the elderly, and infants.

When influenza progresses to pneumonia, radiographic findings include segmental areas of consolidation that may be homogeneous or patchy and unilateral or bilateral (**Fig. 1**). Serial radiographs show poorly defined, patchy areas of air-space consolidation that rapidly becomes confluent. Pleural effusion is rare.[10] The radiologic abnormalities usually resolve in 3 weeks. CT demonstrates diffuse or patchy areas of ground-glass attenuation mixed with consolidation and small centrilobular nodules.[11]

Avian influenza is caused by the H5N1 subtype of the influenza A virus. Human transmission occurs via close contact with infected birds/poultry. Avian influenza can cause either a mild influenza type illness, which is indistinguishable from seasonal influenza, or more commonly a rapidly progressive community-acquired pneumonic illness, resulting in respiratory and multiorgan failure.[12] Several outbreaks have been reported in countries including Vietnam, Thailand, and Indonesia. The most common radiographic finding is multifocal consolidation. CT findings include focal, multifocal, or diffuse ground glass opacities and areas of consolidation. Centrilobular nodules, pseudocavitation, cavitation, pneumatocele formation, lymphadenopathy, and pleural effusions have been reported.[12]

Cytomegalovirus
Cytomegalovirus (CMV) is a double-stranded deoxyribonucleic acid virus from the herpesvirus family.[13] It is distributed worldwide, with seroprevalence highest in South America, Africa, and Asia and lowest in Western Europe and United States.[14] CMV infection is mostly asymptomatic

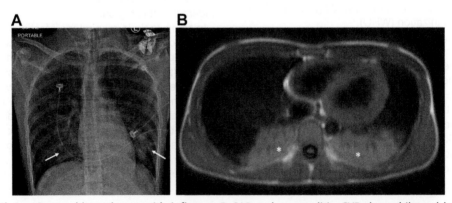

Fig. 1. (*A*) An 18-year-old gentleman with influenza B CAP and myocarditis. CXR shows bilateral lower-zone consolidation (*white arrows*). Endotracheal tube, extracorporeal membrane oxygenation (ECMO) catheters, and feeding tube are present. (*B*) Half-Fourier-acquisition single-shot turbo-spin-echo image from cardiovascular MR imaging (obtained as evaluation for myocarditis) shows bilateral lower lobe consolidation (*). Not pictured here was extensive subepicardial late gadolinium enhancement (LGE) of the anterior, lateral, and inferior left ventricular wall and midwall LGE of the ventricular septum, from basal to apical levels, with corresponding myocardial edema on T2-weighted short tau inversion recovery images, in keeping with acute myocarditis.

in immunocompetent hosts, although transient infectious mononucleosis–like syndrome has been described.[15] CMV can cause life-threatening pulmonary infection in immunocompromised patients due to reactivation of the latent virus or due to infusion of CMV-seropositive marrow or blood products.[7] Person-to-person transmission is via contact with bodily secretions of infected persons.[16] Imaging demonstrates bilateral asymmetrical ground-glass opacities, consolidation, linear opacities, nodules, and masses[7,17–19] **(Fig. 2)**. The nodules are usually in the centrilobular distribution,[11,17,19] although subpleural and random locations have been described.[18]

Bacterial

The most common bacterial causes for CAP in Asia are *Streptococcus pneumoniae* (29.2%), *Klebsiella pneumoniae* (15.4%), *Hemophilus influenzae* (15.1%), *Chlamydia pneumoniae* (13.4%), and *Mycoplasma pneumoniae* (11.0%).[20] Important bacterial pathogens in SEA also include *Burkholderia pseudomallei* and *Mycobacterium tuberculosis*.[6,21]

Tuberculosis

Tuberculosis (TB) is a communicable disease of public health importance globally, with high burden in certain countries. The 2020 WHO Global Tuberculosis Report showed that an estimated 10.0 million people fell ill with TB in 2019. Most cases were in the WHO regions of SEA (44%), Africa (25%), and Western Pacific (18%), with smaller percentages in Eastern Mediterranean (8.2%), the Americas (2.9%), and Europe (2.5%).[22]

Drug-resistant TB is an emerging problem. Globally in 2019, an estimated 3.3% (95%

confidence interval [CI]: 2.3% to 4.3%) of new cases and 18% (95% CI: 9.7%–27%) of previously treated cases had multidrug-/rifampicin-resistant tuberculosis (MDR/RR-TB).[22] Indonesia, Myanmar, The Philippines, Thailand, and Vietnam are listed among the 30 high MDR-TB burden countries. According to WHO guidelines, detection of MDR/RR-TB requires bacteriologic confirmation of TB and testing for drug resistance using rapid molecular tests, culture methods, or sequencing technologies.

Tuberculosis is mostly caused by *M tuberculosis*, one of several mycobacterial species belonging to the *M tuberculosis* complex. Transmission is via airborne respiratory droplets.[23]

Pulmonary TB is classically divided into primary and postprimary patterns.[24] Primary TB manifests as mediastinal lymphadenopathy, consolidation, pleural effusion, and miliary nodules. Lymphadenopathy typically involves right paratracheal and hilar nodes, which demonstrate central low attenuation with peripheral enhancing rims.[25] Postprimary TB characteristically demonstrates consolidation with cavitation centered in the apical and posterior segments of the upper lobes and apical segments of the lower lobes.[26] The predominant upper lobe distribution of tuberculosis is due to relative overventilation, regional high oxygen tension, and delayed lymphatic clearance in the apices.[27]

The clinical and radiological features of primary and postprimary TB may overlap, and clinically, it is now more important to differentiate active TB from latent TB, given differences in management. Active TB can occur as primary tuberculosis, developing shortly after infection, or postprimary tuberculosis, developing after a long period of latent infection. Imaging features that suggest active TB include cavitation, consolidation, centrilobular tree-in-bud nodules, miliary nodules, necrotic nodes, and pleural effusion[23] **(Figs. 3 and 4)**. Latent TB broadly encompasses latent tuberculosis infection and previous (inactive) tuberculosis. Latent TB (narrow definition) refers to positive findings on laboratory screening tests in the absence of radiographic or clinical evidence of active disease. Inactive tuberculosis is characterized by stable (≥6 months) fibronodular changes, including scarring (peribronchial fibrosis, bronchiectasis, and architectural distortion) and nodular opacities and pleural thickening in the lung apices. Fibronodular change is associated with considerably higher risk of developing tuberculosis reactivation. Calcified granulomas and calcified lymph nodes are associated with low risk of reactivation. Healed tuberculous cavities may

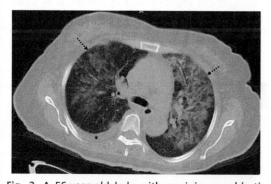

Fig. 2. A 56-year-old lady with angioimmunoblastic T-cell lymphoma and cytomegalovirus pneumonia. Axial CT image of the thorax in lung window shows bilateral asymmetrical ground glass opacities (dotted *arrows*) and a small right pleural effusion (*). Scattered subcentimeter nodules are also seen in the right lung.

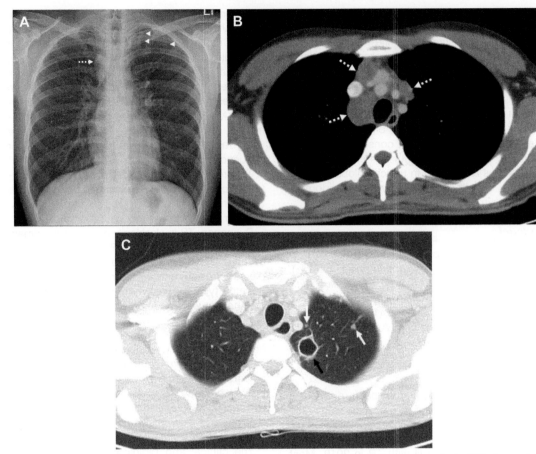

Fig. 3. (A) A 26-year-old gentleman with right neck mass due to *Mycobacterium tuberculosis*. CXR shows right paratracheal mass (*dotted arrow*) and nodularities (*arrowheads*) in the left lung apex. (B, C) CT shows necrotic enlarged mediastinal nodes (*white dotted arrows*), with cavitary lesion (*black solid arrow*) and centrilobular nodules (*white solid arrows*) in left lung apex. This case demonstrates an overlap of imaging findings between primary and postprimary TB.

persist and can be complicated by hemoptysis, bacterial infection, or mycetoma.[23]

The presence of cavities in the initial CXR has implications on the length of treatment of active TB, requiring a longer duration of treatment.[23] Radiographic improvement at 2 months of treatment (ie, end of intensive phase) provides evidence of treatment response. Pulmonary

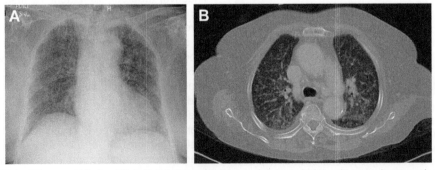

Fig. 4. (A, B) An 81-year-old lady with ischemic heart disease and chronic kidney disease, diagnosed with miliary tuberculosis. CXR (A) and CT (B) show extensive miliary nodules.

tuberculosis lesions usually heal with sequelae of fibrosis and scarring. The end-of-treatment CXR is useful to serve as a new baseline for future comparison. The presence of cavitation in the end-of-treatment CXR has been shown to be associated with increased risk of relapse.[28] Besides the use of radiographs, treatment response is monitored clinically (decrease in cough and systemic symptoms and increase in weight) and bacteriologically. If sputum cultures remain positive after 3 months of treatment, or if there is bacteriologic reversion from negative to positive at any time, drug susceptibility testing should be repeated.[29,30]

Melioidosis

Melioidosis is a potentially life-threatening condition caused by gram-negative necrotic bacillus *B pseudomallei*, endemic to SEA, Northern Australia, and parts of Oceania.[31,32] Infection in humans is typically caused by percutaneous inoculation with contaminated soil/water and occasionally by inhalation.[33] Pulmonary melioidosis manifestations range from acute disseminated septicemia,

subacute or localized pneumonia, to chronic infection.[33] Imaging features include lung nodules and consolidation. The lung lesions may coalesce and cavitate, resulting in pneumothorax (**Fig. 5**) and bronchopleural fistula.[34] Simultaneous involvement of other organs with abscesses is common. The aforementioned figure notwithstanding, pleural effusion, empyema, and mediastinal lymphadenopathy are relatively rare in melioidosis. These findings can be useful in differentiating melioidosis from TB,[34] given that both infections preferentially involve the upper lobes. Also note that confluent consolidation (**Fig. 6**) occurs more commonly in melioidosis compared with TB[35] (**Table 1**).

Streptococcus pneumoniae

S pneumoniae are gram-positive, lancet-shaped facultative anaerobic organisms that typically occur in pairs or short chains. It colonizes the human nasopharynx. Transmission is via droplets/aerosols from infected persons.[36,37] *S pneumoniae* is the most common cause of CAP in Asia.[20,21]

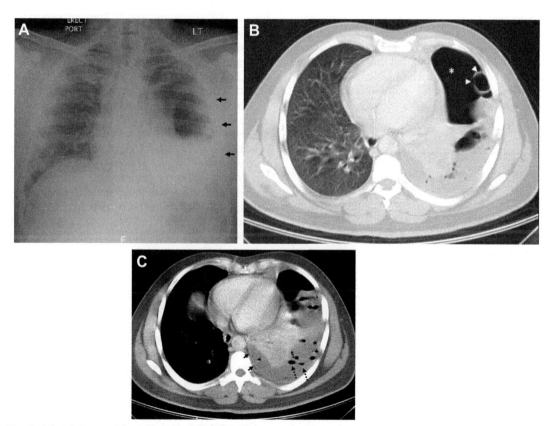

Fig. 5. (*A*) A 32-year-old gentleman with fever due to melioidosis. CXR shows a large left hydropneumothorax (*black arrows*) with left lung collapse. (*B, C*) CT shows a large left pneumothorax (*). Gas pockets (*black dotted arrows*) within the left pleural fluid, with pleural thickening (*black solid arrows*), suggest left pyopneumothorax. Hypodense areas within the collapsed left lung may represent necrosis.

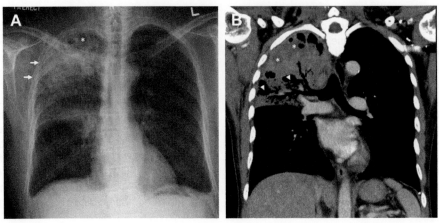

Fig. 6. (*A*) A 64-year-old gentleman with psoriasis, diagnosed with melioidosis. CXR shows consolidation (*arrows*) with cavitation (*) in the right upper lobe. (*B*) CT shows right upper lobe pneumonia with cavitation (*arrowheads*) and necrosis (*).

Four types of radiographic appearances have been described: classic lobar pneumonia, patchy bronchopneumonia, interstitial (irregular linear) pneumonia, and a mixture of the latter 2 types[38] (**Fig. 7**). Occasionally, it may present as round pneumonia, more commonly seen in children. Centrilobular nodules, bronchial wall thickening, bilateral pleural effusions, cavitation, gangrene, and pneumatocele formation are unusual but when present suggest polymicrobial infection.[39,40] Parapneumonic pleural effusions are not uncommon.[41]

Table 1
Imaging features of tuberculosis and melioidosis

Imaging Features	Tuberculosis	Melioidosis
Location	Upper lobes	Upper lobes
Branching tree in bud opacities	+	−
Lung nodules	+	+
Consolidation	+	+, more confluent
Cavitation	+	+
Bronchopleural fistula	+	+
Pneumothorax	+	+
Pleural effusion/ empyema	+	Rare
Mediastinal lymphadenopathy	+	Rare

(+): may be present; (−): not present.

Staphylococcus aureus

Staphylococcus aureus are gram-positive, nonmotile, non–spore-forming, coagulase-producing facultative anaerobes that are cocci-shaped and arranged in clusters. They colonize the nasal passage and skin.[42] Transmission is via contact.[43] *S aureus* is one of the top common causes of CAP in Asia.[20,21] It is an important cause of nosocomial pneumonia, especially in the intensive care unit.[4]

Radiographic features that suggest staphylococcal pneumonia include bilateral patchy bronchopneumonia (lobular pneumonia), together with cavitation, pneumatoceles, and spontaneous pneumothorax[44] (**Fig. 8**). Pneumatoceles tend to resolve spontaneously in weeks or a few months following infection. Lobar enlargement with bulging of the interlobar fissures can be seen in severe cases. Pleural effusions occur in 30% to 50% of patients; of these, approximately half represent empyemas. Abscesses develop in 15% to 30% of patients.[39,45]

Klebsiella pneumoniae

K pneumoniae is a gram-negative, encapsulated, nonmotile facultative anaerobic bacterium found in the environment. It colonizes human mucosal surfaces of the nasopharynx and gastrointestinal tract.[46] Transmission is via contact. *K pneumoniae* is one of the top common causes of CAP in Asia.[20] *K pneumonia* tends to affect people with underlying diseases, such as alcoholism, diabetes, and chronic lung disease.

Radiographic features are similar to streptococcal pneumonia, presenting as lobar consolidation with air bronchograms. However, there is greater tendency for lobar expansion with bulging

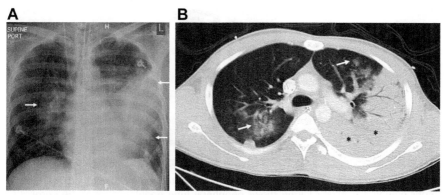

Fig. 7. (*A*) A 26-year-old gentleman with *Streptococcus pneumoniae* CAP. CXR shows bilateral patchy consolidation (*arrows*). Endotracheal tube, right central catheter, and feeding tube are present. (*B*) CT shows extensive lobar and segmental consolidation (*) in the left lung and patchy ill-defined airspace opacities (*arrows*) in both lungs.

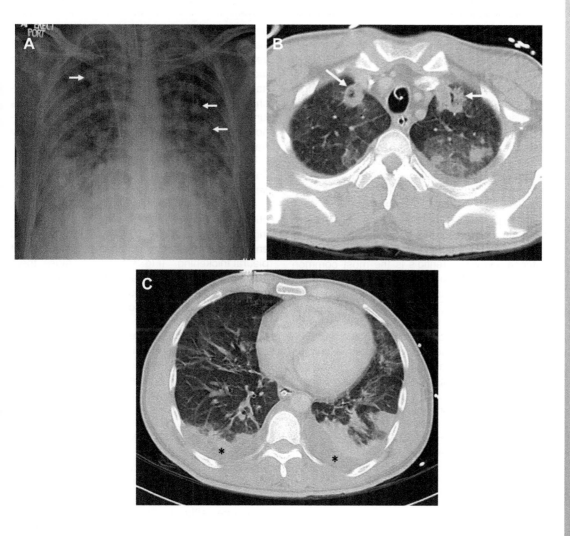

Fig. 8. (*A*) A 33-year-old gentleman with staphylococcal osteomyelitis and paraspinal abscesses and severe CAP. CXR shows bilateral patchy consolidation and nodular opacities (*arrows*). (*B*, *C*) CT shows bilateral nodular lesions (some with cavitation [*white arrows*]), patchy ground-glass opacities, consolidation, and pleural effusions (*).

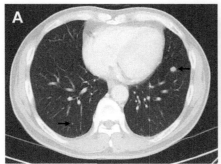 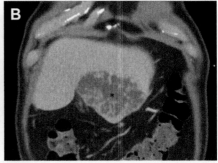

Fig. 9. A 70-year-old gentleman with *Klebsiella pneumoniae* bacteraemia with hepatic abscess and presumed pulmonary septic emboli. (*A*) Axial CT lung shows peripheral lung nodules (*arrows*). (*B*) Coronal CT abdomen shows left hepatic lobe abscess (*asterisk*).

of the fissures due to formation of voluminous inflammatory exudate. Abscesses, cavity formation, and pleural effusions are also more common.[4] Rupture of a lung abscess can result in formation of empyema, bronchopleural fistula, and pneumothorax.[39] The most common CT findings of acute *K pneumonia* are ground-glass attenuation, followed by consolidation and intralobular reticular opacities, predominantly in the periphery of the lungs, with pleural effusion.[47] Septic pulmonary emboli can also be seen in patients with *K pneumoniae* liver abscess and manifest as multiple nodules (**Fig. 9**) and wedge-shaped lesions distributed diffusely within the peripheral lung regions and consolidation within the lower lobes.[48]

Salmonella enteritidis

Salmonella species are worldwide rod-shaped, gram-negative facultative anaerobes that belong to the Enterobacteriaceae family.[49] Salmonella enterica serovar Enteritidis is the most common serotype reported from human isolates globally.[50] Infections usually start from ingestion of contaminated food or water. Person-to-person transmission can also occur through the fecal-oral route. Five clinical manifestations have been described: gastroenteritis, enteric fever, bacteraemia, chronic carrier state, and localized infections.[51] Pulmonary infections may be due to hematogenous spread from the gastrointestinal tract, aspiration of infected gastric contents, or direct extension from a nearby site. Pulmonary involvement in salmonella infections may present as lobar pneumonia or bronchopneumonia (**Fig. 10**). Empyemas, pleural effusions, lung abscesses, and bronchopleural fistulas may be seen in complicated cases.[51–53]

Actinomycosis

Actinomycosis is an uncommon, chronic suppurative bacterial infection caused by actinomyces species, especially *Actinomyces israeli*.

Actinomycetes are branching gram-positive anaerobic bacteria belonging to the Actinomycetaceae family and are commensal in the human oropharynx, gastrointestinal tract, and female genitalia.[54] Thoracic infection is believed to occur via aspiration of oropharyngeal or gastrointestinal secretions into the respiratory tract. It is seen more frequently in patients with underlying pulmonary disease, such as emphysema, chronic bronchitis, or bronchiectasis, and those with previous lung damage. Other risk factors include alcoholism, poor oral hygiene, dental disease, dental trauma, and facial trauma.[55]

The disease is characterized by suppuration, sinus tract formation, and purulent discharge containing yellowish "sulfur granules."[56]

Pulmonary involvement usually appears as chronic segmental airspace consolidation containing necrotic low-attenuation areas with peripheral enhancement, often accompanied by adjacent pleural thickening[57] (**Fig. 11**). In later stages, there is destruction of lung parenchyma, and the infection may extend across fissures to a neighboring pulmonary lobe, pleura, or chest wall, with abscess formation in these areas.[55] The condition may also present as a mass that may mimic lung cancer.[56] Associated findings include interlobular septal thickening, bronchiectasis, mediastinal lymphadenopathy, adjacent pleural thickening, pleural effusion, and empyema.

Nocardiosis

Nocardiosis is caused by Nocardia species, which are a group of aerobic, gram-positive, partially acid-fast bacteria that are ubiquitous in soil worldwide, not considered part of normal human flora nor a common laboratory contaminant.[58] Infection is acquired either by cutaneous inoculation or by inhalation. Most infections affect immunocompromised patients or patients with preexisting pulmonary disease, although infections have also been reported in immunocompetent patients.[59,60] The

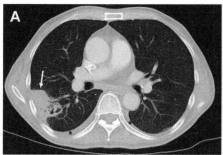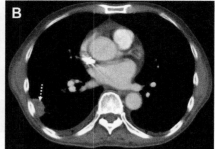

Fig. 10. (*A, B*) A 62-year-old gentleman with chronic hepatitis B and retroviral infection who presented with salmonella enteritidis bacteraemia and pulmonary infection. CT shows peripheral masslike consolidation (*solid arrow*) in the right lower lobe with internal hypodense areas that indicate necrosis (*dotted arrow*) and bilateral pleural effusions (*).

clinical spectrum of Nocardiosis can be divided into cutaneous, pulmonary and disseminated forms. Disseminated Nocardiosis occurs through hematogenous spread from the lungs most commonly to the central nervous system, skin, and joints.[61]

Imaging features for pulmonary Nocardiosis include multifocal consolidation, nodules/masses, and pleural effusion.[62] Cavitation and abscess formation can be seen in the areas of consolidation and nodules/masses (**Fig. 12**). Most nodules and masses have poorly defined margins and peripheral predominance,[63] with perilesional interlobular septal thickening and ground glass opacities.[64] Infection can spread to the chest wall, resulting in chest wall abscesses.

Fungal

The epidemiology of fungal infections is not well described in Asia. Some of the most clinically significant opportunistic mold and yeast infections in the Asia-Pacific region include aspergillosis, mucormycosis, pythiosis, scedosporiosis, fusariosis, candidiasis, trichosporonosis, and cryptococcosis.[65]

Aspergillosis

Aspergillus is a ubiquitous soil-dwelling organism found in both indoor and outdoor environment.[66,67] Pulmonary disease is caused mainly by *Aspergillus fumigatus* and has a spectrum of clinical syndromes. The clinical spectrum ranges from allergic bronchopulmonary aspergillosis in asthmatic patients, aspergilloma in patients with chronic cavitatory lung disease, and chronic necrotizing aspergillosis in chronic lung disease patients, to invasive pulmonary aspergillosis in immunocompromised hosts.[67] Aspergilloma is the most common and best-recognized clinical manifestation. The aspergilloma (fungal ball) consists of masses of fungal mycelia, inflammatory cells, fibrin, mucus, and tissue debris, usually developing in a preexisting lung cavity, most

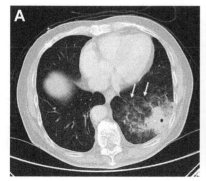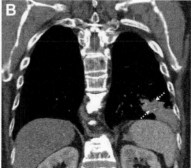

Fig. 11. (*A*) A 61-year-old gentleman with metastatic colon cancer and hemoptysis due to actinomycosis. CT demonstrates masslike consolidation (*) in the left lower lobe, with adjacent ground-glass opacities and interstitial thickening (*arrows*). (*B*) CT shows tiny calcified foci and internal hypodense foci (*dotted arrows*) within the masslike consolidation, suggesting necrosis.

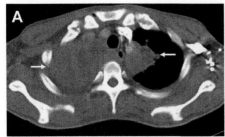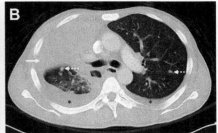

Fig. 12. (*A, B*) A 42-year-old gentleman with myelodysplastic syndrome and pulmonary nocardiosis. CT shows bilateral cavitary masslike consolidation (*solid arrows*) containing foci of low attenuation likely representing necrosis. Irregular nodules (*dotted arrows*) and pleural effusions (*) are also present.

commonly, tuberculous cavities.[66,68] Imaging classically demonstrates a mobile intracavitary mass within an upper-lobe cavity (**Fig. 13**). Crescentic air lucency can be seen between the fungus ball and the wall of the cavity, termed "Monod's Sign".[69,70] The adjacent pleura may be thickened.[71] Thick-walled, slowly expanding cavities surrounded by dense consolidation with pleural thickening, abnormal enhancement of extrapleural fat, parenchymal destruction, and empyema can be seen in chronic cavitary pulmonary aspergillosis (CCPA).[72] The cavities may or may not contain an aspergilloma. When CCPA is left untreated, severe fibrotic destruction of at least 2 lobes of lung leads to development of chronic fibrosing pulmonary aspergillosis. Subacute invasive aspergillosis, previously termed chronic necrotizing or semiinvasive aspergillosis, is usually seen in mildly immunocompromised patients, occurring over 1 to 3 months, with variable radiological features including cavitation, nodules, and progressive consolidation with "abscess formation."[73]

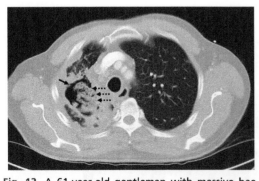

Fig. 13. A 61-year-old gentleman with massive haemoptysis secondary to right upper lobe aspergilloma, on background of cavitary pulmonary TB. CT shows irregular mass (*dotted arrows*) within a right upper lobe cavity with adjacent parenchymal changes in keeping with chronic pulmonary aspergillosis with an accompanying aspergilloma (*solid arrow*).

Cryptococcosis

Cryptococcosis is caused by pathogenic encapsulated yeasts in the genus Cryptococcus. The 2 main pathogenic cryptococcal species for humans and animals are *Cryptococcus neoformans* and *Cryptococcus gattii*, sometimes considered together as part to the *C neoformans* species complex.[74] *C neoformans* is found worldwide in association with excreta from certain birds such as pigeons and in a variety of tree species in their hollows. *C gattii* is commonly associated with several species of eucalyptus trees in tropical and subtropical climates.[74,75] Transmission is via inhalation of cryptococcal particles, with subsequent hematogenous dissemination to the central nervous system, skin, and bones, depending on the host immune status[76,77] (see also Ryzdak in this issue). Cryptococcosis occurs predominantly in immunocompromised patients but also occurs occasionally in immunocompetent hosts.[78] Cryptococcal pulmonary involvement ranges from asymptomatic colonization or infection to severe pneumonia with respiratory failure.[79]

Imaging findings include solitary or multiple nodules, segmental or lobar consolidation, cavitation within nodules (10%–15%), hilar and mediastinal lymphadenopathy, and pleural effusion[80,81] (**Figs. 14 and 15**). The nodules tend to be peripherally located[76,77,82] and may show smooth or irregular margins with spiculations.[77]

Parasites

The clinical and radiological findings of some parasitic thoracic infections may mimic tuberculosis and malignancy. It is thus important to consider parasitic infections in the differential diagnosis, as most are curable if identified early. Amebiasis, strongyloidiasis, lymphatic filariasis, malaria, and paragonimiasis are more commonly seen in SEA.

Strongyloidiasis

Strongyloidiasis is a chronic parasitic infection caused by *Strongyloides stercoralis*, endemic in

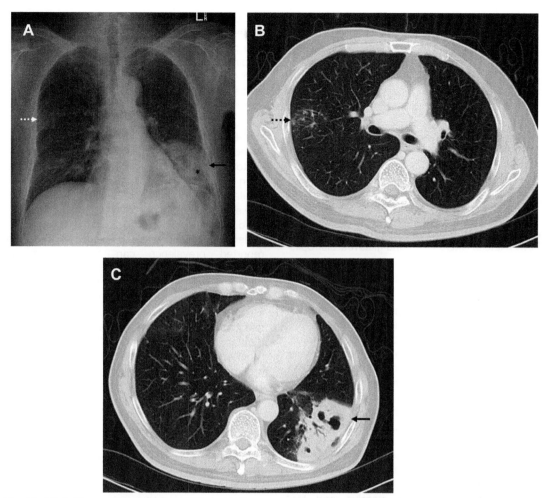

Fig. 14. (*A*) A 63-year-old gentleman with multiple comorbidities and cryptococcal pneumonia. CXR shows mass-like consolidation in the left lower lobe (*black solid arrow*) with areas of cavitation (*), and small nodularities in the right midzone (*dotted white arrow*). (*B, C*) CT shows centrilobular nodules in the right upper lobe (*dotted arrow*) and cavitary masslike consolidation in the left lower lobe (*solid arrow*).

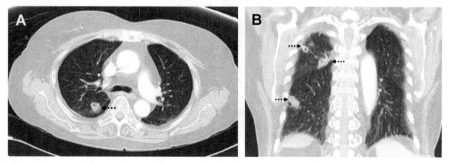

Fig. 15. (*A, B*) A 76-year-old lady with autoimmune hepatitis and primary biliary cirrhosis on immunosuppressant therapy, diagnosed with cryptococcosis. CT shows bilateral lung nodules with internal cavitation (*dotted arrows*).

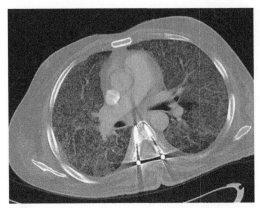

Fig. 16. A 63-year-old gentleman with multiple co-morbidities and disseminated strongyloidiasis. CT shows bilateral extensive ground-glass/reticular opacities and miliary nodules.

tropical and subtropical regions of the world.[83] Studies have reported prevalence of up to 57.0% in Thailand, 44.7% in Cambodia, 41.0% in Laos, and 39.0% in Malaysia.[84] Initial infection occurs when infective larvae in the soil penetrate the skin. The larvae invade the lungs, migrate to the pharynx, and are swallowed into the small intestine, where eggs are laid.[85] The larvae can reinfect their host via the intestinal mucosa or perianal skin.

This reinfection process is termed autoinfection and allows S stercoralis to complete its life cycle and proliferate within a single host. In immunocompromised patients, uncontrolled proliferation of larvae can lead to a massive and life-threatening parasitic infestation (hyperinfection syndrome), and disseminated strongyloidiasis, characterized by dissemination to other organs not involved in the life cycle of S stercoralis[85,86] (see also Restrepo in this issue).

Imaging findings include ill-defined, patchy, migratory airspace consolidation, miliary nodules, and diffuse reticular interstitial opacities (Fig. 16). Hyperinfection syndrome can manifest with extensive pneumonia, alveolar hemorrhage, and adult respiratory distress syndrome. Pleural effusion, cavitation, and abscess formation can be seen with superimposed bacterial infection.

Amebiasis

Amebiasis is caused by Entamoeba histolytica, a protozoan found worldwide, most commonly seen in tropical and subtropical regions with poor sanitation and poor socioeconomic condition.[86,87] The exact burden of amebiasis is difficult to quantify due to limited diagnostic capabilities and surveillance in many endemic places.[88] Also, the reported prevalence can be affected by geographic region, study design, sample size, and the sensitivity of the diagnostic modality used. For instance, the reported prevalence in Malaysia ranged from 1% to 83%.[89] E histolytica infection incidence of 11% has been reported in Vietnam.[90] The prevalence in Thailand has been reported to be 7.1%.[91] Transmission is via fecal-oral route ingestion of amebic cysts. The trophozoites may invade bowel wall mucosa to enter the portal circulation. Liver abscesses and pleuropulmonary involvement are the most common extraintestinal manifestations. Pleuropulmonary involvement is most commonly due to direct extension from a liver abscess (tertiary route),[92] followed by hematogenous spread (secondary route) and, less frequently, aspiration (primary route).[92] Imaging features include pleural effusion/empyema, elevation of the right hemidiaphragm, and pulmonary consolidation with or without cavitation (Fig. 17). A hepatobronchial or bronchobiliary fistula can form if the abscess drains through a bronchus. In rare cases, invasion of inferior vena cava occurs and may result in pulmonary thromboembolism.[93]

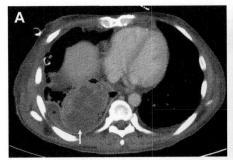
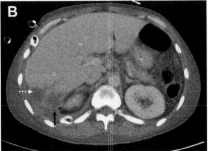

Fig. 17. (A, B) A 54-year-old gentleman with hepatic and pleuroparenchymal amebiasis. CT shows necrotic appearance of right lower pulmonary lobe (white solid arrow). The right empyema (*) is contiguous with a right subphrenic collection (dotted white arrow), via a right hemidiaphragmatic defect (black solid arrow).

SUMMARY

The burden of pneumonia in SEA remains high, especially when coupled with global warming and climate change. The common pathogens endemic in SEA and their typical radiological features have been discussed. Global migration and international tourism blur the geographic boundaries of these tropical infectious agents, and it is important for physicians to recognize and diagnose them early, as many of these diseases can be easily treated by instituting the correct therapy.

CLINICS CARE POINTS

- Chest x-ray is the first line imaging modality for suspected thoracic infections.In complicated cases of severe pneumonia and in febrile neutropenic patients, Chest CT may be warranted.

- Classical imaging features for certain respiratory pathogens have been described in this article.

- Imaging features for various thoracic infections can overlap and a combination of clinical, radiological and microbiological findings are needed to arrive at the final diagnosis.

- Common clincially significant respiratory pathogens in SEA are tuberculosis and meliodosis.

DISCLOSURE

C.C. Ong and L.L.S. Teo declare that they have no conflict of interest. This review article has been approved by the local institutional review board (2021/00324), with waiver of informed consent.

REFERENCES

1. WHO The top 10 causes of death. World Health Organisation. 2020. Available at: https://www.who.int/news-room/fact-sheets/detail/the-top-10-causes-of-death. Accessed June 28 2021.
2. Subregions in Asia by population. 2021. Available at: https://www.worldometers.info/world-population/population-by-asia-subregion/. Accessed 29 June 2021.
3. Washington L, Khan A, Mohammed TL, et al. ACR Appropriateness Criteria on acute respiratory illness. J Am Coll Radiol 2009;6(10):675–80.
4. Tarver RD, Teague SD, Heitkamp DE, et al. Radiology of community-acquired pneumonia. Radiol Clin North Am 2005;43(3):497–512, viii.
5. Vilar J, Domingo ML, Soto C, et al. Radiology of bacterial pneumonia. Eur J Radiol 2004;51(2):102–13.
6. Song JH, Huh K, Chung DR. Community-Acquired Pneumonia in the Asia-Pacific Region. Semin Respir Crit Care Med 2016;37(6):839–54.
7. Koo HJ, Lim S, Choe J, et al. Radiographic and CT Features of Viral Pneumonia. Radiographics 2018; 38(3):719–39.
8. Simonsen L. The global impact of influenza on morbidity and mortality. Vaccine 1999;17:S3–10.
9. Tamerius JD, Shaman J, Alonso WJ, et al. Environmental predictors of seasonal influenza epidemics across temperate and tropical climates. Plos Pathog 2013;9(3):e1003194.
10. Oikonomou A, Muller NL, Nantel S. Radiographic and high-resolution CT findings of influenza virus pneumonia in patients with hematologic malignancies. AJR Am J Roentgenol 2003;181(2):507–11.
11. Kim EA, Lee KS, Primack SL, et al. Viral pneumonias in adults: radiologic and pathologic findings. Radiographics 2002;S137–49, 22 Spec No.
12. Qureshi NR, Hien TT, Farrar J, et al. The radiologic manifestations of H5N1 avian influenza. J Thorac Imaging 2006;21(4):259–64.
13. Pomeroy C, Englund JA. Cytomegalovirus: Epidemiology and infection control. Am J Infect Control 1987;15(3):107–19.
14. Cannon MJ, Schmid DS, Hyde TB. Review of cytomegalovirus seroprevalence and demographic characteristics associated with infection. Rev Med Virol 2010;20(4):202–13.
15. Horwitz CA, Henle W, Henle G, et al. Clinical and laboratory evaluation of cytomegalovirus-induced mononucleosis in previously healthy individuals. Report of 82 cases. Medicine (Baltimore) 1986; 65(2):124–34.
16. Forbes BA. Acquisition of cytomegalovirus infection: an update. Clin Microbiol Rev 1989;2(2):204–16.
17. Moon JH, Kim EA, Lee KS, et al. Cytomegalovirus pneumonia: high-resolution CT findings in ten non-AIDS immunocompromised patients. Korean J Radiol 2000;1(2):73–8.
18. Franquet T, Lee KS, Muller NL. Thin-section CT findings in 32 immunocompromised patients with cytomegalovirus pneumonia who do not have AIDS. AJR Am J Roentgenol 2003;181(4):1059–63.
19. Horger MS, Pfannenberg C, Einsele H, et al. Cytomegalovirus pneumonia after stem cell transplantation: correlation of CT findings with clinical outcome in 30 patients. AJR Am J Roentgenol 2006;187(6):W636–43.
20. Song JH, Oh WS, Kang CI, et al. Epidemiology and clinical outcomes of community-acquired pneumonia in adult patients in Asian countries: a prospective study by the Asian network for surveillance of resistant pathogens. Int J Antimicrob Agents 2008;31(2):107–14.

21. Peto L, Nadjm B, Horby P, et al. The bacterial aetiology of adult community-acquired pneumonia in Asia: a systematic review. Trans R Soc Trop Med Hyg 2014;108(6):326–37.

22. Global Tuberculosis Report 2020. World Health Organisation.

23. Nachiappan AC, Rahbar K, Shi X, et al. Pulmonary Tuberculosis: Role of Radiology in Diagnosis and Management. Radiographics 2017;37(1):52–72.

24. Burrill J, Williams CJ, Bain G, et al. Tuberculosis: a radiologic review. Radiographics 2007;27(5):1255–73.

25. Im JG, Song KS, Kang HS, et al. Mediastinal tuberculous lymphadenitis: CT manifestations. Radiology 1987;164(1):115–9.

26. Leung AN. Pulmonary tuberculosis: the essentials. Radiology 1999;210(2):307–22.

27. Nemec SF, Bankier AA, Eisenberg RL. Upper lobe-predominant diseases of the lung. AJR Am J Roentgenol 2013;200(3):W222–37.

28. Hamilton CD, Stout JE, Goodman PC, Mosher A, et al. Tuberculosis Trials Consortium. The value of end-of-treatment chest radiograph in predicting pulmonary tuberculosis relapse. Int J Tuberc Lung Dis 2008;12(9):1059–64.

29. Nahid P, Mase SR, Migliori GB, et al. Treatment of Drug-Resistant Tuberculosis. An Official ATS/CDC/ERS/IDSA Clinical Practice Guideline. Am J Respir Crit Care Med 2019;200(10):e93–142.

30. Nahid P, Dorman SE, Alipanah N, et al. Official American Thoracic Society/Centers for Disease Control and Prevention/Infectious Diseases Society of America Clinical Practice Guidelines: Treatment of Drug-Susceptible Tuberculosis. Clin Infect Dis 2016;63(7):e147–95.

31. White NJ. Melioidosis. Lancet 2003;361(9370):1715–22.

32. Ip M, Osterberg LG, Chau PY, et al. Pulmonary melioidosis. Chest 1995;108(5):1420–4.

33. Ko SF, Kung CT, Lee YW, et al. Imaging spectrum of thoracic melioidosis. J Thorac Imaging 2013;28(3):W43–8.

34. Lim KS, Chong VH. Radiological manifestations of melioidosis. Clin Radiol 2010;65(1):66–72.

35. Harvey J, Boles B, Brown D. A review of imaging findings in melioidosis: revealing the tropics' dirty secret. Radiol Infect Dis 2020;7(4):176–85.

36. Henriques-Normark B, Tuomanen EI. The pneumococcus: epidemiology, microbiology, and pathogenesis. Cold Spring Harb Perspect Med 2013;3(7).

37. Weiser JN, Ferreira DM, Paton JC. Streptococcus pneumoniae: transmission, colonization and invasion. Nat Rev Microbiol 2018;16(6):355–67.

38. Kantor HG. The many radiologic facies of pneumococcal pneumonia. AJR Am J Roentgenol 1981;137(6):1213–20.

39. Gharib AM, Stern EJ. Radiology of Pneumonia. Med Clin North Am 2001;85(6):1461–91.

40. Okada F, Ando Y, Matsushita S, et al. Thin-section CT findings of patients with acute Streptococcus pneumoniae pneumonia with and without concurrent infection. Br J Radiol 2012;85(1016):e357–64.

41. Taryle DA, Potts DE, Sahn SA. The incidence and clinical correlates of parapneumonic effusions in pneumococcal pneumonia. Chest 1978;74(2):170–3.

42. Williams RE. Healthy carriage of Staphylococcus aureus: its prevalence and importance. Bacteriol Rev 1963;27:56–71.

43. Lowy FD. Staphylococcus aureus infections. N Engl J Med 1998;339(8):520–32.

44. Macfarlane J, Rose D. Radiographic features of staphylococcal pneumonia in adults and children. Thorax 1996;51(5):539–40.

45. Franquet T. Imaging of Community-acquired Pneumonia. J Thorac Imaging 2018;33(5):282–94.

46. Podschun R, Ullmann U. Klebsiella spp. as nosocomial pathogens: epidemiology, taxonomy, typing methods, and pathogenicity factors. Clin Microbiol Rev 1998;11(4):589–603.

47. Okada F, Ando Y, Honda K, et al. Clinical and pulmonary thin-section CT findings in acute Klebsiella pneumoniae pneumonia. Eur Radiol 2009;19(4):809–15.

48. Chang Z, Gong Z, Zheng J, et al. Computed Tomography Features of Septic Pulmonary Embolism Caused by Klebsiella pneumoniae Liver Abscess Associated With Extrapulmonary Metastatic Infection. J Comput Assist Tomogr 2016;40(3):364–9.

49. Coburn B, Grassl GA, Finlay BB. Salmonella, the host and disease: a brief review. Immunol Cell Biol 2007;85(2):112–8.

50. Galanis E, Lo Fo Wong DM, Patrick ME, et al. Web-based surveillance and global Salmonella distribution, 2000-2002. Emerg Infect Dis 2006;12(3):381–8.

51. Cohen JI, Bartlett JA, Corey GR. Extra-intestinal manifestations of salmonella infections. Medicine (Baltimore) 1987;66(5):349–88.

52. Saeed NK. Salmonella pneumonia complicated with encysted empyema in an immunocompromised youth: Case report and literature Review. J Infect Dev Ctries 2016;10(4):437–44.

53. Casado JL, Navas E, Frutos B, et al. Salmonella lung involvement in patients with HIV infection. Chest 1997;112(5):1197–201.

54. Yildiz O, Doganay M. Actinomycoses and Nocardia pulmonary infections. Curr Opin Pulm Med 2006;12(3):228–34.

55. Han JY, Lee KN, Lee JK, et al. An overview of thoracic actinomycosis: CT features. Insights Imaging 2013;4(2):245–52.

56. Hsieh MJ, Liu HP, Chang JP, et al. Thoracic actinomycosis. Chest 1993;104(2):366–70.

57. Cheon JE, Im JG, Kim MY, et al. Thoracic actinomycosis: CT findings. Radiology 1998;209(1):229–33.

58. McNeil MMBJ. The Medically Important Aerobic Actinomycetes: Epidemiology and Microbiology. Clin Microbiol Rev 1994;357–417.

59. Lederman ER, Crum NF. A case series and focused review of nocardiosis: clinical and microbiologic aspects. Medicine (Baltimore) 2004;83(5):300–13.

60. Hui CH, Au VW, Rowland K, et al. Pulmonary nocardiosis re-visited: experience of 35 patients at diagnosis. Respir Med 2003;97(6):709–17.

61. Ambrosioni J, Lew D, Garbino J. Nocardiosis: updated clinical review and experience at a tertiary center. Infection 2010;38(2):89–97.

62. Kanne JP, Yandow DR, Mohammed TL, et al. CT findings of pulmonary nocardiosis. AJR Am J Roentgenol 2011;197(2):W266–72.

63. Chen J, Zhou H, Xu P, et al. Clinical and radiographic characteristics of pulmonary nocardiosis: clues to earlier diagnosis. PLoS One 2014;9(3): e90724.

64. Sato H, Okada F, Mori T, et al. High-resolution Computed Tomography Findings in Patients with Pulmonary Nocardiosis. Acad Radiol 2016;23(3): 290–6.

65. Slavin MA, Chakrabarti A. Opportunistic fungal infections in the Asia-Pacific region. Med Mycol 2012;50(1):18–25.

66. Soubani AO, Chandrasekar PH. The clinical spectrum of pulmonary aspergillosis. Chest 2002; 121(6):1988–99.

67. Kousha M, Tadi R, Soubani AO. Pulmonary aspergillosis: a clinical review. Eur Respir Rev 2011;20(121): 156–74.

68. Aquino SL, Kee ST, Warnock ML, et al. Pulmonary aspergillosis: imaging findings with pathologic correlation. AJR Am J Roentgenol 1994;163(4):811–5.

69. Gefter WB. The spectrum of pulmonary aspergillosis. J Thorac Imaging 1992;7(4):56–74.

70. Pesle GD, Monod O. Bronchiectasis due to aspergilloma. Dis Chest 1954;25(2):172–83.

71. Panse P, Smith M, Cummings K, et al. The many faces of pulmonary aspergillosis: Imaging findings with pathologic correlation. Radiol Infect Dis 2016; 3(4):192–200.

72. Hayes GE, Novak-Frazer L. Chronic Pulmonary Aspergillosis-Where Are We? and Where Are We Going? J Fungi (Basel) 2016;2(2).

73. Denning DW, Cadranel J, Beigelman-Aubry C, et al. Chronic pulmonary aspergillosis: rationale and clinical guidelines for diagnosis and management. Eur Respir J 2016;47(1):45–68.

74. Setianingrum F, Rautemaa-Richardson R, Denning DW. Pulmonary cryptococcosis: A review of pathobiology and clinical aspects. Med Mycol 2019;57(2):133–50.

75. Herkert PF, Hagen F, Pinheiro RL, et al. Ecoepidemiology of Cryptococcus gattii in Developing Countries. J Fungi (Basel) 2017;3(4).

76. Lacomis JM, Costello P, Vilchez R, et al. The radiology of pulmonary cryptococcosis in a tertiary medical center. J Thorac Imaging 2001;16(3):139–48.

77. Kishi K, Homma S, Kurosaki A, et al. Clinical features and high-resolution CT findings of pulmonary cryptococcosis in non-AIDS patients. Respir Med 2006; 100(5):807–12.

78. Song KD, Lee KS, Chung MP, et al. Pulmonary cryptococcosis: imaging findings in 23 non-AIDS patients. Korean J Radiol 2010;11(4):407–16.

79. Shirley RM, Baddley JW. Cryptococcal lung disease. Curr Opin Pulm Med 2009;15(3):254–60.

80. Chong S, Lee KS, Yi CA, et al. Pulmonary fungal infection: imaging findings in immunocompetent and immunocompromised patients. Eur J Radiol 2006;59(3):371–83.

81. Zavala S, Baddley JW. Cryptococcosis. Semin Respir Crit Care Med 2020;41(1):69–79.

82. Lindell RM, Hartman TE, Nadrous HF, et al. Pulmonary cryptococcosis: CT findings in immunocompetent patients. Radiology 2005;236(1):326–31.

83. Woodring JH, Halfhill H 2nd, Reed JC. Pulmonary strongyloidiasis: clinical and imaging features. AJR Am J Roentgenol 1994;162(3):537–42.

84. Schar F, Giardina F, Khieu V, et al. Occurrence of and risk factors for Strongyloides stercoralis infection in South-East Asia. Acta Trop 2016;159:227–38.

85. Nabeya D, Haranaga S, Parrott GL, et al. Pulmonary strongyloidiasis: assessment between manifestation and radiological findings in 16 severe strongyloidiasis cases. BMC Infect Dis 2017;17(1):320.

86. Martinez S, Restrepo CS, Carrillo JA, et al. Thoracic manifestations of tropical parasitic infections: a pictorial review. Radiographics 2005;25(1):135–55.

87. Kunst H, Mack D, Kon OM, et al. Parasitic infections of the lung: a guide for the respiratory physician. Thorax 2011;66(6):528–36.

88. Shirley DT, Farr L, Watanabe K, et al. A Review of the Global Burden, New Diagnostics, and Current Therapeutics for Amebiasis. Open Forum Infect Dis 2018;5(7):ofy161.

89. Tengku SA, Norhayati M. Public health and clinical importance of amoebiasis in Malaysia: a review. Trop Biomed 2011;28(2):194–222.

90. Blessmann J, Van Linh P, Nu PA, et al. Epidemiology of amebiasis in a region of high incidence of amebic liver abscess in central Vietnam. Am J Trop Med Hyg 2002;66(5):578–83.

91. Sirivichayakul CP-aC, Wisetsing P, Siripanth C, et al. Prevalence of intestinal parasitic infection among Thai people with mental handicaps. Southeast Asian J Trop Med Public Health 2003;34(2):259–63.

92. Shamsuzzaman SM, Hashiguchi Y. Thoracic amebiasis. Clin Chest Med 2002;23(2):479–92.

93. Rodriguez Carnero P, Hernandez Mateo P, Martin-Garre S, et al. Unexpected hosts: imaging parasitic diseases. Insights Imaging 2017;8(1):101–25.

Endemic Thoracic Infections in Sub-Saharan Africa

Chara E. Rydzak, MD, PhD[a],*, Ana Santos Lima, MD[a],
Gustavo S.P. Meirelles, MD[b]

KEYWORDS

• Pulmonary infections • Infectious disease • Sub-Saharan Africa • Thoracic radiology

KEY POINTS

- Emerging viral and bacterial infections impacting sub-Saharan Africa include measles, dengue, Ebola, and plague, which are exacerbated by limited vaccination, exposure to disease vectors and reservoirs, and limited sanitation.
- Endemic fungal infections have overlapping features including nodules, consolidation, cavitation, and lymphadenopathy and may present as miliary disease in immunocompromised patients.
- Parasitic infections in sub-Saharan Africa may have numerous imaging manifestations, including eosinophilic pneumonia, nodules, pleural disease, and ARDS.
- High HIV/AIDS prevalence in sub-Saharan Africa results in many immunocompromised individuals at increased risk for less typical and more severe sequelae of endemic infections.

INTRODUCTION

Pulmonary infections are a leading contributor to morbidity and mortality globally, particularly in resource-poor regions of sub-Saharan Africa where access to health care is limited.[1] Before the coronavirus disease 2019 (COVID-19) pandemic, an estimated 2.3 million deaths occurred annually due to respiratory infections.[1] Sub-Saharan Africa has some of the highest burden of disease due to pulmonary infections across all age groups[1]; this is compounded by high rates of human immunodeficiency virus (HIV)/AIDS infection in the region, predisposing immunocompromised individuals to thoracic infections with more serious sequelae.[2,3]

The COVID-19 pandemic has demonstrated that the impact of transmissible pulmonary infections is not only borne by the individual or local community. The effects of these infections can be far reaching as global travel, migration, and commerce are disrupted. Climate change is quickly altering our environment and thereby changing the epidemiology and geographic profile of these diseases.[4–8] In addition, breakdowns in government due to political unrest can lead to loss of basic infrastructure and services such as sanitation and health care, contributing to reemergence of infections.[4–8] These factors highlight the importance of understanding endemic thoracic infections in sub-Saharan Africa and their radiologic and clinical correlates to aid in timely diagnosis and treatment.

Emerging Viral

Measles

Measles is one of the most contagious infectious pathogens, requiring a herd immunity threshold of 89% to 94% to stop transmission with significant outbreaks occurring even in populations in which less than 10% of individuals are

[a] Department of Diagnostic Radiology, Oregon Health & Science University, 3181 SW Sam Jackson Park Road, Mail Code L340 Portland, OR 97239, USA; [b] Alliar Group, Rua Ernesto Nazaré, 389 - Alto de Pinheiros, São Paulo, São Paulo 05462-000, Brazil
* Corresponding author.
E-mail address: rydzak@ohsu.edu

Radiol Clin N Am 60 (2022) 461–479
https://doi.org/10.1016/j.rcl.2022.01.003
0033-8389/22/© 2022 Elsevier Inc. All rights reserved.

susceptible.[9] Measles is typically a childhood infection characterized by fever, cough, maculopapular skin rash, coryza, and/or conjunctivitis, but severe disease can cause pneumonia, gastroenteritis, severe desquamation, blindness, encephalitis, subacute sclerosing panencephalitis, and death.[9,10] More serious complications occur in vulnerable immunocompromised patients, malnourished children, and pregnant women, as well as in young adults experiencing infection at an older age.[9–11] Although vaccination programs exist worldwide, many individuals in resource-poor areas go unvaccinated with frequent measles outbreaks.[9,10]

On chest radiograph, air space consolidation and reticular opacities are often present as well as hilar lymphadenopathy.[12] On computed tomography (CT), manifestations can include nodular peribronchial infiltrates; interlobular septal thickening; reticulonodular, micronodular, and/or ground-glass opacities; as well as pleural effusions (**Fig. 1**).[10–12] In severe cases, more extensive consolidation can occur and acute respiratory distress syndrome (ARDS) may develop with fibrotic changes.[10,11] Superimposed bacterial infection is common.[11,12]

Dengue fever

Dengue infection occurs worldwide in tropical and subtropical regions and is a vector-borne viral disease transmitted by mosquito.[13] Although the greatest burden of disease is in Asia, dengue is endemic to Africa and the geographic range is expected to expand due to climate change and urbanization.[13,14] Approximately one-fifth of Africa's population is now seropositive for dengue.

Dengue infection can range from mild fever to severe dengue hemorrhagic fever or dengue shock syndrome.[14,15] Pulmonary involvement in severe disease commonly includes pleural effusions, pneumonitis, noncardiogenic pulmonary edema (ARDS), bronchiolitis, hemorrhage, and hemoptysis.[14–16] On imaging, pulmonary infection can present as ground-glass opacities, consolidation, airspace nodules, and septal line thickening. Pleural and pericardial effusions can also be seen (**Fig. 2**).[16]

Ebola

Ebola virus is a zoonotic infection, with several species acting as reservoirs, whereas humans, monkeys, and apes are end hosts.[17] Although primarily endemic to regions of central Africa, cases have been reported outside these regions, including the United States, Italy, and the Philippines, due to international travel or care of infected individuals by health care works.[17,18] Infection is through direct contact and results in a hemorrhagic fever with multisystem involvement and high case fatality rate.[17–20] Symptoms initially include malaise, myalgias, high fevers, and chills progressing to abdominal pain, diarrhea, nausea, and vomiting as well as confusion, seizures, and coma.[17–20] Pulmonary symptoms include cough, chest pain, shortness of breath, and nasal discharge.[17–20] As the disease progresses, bruising, oozing from wounds and puncture sites, and visceral hemorrhage arise, culminating in severe diffuse coagulopathy, metabolic abnormalities, shock, and potentially death.[17–20]

Given that most infections occur in remote resource-poor regions, imaging data are limited.[21] Future outbreaks are likely to occur both in and outside of sub-Saharan Africa. If imaging is performed in those settings, the risk of transmission necessitates rigorous protocols to protect health care works and patients during imaging and subsequent decontamination of equipment.[17,18,20,21]

Emerging Bacterial

Plague

Plague due to *Yersinia pestis* infection is a zoonosis transmitted by flea vectors from rodent hosts to humans and has reemerged in multiple regions, including areas of sub-Saharan Africa with heavy endemic disease burden in Uganda, Democratic Republic of Congo, Mozambique, and Tanzania.[22–25] Of particular note, Madagascar has faced multiple endemic plague outbreaks, most recently in the face of the COVID-19 pandemic, straining the health care system.[25]

Several forms of plague exist, including bubonic (most common), septicemic, and pneumonic plague (primary or secondary).[22,23] The most recent outbreak of primarily bubonic plague in Madagascar has been facilitated by the limited

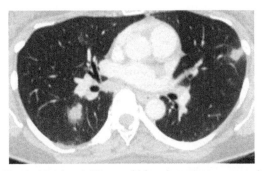

Fig. 1. Measles. A 39-year-old female patient presented with chest pain and fever for 4 days at the time of a local measles outbreak. Axial unenhanced CT image of the chest demonstrates nodular areas of consolidation with mild ground-glass opacities also present. (*Courtesy of Dr Gilberto Szarf.*)

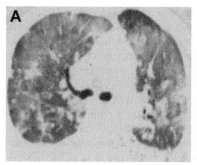 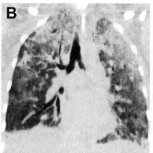 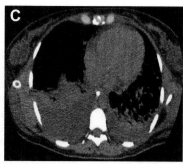

Fig. 2. Dengue hemorrhagic fever. A 40-year-old female patient presented with severe headache, myalgia, fever, worsening dyspnea, and nasal discharge for 1 week. Axial (*A*) unenhanced CT image of the chest shows diffuse areas of ground glass and consolidation with some areas of septal line thickening. Coronal (*B*) unenhanced CT image of the chest demonstrates extensive consolidation in the upper lungs with more patchy areas of ground glass in the lower lungs. Axial (*C*) unenhanced CT image of the chest shows bilateral pleural effusions with areas of consolidation and atelectasis.

public health system overtaxed by the concurrent COVID-19 pandemic as well as limited health care access in rural areas leading to delayed care; this results in particularly high mortality rates for bubonic plague of 40% to 70% versus 20.8% with treatment.[25] Primary pneumonic plague is less common but can be rapidly fatal, occurring through inhalation of infected respiratory secretions or droplets, making the potential for direct human-to-human transmission and spread to other populations a significant public health risk.[22,23,25] Symptoms include dyspnea, high fever, pleuritic chest pain, and cough sometimes with bloody sputum, whereas disseminated infection can cause meningitis and gastrointestinal involvement.[23] Secondary pneumonic plague is more common and develops due to hematogenous spread of infection.[22,23] Many symptoms of

pneumonic plague are similar to those found with COVID-19 infection, leading to misdiagnosis and an increased fatality rate of nearly 100% without appropriate treatment versus 60.5% with treatment.[25]

On imaging, lobar pneumonia, extensive consolidations, and alveolar infiltrates can rapidly progress to diffuse bilateral pneumonitis and findings compatible with ARDS (**Fig. 3**).[23] Pleural effusions and cavitation may occur.[23]

Leptospirosis

Leptospirosis is a spirochetal zoonosis transmitted to humans via contact of mucous membranes or skin abrasion with water or soil contaminated with urine from infected animals.[26,27] Fever, chills, headache, conjunctival hemorrhage, epistaxis, and myalgia occur in mild

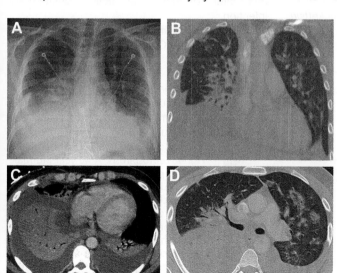

Fig. 3. *Y pestis* infection. A 32-year-old outdoorsman presented with fevers, chills, headache, severe myalgias, jaundice, and transaminitis after returning from a hunting trip. Chest radiograph (*A*) and contrast-enhanced coronal (*B*) and axial (*C, D*) chest CT images of *Y pestis* infection (plague) show pleural effusions and area of dense lobar consolidation in the right lower lobe with additional scattered ground-glass opacities and areas of consolidation.

disease, whereas severe disease can manifest as cough with hemoptysis, respiratory compromise, jaundice, and renal failure (known as Weil syndrome).[26–28] Pulmonary symptoms include chest pain, cough, and dyspnea as well as mild to severe hemoptysis in the setting of hemorrhagic pneumonitis and respiratory failure.[26,27] Severe pulmonary involvement may rapidly progress and cause massive pulmonary hemorrhage leading to respiratory insufficiency, ARDS, and death.[26,27]

Imaging findings may resemble viral pneumonia, bronchopneumonia, tuberculosis (TB), ARDS, or other causes of pulmonary hemorrhage.[26] Chest radiographs can initially be normal despite clinical symptoms.[26] Imaging may show ill-defined airspace nodules, bilateral consolidations, and ground-glass opacities as well as crazy-paving patterns with interlobular septal thickening with greater involvement in the peripheral, posterior, and lower lungs (**Fig. 4**).[26,28] Pleural and pericardial effusions may be present.[26,28]

Rickettsioses and other intracellular bacterial infections of sub-Saharan Africa

Rickettsial diseases are vector-borne zoonoses caused by obligate intracellular bacteria in the order Rickettsiales transmitted to humans by tick or flea bites, a number of which are endemic to sub-Saharan Africa.[29,30] Rickettsioses often present as nonspecific febrile illnesses that are difficult to distinguish from other common fever-causing etiologies.[31] Although not all rickettsioses cause pulmonary disease, a common feature is development of increased microvascular permeability causing cerebral and noncardiogenic pulmonary edema with severe cases leading to respiratory failure and death.[32]

On imaging, untreated infection with *Rickettsia typhi* is reported to cause hemorrhagic bronchopneumonia, lung abscess formation and ARDS with pleural effusions, diffuse opacities, pulmonary edema, and interstitial abnormalities.[33,34] Diffuse micronodular opacities, ground-glass opacities, interstitial infiltration and consolidation, as well as pleural effusions have been reported in infections with *Rickettsia felis* and *R typhi*.[34]

Q fever is caused by infection with *Coxiella burnetii*, also an intracellular bacterium only recently removed from the order Rickettsiales.[30,35] Goats, sheep, and cattle play important roles in the livestock economy in many regions of sub-Saharan Africa, but these ruminants are also the main reservoirs for *C burnetii* with infection. Data are limited; however, Q fever is estimated to account for 2% to 9% of hospitalizations due to febrile illness and 1% to 3% of infective endocarditis cases in Africa.[35]

On imaging, segmental, patchy, lobar, or multilobar opacities are most common as well as rounded opacities and pleural effusions.[36–38] Consolidations can appear masslike, and nonspecific nodules may be present along with lymphadenopathy.[37,38] A nodular pattern with a halo of ground-glass opacities is sometimes seen with a connecting vessel.[37,38] In immunocompromised patients, necrotizing pneumonia may occur.[37]

Mycobacterial

TB due to *Mycobacterium tuberculosis* plays a significant role in morbidity and mortality in sub-Saharan Africa where coinfection with HIV/AIDS is common and multidrug-resistant TB (MDR-TB) and extensively drug-resistant TB (XDR-TB) are prevalent.[39,40] Chest radiographs are often used for screening and diagnosis as well as monitoring response to treatment as an adjunct to microbiology tests and clinical assessment, particularly in the setting with limited laboratory culture and testing resources.[40] Infection can manifest as active infection as either primary or postprimary TB, or as an asymptomatic latent infection that can later develop into active postprimary infection.[39]

TB infection manifests a wide range of imaging presentations (see Ching Ching Ong and Lynette L.S. Teo's article, "Endemic Thoracic Infections in Southeast Asia," in this issue) in its role as an endemic infection in the sub-Saharan Africa region. Common features of active disease include often upper and midlung-predominant cavitary disease, tree-in-bud opacities, consolidation,

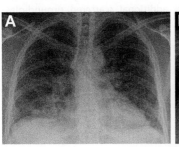
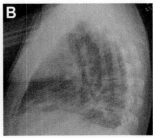

Fig. 4. Leptospirosis. A 40-year-old male traveler presented with persistent fevers for 5 days, headache, photophobia, body aches, nausea, abdominal pain, sore throat, and conjunctivitis. Posteroanterior (*A*) and lateral (*B*) chest radiograph show bilateral airspace opacities in the lower lungs with some areas of ill-defined nodularity. Airspace opacities become more confluent and consolidative in the lung base.

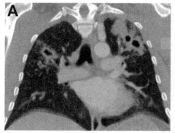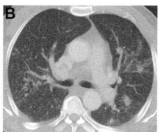

Fig. 5. Postprimary active tuberculosis. A 55-year-old male patient presented with chest pain and cough for 4 months with bloody sputum. Coronal (A) and axial (B) contrast-enhanced CT images of the chest show multiple areas of cavitation in the upper lungs in addition to areas of tree-in-bud opacities, larger nodules, and areas of nodular consolidation.

bronchiectasis, and bulky lymphadenopathy that can mimic malignancy, as well as miliary disease particularly in immunocompromised patients (**Figs. 5–7**).[39,41–43] Pleural effusions and empyemas can occur, as well as cardiac and chest wall involvement in addition to extrathoracic sites of disease.[39,42] Extent of lung involvement and cavities on chest radiography are associated with higher bacterial load in sputum, delayed clearance, and higher risk of treatment failure; lack of improvement on imaging with adherence to standard treatment regimens is concerning for MDR/XDR-TB.[40,44] Although data are limited regarding chest imaging and MDR/XDR-TB specifically, radiologic disease extent and cavities may be independent risk factors for poorer outcomes in these patients.[40,44] Similarly, CT chest imaging of patients with TB shows higher frequency of multiple cavities, nodules, and bronchiectasis in patients with MDR/XDR-TB compared with drug-sensitive TB.[43] Inactive TB in patients with significant prior infection is characterized by chronic fibronodular changes, including bronchiectasis, peribronchial fibrosis, architectural distortion, and scarring and nodular opacities in the apical and upper lungs.[39,42]

Fungal

Histoplasmosis

Pulmonary histoplasmosis is caused by infection with the fungal genus *Histoplasma*, most commonly *Histoplasma capsulatum*[45,46] (see Jeffrey P. Kanne's article, "North American Endemic Fungal Infections," in this issue). In Southern Africa, *H capsulatum* var. *capsulatum* comprises most of the cases, whereas in regions of Central and West Africa, *H capsulatum* var. *dubuosii* makes up most of the cases. Infection occurs via inhalation usually due to disturbance of soil containing the fungus or material contaminated with bird or bat guano harboring the fungus.[45–47] HIV/AIDS and the increasing use of immunosuppressive medications has led to a growing number of vulnerable individuals and increased incidence of histoplasmosis, particularly in Africa where HIV/AIDS prevalence is high.[46–48]

Pulmonary histoplasmosis presents with nonspecific symptoms and varied imaging, ranging from asymptomatic to severe disease depending on host factors, inoculum size, and virulence of the fungal strain with acute, subacute, and chronic forms.[46,47] Radiologic appearance can mimic TB, and misdiagnosis is a problem

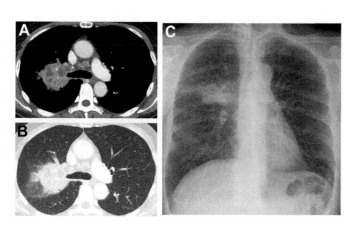

Fig. 6. Active TB. Axial (A, B) CT of the chest with contrast and frontal radiograph (C) of the chest shows a large right hilar mass in this 70-year-old female patient presenting with cough and fever for several weeks. CT images show enhancing areas with low-attenuation regions in keeping with necrosis; multiple necrotic lymph nodes were also demonstrated.

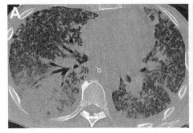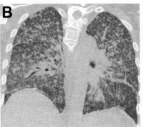

Fig. 7. Miliary TB. Axial (*A*) and coronal (*B*) unenhanced CT images of the chest in a 63-year-old patient with HIV/AIDS demonstrating extensive miliary TB with numerous small nodules throughout the lungs as well as areas of coalescing consolidation and small pleural effusions.

particularly in regions such as sub-Saharan Africa where TB prevalence is high and access to diagnostic facilities is limited.[48] Acute infection manifests as unilateral or bilateral nodules and/or diffuse bilateral patchy opacities with lymphadenopathy (**Fig. 8A**).[46,47] Miliary disease and ARDS may occur (**Fig. 8B**). Subacute disease often shows lymphadenopathy, whereas airspace disease tends to be less diffuse and more focal or patchy.[46,47] Imaging findings of chronic disease include calcified lymph nodes and nodules, upper lobe-predominant cavitation and fibrosis, broncholithiasis, and rarely fibrosing mediastinitis (see Jeffrey P. Kanne's article, "North American Endemic Fungal Infections," in this issue).[46,47]

Blastomycosis

Blastomycosis typically results from *Blastomyces dermatitidis* infection acquired by inhalation of spores aerosolized during activities causing disruption of soil[4,49,50] (see Jeffrey P. Kanne's article, "North American Endemic Fungal Infections," in this issue). *Blastomyces* species are endemic to sub-Saharan Africa as well as the United States, Canada, India, and the Middle East.[4,50,51] There is, however, debate whether disease caused by *Blastomyces* species in Africa and the Middle East are the same taxa as species in North America and whether they result in distinct clinicopathologic patterns.[4,50,51] In Africa and the Middle East, *Blastomyces percursus* and *Blastomyces emzantsi* predominate over *B dermatitidis*.[50] Cutaneous disease is most common, followed by pulmonary infection and then

osteoarticular disease.[50] Pulmonary infection may be asymptomatic or present with mild to severe symptoms ranging from chronic cough to ARDS.[51]

Image findings are variable including consolidation with air bronchograms, reticulonodular opacities, nodules, masses, interstitial abnormalities, cavitary lesions, and miliary disease (**Fig. 9**).[50,51.51] Airspace consolidations are the most frequent abnormality and tend to be more central compared with other fungal infections.[51,52] Multiple nodules and well-defined masses with irregular borders are common, mimicking lung malignancy.[51,52] Infection can also mimic community-acquired pneumonia, histoplasmosis, and TB clinically, but can rapidly progress to diffuse consolidations.[50,51] Rarely, fibrotic changes can occur, usually in the upper lungs with chronic disease.[51] Unlike histoplasmosis, lymphadenopathy, nodal calcification, chest wall invasion, and pleural effusions are less common but may occur.[51,53]

Cryptococcosis

Cryptococcus infection is endemic to sub-Saharan Africa, often affecting multiple organ systems with high morbidity and mortality, particularly with HIV/AIDS with meningitis often being the primary presentation.[54] *Cryptococcus neoformans* mainly infects immunosuppressed individuals, whereas *Cryptococcus gattii* typically infects immunocompetent individuals.[54] Infection occurs via inhalation of fungal particles from the environment, particularly soil contaminated with avian droppings or rotting wood.[55] Patients with

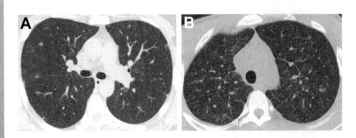

Fig. 8. Histoplasmosis. Axial (*A*) contrast-enhanced CT image of the chest shows multiple nodules in the lungs, some with hazy surrounding ground-glass opacity in a 36-year-old immunocompetent patient with histoplasmosis. Axial (*B*) noncontrast CT image shows disseminated histoplasmosis in a 32-year-old immunocompromised patient with HIV/AIDS with numerous small nodules in a miliary pattern.

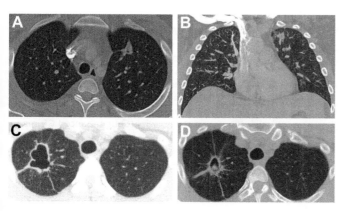

Fig. 9. Blastomycosis. Axial (*A*) and coronal (*B*) contrast-enhanced CT images of the chest show a solitary nodular consolidation in the left upper lobe due to blastomycosis in a 31-year-old patient with ulcerative colitis. Axial unenhanced CT images (*C, D*) of a different patient presenting with hemoptysis show a cavitary lesion due to blastomycosis (*C*) with subsequent decrease in the size of the cavity but interval development of a mycetoma (*D*).

pulmonary cryptococcal infection may be asymptomatic or have fever, dry cough, dyspnea, chest pain, or malaise.[54]

Risk factors such as lung disease and immunodeficiency impact clinical and imaging manifestations.[54] Typical imaging findings include single or multiple pulmonary nodules, consolidation, masses, nodular or reticular interstitial pattern, ground-glass opacities, lymphadenopathy, and pleural effusions (**Fig. 10**).[54,56,57] Solitary or multiple pulmonary nodules, consolidation, and masses are most common in immunocompetent individuals.[54,56,57] Nodules and masses can have surrounding ground-glass opacities.[56,57] Immunosuppressed individuals more often have pleural effusions, reticular or reticulonodular interstitial changes, cavitation, or miliary disease.[54,56,57]

Uncommon Endemic Fungal Infections

Although less common, mucormycosis and emergomycosis are important endemic and emerging fungal infections in sub-Saharan Africa. Pulmonary mucormycosis is an aggressive fungal infection that is frequently fatal with a mortality rate of approximately 45% and typically affects immunocompromised and diabetic patients, especially those with uncontrolled diabetes (see Godoy and colleagues' article, "Invasive Fungal Pneumonia in Immunocompromised Patients," in this issue).[52,58,59] Uncontrolled diabetes and HIV/AIDS infection are common in resource-poor regions such as sub-Saharan Africa and pose increased risk for mucormycosis.[59] Infection is usually by inhalation of fungi found in soil, animal excrement, and rotting food.[58]

On imaging, mucormycosis often presents with lobar or multifocal consolidations, nodules, or masslike opacities with relatively rapid progression compared with other entities (**Fig. 11**).[52,58] Surrounding ground-glass opacities resulting from hemorrhage may occur as well as central necrosis, cavitation, abscess formation, and in some instances, air crescent sign.[52,58] Lymphadenopathy and pleural effusions may also be present.[52,58] An endobronchial mass with bronchial occlusion is seen in airway involvement.[52,58] Invasion of the pulmonary artery with thrombosis and infarction can occur or development of pulmonary artery pseudoaneurysm, increasing the risk of fatal hemoptysis.[58] The heart, mediastinum, pleura, chest wall, and diaphragm can be involved with soft tissue gas worrisome for chest wall extension.[58]

Emergomycosis, although less common, is a globally emerging systemic fungal infection endemic to sub-Saharan Africa caused by novel *Emergomyces* species.[60] Emergomycosis is

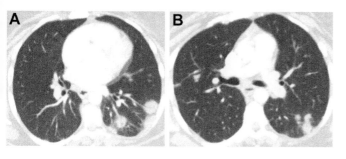

Fig. 10. Cryptococcosis. Axial unenhanced CT images of the chest (*A, B*) show multiple nodules and nodular consolidations in a 33-year-old patient with diabetes presenting with ~6 weeks of dry cough unimproved with antibiotic treatment. Some nodules demonstrate mild surrounding ground-glass opacity, for example, in the left lower lobe. Other nodular areas of consolidation in the right upper and left lower lobes have air bronchograms.

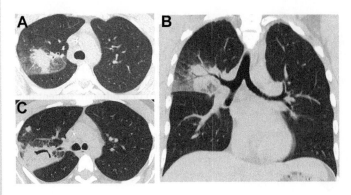

Fig. 11. Mucormycosis. Axial (*A*) and coronal (*B*) unenhanced CT images of the chest show dense consolidation with areas of surrounding ground-glass opacities in a 31-year-old neutropenic patient with acute myeloid leukemia. Air bronchograms are also seen to best advantage on the coronal images. On follow-up study, axial (*C*) unenhanced CT image shows interval cavitation within the area of consolidation with additional focal nodule.

typically seen in immunocompromised individuals, and the burden of disease is greatest in sub-Saharan Africa where HIV/AIDS prevalence is high.[60,61] Inhalation of fungi in soil is the primary route of infection leading to extrapulmonary dissemination.[60,61] Emergomycosis is a multisystem disease involving skin, lungs, spleen, liver, bone marrow, lymph nodes, gastrointestinal tract, and brain.[60]

Pulmonary disease is common with approximately 86% of patients having abnormal chest radiographs.[60,61] Emergomycosis imaging findings can mimic other fungal infections and manifests as areas of consolidation, diffuse and focal reticulonodular infiltrates, lobar atelectasis, pleural effusions, and lymphadenopathy.[60,61]

Parasitic Infections

Malaria
Malaria is a vector-borne parasitic disease transmitted by *Anopheles* mosquito bite and caused by 5 *Plasmodium* species—*Plasmodium falciparum*, *Plasmodium vivax*, *Plasmodium ovale*, *Plasmodium malariae*, and the primarily zoonotic monkey malaria, *Plasmodium knowlesi*[7,62,63] (see Restrepo and colleagues' article, "Endemic Thoracic Infections in Latin America and the Caribbean,"in this issue). Although found worldwide, the greatest burden of disease from malaria is in sub-Saharan Africa where most cases of *P falciparum* infections occur.[62,63] Fever, chills,

profuse sweating, anemia, leukopenia, and splenomegaly are the most common symptoms.[7,62–64] Pulmonary involvement manifests as dry cough and tachypnea and can result in ARDS.[7,62–64] Severe infection may also cause cerebral involvement, renal failure, shock, and spontaneous bleeding with disseminated intravascular coagulation.[65]

On imaging, features of severe pulmonary edema, pleural effusion, and areas of consolidation can be seen depending on severity of illness (**Fig. 12**).[7,64,65] Findings of ARDS are most commonly associated with *P falciparum* infection.[66] Constrictive bronchiolitis and bilateral patchy consolidations consistent with eosinophilic pneumonia have been described with pyrimethamine in the past.[64]

Amebiasis
Entamoeba histolytica infection (amebiasis) is endemic to sub-Saharan Africa and is a leading cause of morbidity and mortality due to a parasitic protozoan infection.[7,67–69] The limited data for sub-Saharan Africa shows amebiasis is widespread with approximately one-third of the population in Vhembe, South Africa, having reactive serology.[68,69] Infection is via fecal-oral transmission typically in settings where there is resource-limited sanitation and hygiene leading to contamination of food and water, but it can also be spread from person to person via sexual transmission.[7,64,66,68,69]

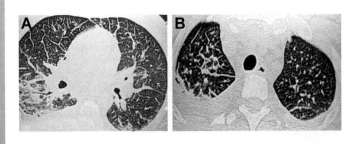

Fig. 12. Malaria. A 38-year-old patient presented with fever, headache, rhinorrhea, dyspnea, hematuria, and sore throat. Axial CT images (*A*, *B*) of the chest without contrast show extensive septal line thickening with several areas of ground-glass opacities and consolidations as well as bilateral pleural effusions consistent with pulmonary edema. This patient met criteria for ARDS.

Pleuropulmonary involvement is the second most common site of disease after liver abscess.[7,64,67] Direct extension of liver disease through the diaphragm can result in pleural, pericardial, and lung involvement including reactive pleural effusion, pneumonitis, empyema, and bronchopleural fistula; rupture into the pericardial space can also occur.[7,64,67]

On imaging, an elevated right hemidiaphragm often precedes evidence of pleural effusion, empyema, or consolidation (**Fig. 13**).[7,64] Consolidation and cavitation are common, and lung abscess can be seen with direct communication with an amebic liver abscess.[7,64] Mediastinal involvement and pericarditis can occur with pericardial effusion due to inflammatory reaction or drainage of liver abscess to the pericardium.[7,64]

Hydatid disease

Echinococcus granulosus infection (hydatid disease) is caused by the larval stage of the *Echinococcus* tapeworm with *E granulosus sensu lato* usually manifesting as cystic echinococcosis (see Restrepo and colleagues' article, "Endemic Thoracic Infections in Latin America and the Caribbean,"in this issue). Disease most commonly affects the liver and lungs, although nearly any organ can be involved.[70,71] Endemic disease is found in countries where raising sheep, cattle, and other pastural livestock with close contact with dogs is common, including regions of sub-Saharan Africa.[8,70,71] Members of the Canidae family are the definitive host, whereas sheep, cattle, or horses serve as intermediate hosts.[8,71] Humans are inadvertent intermediate hosts, infected from ingestion of contaminated water or food or via contact with infected animals.[70]

Uncomplicated infections may be asymptomatic for years; infection and compression of adjacent structures can cause symptoms such as chest pain, hemoptysis, coughing, and pneumothorax.[7,8,70] Symptoms related to hypersensitivity reaction, including fever, wheeze, urticaria, and rarely, anaphylaxis can occur if antigenic material from a cyst is released.[7,8] On imaging, uncomplicated hydatid disease presents as round, well-defined homogeneous opacities and may mimic loculated fluid or tumors (**Fig.14**).[70] Erosion of a bronchus can result in introduction of air into cysts leading to an air fluid level or crescentic lucency and suggests impending rupture.[70] Complicated hydatid cyst disease with rupture into the pleural space most commonly leads to pleural effusion or hydropneumothorax with or without floating membranes.[7,70] Invasion of the thoracic wall and pericardium can occur with extension of multiple daughter cysts; the vena cava or pulmonary arteries may be involved, leading to embolization.[70]

Schistosomiasis

Schistosomiasis (or bilharzia) is caused by *Schistosoma* species, with *Schistosoma mansoni* and *Schistosoma haematobium* most frequently causing disease in sub-Saharan Africa.[64,72–74] Schistosomiasis is the second most common cause of mortality due to parasitic infection after malaria and infection in sub-Saharan Africa accounting for 90% of cases.[64,73] Individuals become infected through skin exposure to water contaminated with cercariae excreted by snails with the disease generally endemic in low-income communities with limited access to clean water and adequate health care.[7,64,72,73] Although *S mansoni* and *S haematobium* typically cause intestinal and urogenital schistosomiasis respectively, pulmonary disease also occurs.[64,72–74]

Pulmonary disease is divided into early and late forms.[7,64,72,74] Early or acute disease symptoms include shortness of breath, wheezing, and cough as well as eosinophilia.[64,74] Fever, urticaria, arthralgia, hepatosplenomegaly, and hepatitis

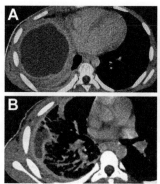
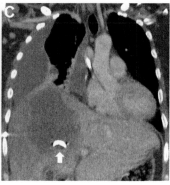

Fig. 13. Amebiasis. Axial (*A, B*) contrast-enhanced CT images of the chest show a rim enhancing abscess in the liver due to *Entamoeba* infection with direct extension into the right lung (*B*), resulting in an empyema with pleural thickening and enhancement in a male patient presenting with right upper quadrant and chest pain. Coronal (*C*) contrast-enhanced CT image of the chest of a different patient presenting with abdominal pain, nausea, vomiting, and bloody diarrhea shows elevation of the right diaphragm and large liver abscess with drain in place (*arrow*) as well as a large complex empyema.

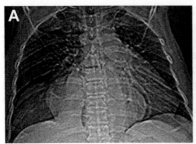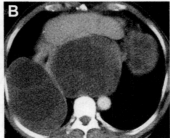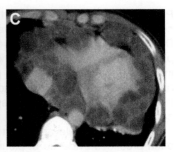

Fig. 14. Hydatid disease. Scout view (A) of a contrast-enhanced CT of the chest shows multiple round well-circumscribed masses in the chest in a 32-year-old-male patient. On axial (B) contrast-enhanced CT image of the chest in the same patient, these masses are found to be extensive hydatid disease with multiple smaller daughter cysts in the larger cysts. The cysts extend from the upper abdomen involving the liver and spleen as well as the lungs. Axial (C) contrast-enhanced CT image of the chest in a different patient shows extensive *Echinococcus* pericarditis due to extension from the liver with numerous hydatid cysts surrounding the heart.

may also occur.[7,64,74] In late or chronic pulmonary disease, deposited eggs in the pulmonary vasculature lead to intimal fibrosis, pulmonary hypertension, and right-sided heart failure; portal hypertension due to liver involvement often precedes chronic lung disease.[7,64,74]

Imaging findings in acute disease include small nodular lesions with ill-defined borders, reticulonodular pattern, bilateral areas of diffuse ground-glass opacities, and findings of eosinophilic pneumonia (Fig. 15).[7,64,72,74] Imaging findings of chronic disease include fibrosis, septal thickening, cardiomegaly, pulmonary arterial enlargement and evidence of pulmonary hypertension with right-sided heart failure.[7,64,74]

Ascariasis
Ascaris lumbricoides infection is endemic to sub-Saharan Africa and one of the most common parasitic infections found worldwide, infecting more than 1.3 billion individuals.[7,64] Infection is through fecal-oral transmission in settings where there is poor sanitation and hygiene.[7,8,64] During larval invasion of the lungs, a portion of patients will become symptomatic when an allergic reaction is triggered resulting in fever, cough, wheezing, expectoration of sputum, hemoptysis, chest pain, and eosinophilia.[7,8,64]

On imaging, migrating ground-glass and consolidative opacities are seen on CT and chest radiograph, typically clearing within 2 weeks, consistent with eosinophilic pneumonia or Löffler syndrome.[7,8,64] Pulmonary nodules may be present.[7,8,64] Chronic eosinophilic pneumonia has also been described.[8] Alveolar hemorrhage, lobar consolidation, pleural effusions, and rarely, pneumothorax can occur (Fig. 16).[7,8,64]

Strongyloidiasis
Strongyloides stercoralis is a parasitic nematode endemic to sub-Saharan as well as South America and South East Asia causing more than 30 million infections globally.[7,75] Infection primarily occurs via the skin through contact with soil contaminated with larvae.[64,75] *Strongyloides* infection can be lifelong given the ability to reinfect the host through the gastrointestinal tract (autoinfection).[75] Chronic autoinfection can result in life-threatening massive

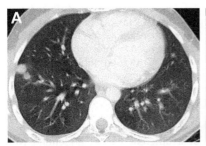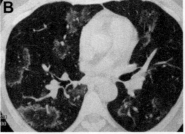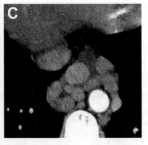

Fig. 15. Schistosomiasis. Axial (A) contrast-enhanced CT image of the chest shows multiple nodules with mild surrounding ground-glass opacity in a 20-year-old man presenting with seizure. Axial (B) unenhanced CT image of the chest in a different patient demonstrates multiple atoll signs with areas of ground-glass opacities with more dense opacities peripherally and relative central clearing. Axial (C) enhanced CT image of the chest of another patient demonstrates extensive varices due to sequalae of chronic schistosomiasis infection.

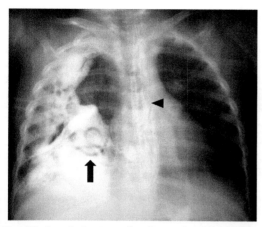

Fig. 16. Ascariasis. Frontal radiograph of a pediatric patient shows a large complex pleural effusion with serpiginous linear filling defects in the pleural fluid and pleural space (*arrow*) as well as linear lucencies in the esophagus (*arrowhead*), which reflect *A lumbricoides*. This is a striking but atypical presentation of ascariasis disease.

infestation, leading to hyperinfection syndrome, particularly in immunocompromised patients.[7,75] During acute infection, a characteristic cutaneous reaction may be seen due to larvae penetrating the skin and causing urticaria.[7,75] Larvae can also migrate intradermally during chronic infection, resulting in intensely itchy red tracts.[75] Peripheral blood eosinophilia and eosinophilic pneumonia, bronchospasm, bronchitis, and abdominal pain or diarrhea can occur.[64]

Imaging findings are similar to ascariasis with migratory, patchy areas of ground-glass opacities and consolidation indicating eosinophilic pneumonia, usually resolving in 2 weeks.[7,64] Severe pneumonia, diffuse alveolar hemorrhage, septal line thickening, pleura effusions, and ARDS can develop in individuals with hyperinfection syndrome, and rarely, a miliary pattern can occur (Fig. 17).[7,64]

Cysticercosis

Cysticercosis from *Taenia solium* infection results from ingesting eggs in contaminated food or water and is most prevalent in resource-poor regions of Africa, South America, Mexico, and Asia.[7,65,76] Infection is usually asymptomatic until degeneration of cysticerci begin and they are no longer able to evade the immune system.[7] Although epileptic seizures due to neurocysticercosis are the most common presentation, cardiopulmonary involvement can occur with disseminated cysticercosis and has been found in 20% to 25% of patients with neurocysticercosis.[7,65,76]

Imaging features of pulmonary cysticercosis include multiple random pulmonary nodules (which may calcify), pleural effusions, and cysticerci in the musculature, including the heart (Fig. 18).[7,76] Nodules are typically well-defined and most often found in skeletal muscles and the central nervous system but can be seen in any body part.[7,76] Nodules initially appear hypoattenuating with a central high-attenuation focus on CT, representing the parasite head, but may calcify and appear as a "rice-grain" or "cigar-shaped" calcification in soft tissues or calcified nodules in the lungs.[7,76]

Less common endemic parasitic diseases

Toxoplasmosis, toxocariasis, and paragonimiasis are less common endemic parasitic infections that can cause pulmonary disease. Pulmonary toxocariasis or larva migrans is caused by infection with the intestinal parasite *Toxocara canis* (canine) or *Toxocara cati* (feline) through ingestion of eggs that hatch in the intestine.[7,66] Endemic to sub-Saharan Africa as well as many other regions, toxocariasis occurs more frequently in settings with close contact with host animals and contaminated soil. Pulmonary involvement is found in 80% of infected individuals, and common presenting respiratory symptoms include severe asthma, cough, wheezing, and bronchiolitis.[7,66] On imaging, findings of eosinophilic pneumonia may be

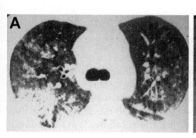
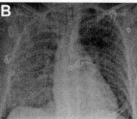

Fig. 17. Strongyloidiasis. Axial (*A*) unenhanced CT of the chest of shows patchy areas of ground-glass opacity and consolidation in the lungs in a 42-year-old patient with hyperinfection syndrome in the setting of AIDS and extensive infection. Frontal chest radiograph (*B*) shows a different patient also with hyperinfection syndrome with extensive opacities, septal thickening, and nodularity in the lungs consistent with pneumonitis and hemorrhage due to *Strongyloides* infection, leading to ARDS.

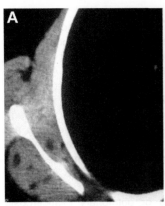
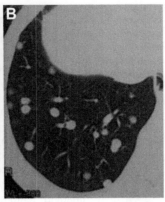

Fig. 18. Cysticercosis. A 49-year-old male patient had dyspnea, seizures, and an abnormality see on initial chest radiograph. Axial (*A*) unenhanced CT image of the chest shows low-attenuation nodules in the skeletal muscle of the chest wall and shoulder, which can calcify, creating "rice-grain" calcifications. Axial (*B*) unenhanced CT image of the chest shows multiple pulmonary nodules.

present with ill-defined ground-glass and consolidative opacities; bilateral involvement is common with the lower lobes and subpleural regions most affected.[7,66] Multiple solid pulmonary nodules and, less often, focal linear opacities can also be seen (**Fig. 19**).[7]

Infection with *Toxoplasma gondii*, a parasite primarily carried by cats, is usually acquired through ingestion of eggs from contaminated cat feces and improperly cooked meat from intermediate hosts.[7,66] Nearly a third of the world's population is infected with *T gondii*, predominantly in developing countries, including many in sub-Saharan Africa.[7] Pulmonary involvement is more common in immunocompromised individuals and is seen with increasing frequency with HIV/AIDS.[7,66] Patients may experience influenza-like illness, fever, myalgia, dyspnea, or lymphadenopathy, whereas neurologic symptoms are more common in immunosuppressed patients with parasite reactivation.[7,66] Imaging findings include nodules and

nodular opacities, ground-glass opacities, and interstitial thickening, as well as pleural effusions and pneumothorax, although less common (**Fig. 20**).[7] Interstitial or lobar pneumonia, diffuse alveolar damage, necrotizing pneumonia, and lymphadenopathy are also seen.[7,66]

Paragonimiasis results from infection with *Paragonimus* species mainly through ingestion of raw or partially cooked freshwater crustaceans.[7,64,77] Endemic areas exist in Asia, Central and South America, as well as Africa with *Paragonimus uterobilateralis*, *Paragonimus africanus*, *Paragonimus gondwanensis*, and *Paragonimus kerberti* found in Africa.[7,64,77] Most documented cases occur in rainforest zones of Central and West Africa with other sporadic areas; however, prevalence in sub-

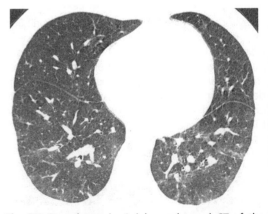

Fig. 19. Toxocariasis. A 14-year-old patient presented with fever, cough tachypnea, and weight loss with no improvement after treatment with antibiotics. Axial unenhanced CT image of the chest shows numerous small nodules and nodular consolidation.

Fig. 20. Toxoplasmosis. Axial unenhanced CT of the chest shows septal thickening, ground-glass opacities, and areas of early consolidation in an immunosuppressed patient presenting with cough, fever, and dyspnea. More severe infections can result in more dense confluent areas of consolidation and ground-glass opacities, which is more commonly seen in immunosuppressed individuals. (*Courtesy of* Dr Dante Escuissato.)

Table 1
Overview of imaging and clinical characteristics of pulmonary infections endemic to sub-Saharan Africa

	Thoracic Imaging Features	Clinical Characteristics	Ref.
Emerging viral			
Measles	• Consolidation • Ground-glass opacity • Reticulonodular & micronodular opacities • Interlobular septal thickening • Pleural effusions	Fever, cough, maculopapular skin rash, coryza, conjunctivitis; may lead to pneumonia, gastroenteritis, severe desquamation, blindness, encephalitis, subacute sclerosing panencephalitis, death	9–12
Dengue fever	• Ground-glass opacities & consolidations • Bronchiolitis • Pleural & pericardial effusions • Noncardiogenic pulmonary edema • Pulmonary hemorrhage	Severe disease causes dengue hemorrhagic fever, dengue shock syndrome, ARDS, death	13–16
Ebola	• Imaging data are limited	Cough, chest pain, shortness of breath, progressive severe coagulopathy, visceral hemorrhage, shock, death	17–21
Emerging bacterial			
Plague (*Y pestis*)	• Lobar pneumonia or alveolar infiltrates • Rapidly progress to diffuse bilateral pneumonitis • Cavitation also seen	Dyspnea, high fever, pleuritic chest pain, cough, hemoptysis, ARDS; primary pneumonic plague can be rapidly fatal but secondary form is more common	22–25
Leptospirosis	• Bilateral consolidations & ground-glass opacities • Interlobular septal thickening, crazy-paving patterns • Nodules • Greater involvement in peripheral, posterior, & lower lungs	Fever, chills, headache, conjunctival hemorrhage, epistaxis, myalgia; can progress to cough with massive hemoptysis, ARDS, jaundice, renal failure	26–28
Rickettsioses (*R typhi*)	• Hemorrhagic bronchopneumonia • Lung abscess • Diffuse micronodular & ground-glass opacities • Consolidation • Pleural effusions	Nonspecific fever, cerebral and noncardiogenic pulmonary edema; severe cases leading to ARDS, death	29–34
Q fever (*C. burnetti*)	• Multilobar, segmental, or patchy consolidations	Fever, rigors, myalgia, cough; can be complicated by pneumonia, endocarditis,	5,30,36–38,78

(continued on next page)

Table 1
(continued)

	Thoracic Imaging Features	Clinical Characteristics	Ref.
	• Nodules • Pulmonary edema • Pleural effusions • Endocarditis & aortitis	myocarditis, hepatitis, and meningoencephalitis	
Mycobacterial			
Tuberculosis	Active disease: • Upper & midlung cavitary disease • Tree-in-bud opacities & consolidation • Bulky lymphadenopathy can mimic malignancy • Miliary disease in immunosuppressed Chronic disease & complications: • Empyema • Cardiac & chest wall involvement • Chronic fibronodular changes (bronchiectasis, peribronchial fibrosis, architectural distortion)	Asymptomatic active and latent infections occur. Symptomatic active disease can present with fever, night sweats, cough with bloody sputum, weight loss, and fatigue	39–44
Fungal			
Histoplasmosis	Acute disease: • Unilateral or bilateral nodules • Bilateral patchy opacities • Lymphadenopathy • Miliary disease can occur Subacute disease: • Lymphadenopathy • Focal or patchy airspace opacities Chronic disease & complications: • Calcified lymph nodes • Broncholiths • Cavitation and fibrosis • Fibrosing mediastinitis	Nonspecific clinical signs and symptoms; acute, subacute and chronic forms of disease and can be asymptomatic	4,45–48
Blastomycosis	• Consolidation • Nodules & masses often central • Cavitation • Miliary disease • Lymphadenopathy & nodal calcification less common	Mild disease presents with cough, whereas severe disease may lead to ARDS; can be asymptomatic	4,49–53
Cryptococcosis	• Single or multiple pulmonary nodules or masses • Solitary nodules (immunocompetent)	Meningitis. Fever, dry cough, dyspnea, chest pain, malaise; immunocompromised at greatest risk of severe infection	54–57,79

	Imaging findings	Clinical	References
	• Miliary disease (immunocompromised) • Consolidation & surrounding ground-glass opacities • Lymphadenopathy • Pleural effusions		
Mucormycosis	• Lobar or multifocal consolidations • Nodules or masslike opacities • Rapid progression • Cavitation • Pulmonary artery thrombosis • Lymphadenopathy • Pleural effusions	Less common infection but aggressive and frequently fatal; affects patients with uncontrolled diabetes or immunosuppression	52,58,59
Emergomycosis	• Consolidation • Diffuse & focal reticulonodular infiltrates • Lobar atelectasis • Pleural effusions • Lymphadenopathy	Multisystem disease involving skin, lungs, spleen, liver, bone marrow, lymph nodes, gastrointestinal tract, brain; more often in immunocompromised individuals	60,61
Parasitic			
Malaria	• Severe pulmonary edema • Pleural effusions • Consolidations	Fever, chills, profuse sweating, anemia, leukopenia, splenomegaly, dry cough; can lead to cerebral edema, renal failure, shock, disseminated intravascular coagulation, ARDS	7,62–66
Amebiasis	• Elevated right hemidiaphragm • Consolidation • Pleural effusion • Empyema, lung abscess, cavitation with direct communication from liver abscess	Cough, dyspnea, chest pain	7,64,67–69
Hydatid disease (*E granulosus*)	Uncomplicated disease: • Round, well-defined opacities mimic loculated fluid or tumor Complicated disease: • Extension into pleural space • Pleural effusion • Hydropneumothorax	Chest pain, hemoptysis, coughing, pneumothorax; hypersensitivity reaction, including fever, wheeze, urticaria, anaphylaxis (rare)	7,8,70,71

(continued on next page)

Table 1
(continued)

	Thoracic Imaging Features	Clinical Characteristics	Ref.
	• Invasion of thoracic wall, pericardium, other structures		
Schistosomiasis	• Small ill-defined nodular lesions • Bilateral diffuse ground-glass opacities • Fibrosis • Eosinophilic pneumonia • Pulmonary hypertension	Shortness of breath, wheezing, cough, eosinophilia, fever, urticaria, arthralgia, hepatosplenomegaly, hepatitis; chronic sequelae of intimal fibrosis, pulmonary hypertension, right sided heart failure	7,64,72–75
Ascariasis	• Migrating ground-glass & consolidative opacities • Pulmonary nodules • Lobar consolidation • Alveolar hemorrhage • Pneumothorax	Symptomatic allergic reaction triggered by larval invasion of lungs resulting in fever, cough, wheezing, expectoration, hemoptysis, chest pain, eosinophilia	7,8,64
Strongyloidiasis	• Migrating ground-glass and consolidative opacities • Septal line • Severe pneumonia and ARDS with hyperinfection syndrome • Miliary pattern (rare)	Characteristic acute cutaneous reaction due to larvae penetrating the skin, causing urticaria; eosinophilia, bronchospasm, bronchitis, abdominal pain, diarrhea	7,8,64,75
Cysticercosis	• Multiple pulmonary nodules • Pleural effusion • Cysticerci in thoracic musculature & myocardium; may calcify ("rice-grain" or "cigar-shaped")	Usually asymptomatic until degeneration of cysticerci with epileptic seizures the most common presentation; pulmonary involvement with disseminated disease	7,65,76
Toxocariasis	• Bilateral ground-glass & consolidative opacities • Lower lobes & subpleural predominance • Nodules • Linear opacities	Severe asthma, cough, wheezing, bronchiolitis, cough, fever, hepatosplenomegaly, lymphadenopathy, abdominal pain, vision, and neurologic issues	7,66
Toxoplasmosis	• Lobar pneumonia • Septal thickening • Nodules and nodular opacities • Lymphadenopathy • Pleural effusions & pneumothorax, less common	Influenzalike illness, myalgia, dyspnea, lymphadenopathy; neurologic symptoms more common in immunocompromised patients	7,66
Paragonimiasis	• Pneumothorax • Pleural effusion or empyema • Patchy consolidation (early) • Cavitation • Nodules (late) • Fluid-filled cysts (late) • Linear opacities from worm migration	Chronic cough, expectoration, hemoptysis, chest pain, fever, malaise	7,64,77

Saharan Africa is likely underestimated due to misdiagnosis as TB and underreporting in resource-poor areas.[77] Pulmonary infection is the primary manifestation of disease and symptoms include chronic cough, hemoptysis, chest pain, and fever.[7,64]

Imaging findings depend on stage of disease and endemic region.[7] When juvenile worms migrate through the diaphragm into the pleural space, this can cause pneumothorax, pleural effusion, or empyema.[7,64] When reaching the lung, infection can produce patchy consolidation due to exudative or hemorrhagic pneumonia and cavitation may occur, which can make distinguishing paragonimiasis from TB challenging in endemic regions.[7,64,77] Low-attenuation fluid-filled cysts can be seen with surrounding consolidation and linear opacities that may reflect worm migration or atelectasis.[7,64] Solitary or multiple nodules can be found reflecting worm cysts; gas-filled cysts suggest communication with the airway.[64]

SUMMARY

A wide range of pulmonary infections are endemic to sub-Saharan Africa, including emerging or reemerging viral and bacterial infections as well as parasitic and fungal infections. This article highlights key imaging and clinical features of disease (Table 1). Ongoing climate change and environmental factors facilitate changes to geographic distribution while increased global commerce and travel increase the likelihood that these endemic diseases will be seen beyond their usual borders. Familiarity with these entities is important for timely diagnosis and treatment to improve patient outcomes.

DISCLOSURE

C. E. Rydzak and A. S. Lima: No disclosures. G.S.P. Meirelles Chief Medical Officer at Alliar Group, Partner at Ambra Saude, Datalife.ai and Bright Photomedicine, President at I2A2, Speaker and member of the advisory board of Boehringer-Ingelheim.

REFERENCES

1. Collaborators GBDLRI. Estimates of the global, regional, and national morbidity, mortality, and aetiologies of lower respiratory infections in 195 countries, 1990-2016: a systematic analysis for the Global Burden of Disease Study 2016. Lancet Infect Dis 2018;18(11):1191–210.
2. Dwyer-Lindgren L, Cork MA, Sligar A, et al. Mapping HIV prevalence in sub-Saharan Africa between 2000 and 2017. Nature 2019;570(7760):189–93.
3. Kharsany AB, Karim QA. HIV infection and AIDS in Sub-Saharan Africa: current status, challenges and opportunities. Open AIDS J 2016;10:34–48.
4. Ashraf N, Kubat RC, Poplin V, et al. Re-drawing the maps for Endemic Mycoses. Mycopathologia 2020; 185(5):843–65.
5. Carugati M, Kilonzo KG, Crump JA. Fever, bacterial zoonoses, and one health in sub-Saharan Africa. Clin Med (Lond) 2019;19(5):375–80.
6. Fenollar F, Mediannikov O. Emerging infectious diseases in Africa in the 21st century. New Microbes New Infect 2018;26:S10–8.
7. Fiorentini LF, Bergo P, Meirelles GSP, et al. Pictorial review of thoracic parasitic diseases: a radiologic guide. Chest 2020;157(5):1100–13.
8. Kunst H, Mack D, Kon OM, et al. Parasitic infections of the lung: a guide for the respiratory physician. Thorax 2011;66(6):528–36.
9. Rota PA, Moss WJ, Takeda M, et al. Measles. Nat Rev Dis Primers 2016;2:16049.
10. Koo HJ, Lim S, Choe J, et al. Radiographic and CT features of viral pneumonia. Radiographics 2018; 38(3):719–39.
11. Rafat C, Klouche K, Ricard JD, et al. Severe measles infection: the spectrum of disease in 36 critically Ill adult patients. Medicine (Baltimore) 2013;92(5): 257–72.
12. Kim EA, Lee KS, Primack SL, et al. Viral pneumonias in adults: radiologic and pathologic findings. Radiographics 2002;22:S137–49.
13. Messina JP, Brady OJ, Golding N, et al. The current and future global distribution and population at risk of dengue. Nat Microbiol 2019;4(9):1508–15.
14. Kumar N, Gadpayle AK, Trisal D. Atypical respiratory complications of dengue fever. Asian Pac J Trop Med 2013;6(10):839–40.
15. Hu T, Liu J, Guan W, et al. CT findings of severe dengue fever in the chest and abdomen. Radiol Infect Dis 2015;2:77–80.
16. Rangari AP, Jayakumar M, Rodriguez MJ. Thoracic computed tomography imaging in dengue fever: a tertiary experience in south indian population. Int J Contemp Med Res 2018;5(6):F4–6.
17. Abi-Jaoudeh N, Walser EM, Bartal G, et al. Ebola and other highly contagious diseases: strategies by the society of interventional radiology for interventional radiology. J Vasc Interv Radiol 2016; 27(2):200–2.
18. Feldmann H, Geisbert TW. Ebola haemorrhagic fever. Lancet 2011;377(9768):849–62.
19. Bluemke DA, Meltzer CC. Ebola virus disease: radiology preparedness. Radiology 2015;274(2): 527–31.
20. Mollura DJ, Palmore TN, Folio LR, et al. Radiology preparedness in ebola virus disease: guidelines and challenges for disinfection of medical imaging

equipment for the protection of staff and patients. Radiology 2015;275(2):538–44.

21. Jardon M, Mohammad SF, Jude CM, et al. Imaging of emerging infectious diseases. Curr Radiol Rep 2019;7(9):25.

22. Prentice MB, Rahalison L. Plague. Lancet 2007; 369(9568):1196–207.

23. Daya M, Nakamura Y. Pulmonary disease from biological agents: anthrax, plague, Q fever, and tularemia. Crit Care Clin 2005;21(4):747–63, vii.

24. Leulmi H, Socolovschi C, Laudisoit A, et al. Detection of Rickettsia felis, Rickettsia typhi, Bartonella Species and Yersinia pestis in Fleas (Siphonaptera) from Africa. PLoS Negl Trop Dis 2014;8(10):e3152.

25. Aborode AT, Dos Santos Costa AC, Mohan A, et al. Epidemic of plague amidst COVID-19 in Madagascar: efforts, challenges, and recommendations. Trop Med Health 2021;49(1):56.

26. Marchiori E, Lourenco S, Setubal S, et al. Clinical and imaging manifestations of hemorrhagic pulmonary leptospirosis: a state-of-the-art review. Lung 2011;189(1):1–9.

27. Gulati S, Gulati A. Pulmonary manifestations of leptospirosis. Lung India 2012;29(4):347–53.

28. Shastri M, Diwanji N, Desai E, et al. Spectrum of radiological findings in leptospirosis on chest radiograph and ultrasonography-study during epidemics in south gujarat region of India. Int J Anat Radiol Surg 2017;6(4):RO07–12.

29. Parola P, Paddock CD, Socolovschi C, et al. Update on tick-borne rickettsioses around the world: a geographic approach. Clin Microbiol Rev 2013; 26(4):657–702.

30. Parola P. Rickettsioses in sub-Saharan Africa. Ann N Y Acad Sci 2006;1078:42–7.

31. Prabhu M, Nicholson WL, Roche AJ, et al. Q fever, spotted fever group, and typhus group rickettsioses among hospitalized febrile patients in northern Tanzania. Clin Infect Dis 2011;53(4):e8–15.

32. Olano JP. Rickettsial infections. Ann N Y Acad Sci 2005;1063:187–96.

33. Doppler JF, Newton PN. A systematic review of the untreated mortality of murine typhus. PLoS Negl Trop Dis 2020;14(9):e0008641.

34. van der Vaart TW, van Thiel PP, Juffermans NP, et al. Severe murine typhus with pulmonary system involvement. Emerg Infect Dis 2014;20(8):1375–7.

35. Vanderburg S, Rubach MP, Halliday JE, et al. Epidemiology of Coxiella burnetii infection in Africa: a one-health systematic review. PLoS Negl Trop Dis 2014; 8(4):e2787.

36. Hartzell J, AL E. Coxiella burnetii infection. BMJ Best Pract 2020;. http://newbp.bmj.com/topics/en-us/1139/pdf/1139/Coxiella%20burnetii%20infection.pdf.

37. Voloudaki AE, Kofteridis DP, Tritou IN, et al. Q fever pneumonia: CT findings. Radiology 2000;215(3): 880–3.

38. Kelm DJ, White DB, Fadel HJ, et al. Pulmonary manifestations of Q fever: analysis of 38 patients. J Thorac Dis 2017;9(10):3973–8.

39. Nachiappan AC, Rahbar K, Shi X, et al. Pulmonary tuberculosis: role of radiology in diagnosis and management. Radiographics 2017;37(1):52–72.

40. Te Riele JB, Buser V, Calligaro G, et al. Relationship between chest radiographic characteristics, sputum bacterial load, and treatment outcomes in patients with extensively drug-resistant tuberculosis. Int J Infect Dis 2019;79:65–71.

41. Jeong YJ, Lee KS. Pulmonary tuberculosis: up-to-date imaging and management. AJR Am J Roentgenol 2008;191(3):834–44. https://doi.org/10.2214/AJR.07.3896.

42. Harisinghani MG, McLoud TC, Shepard JA, et al. Tuberculosis from head to toe. Radiographics 2000;20(2):449–70. quiz 528-9, 532.

43. Cha J, Lee HY, Lee KS, et al. Radiological findings of extensively drug-resistant pulmonary tuberculosis in non-AIDS adults: comparisons with findings of multidrug-resistant and drug-sensitive tuberculosis. Korean J Radiol 2009;10(3):207–16.

44. Manikkam S, Archary M, Bobat R. Chest X-ray patterns of pulmonary multidrug-resistant tuberculosis in children in a high HIV-prevalence setting. South Afr J Radiol 2016;20(1):6–829.

45. Linder KA, Kauffman CA. Current and new perspectives in the diagnosis of blastomycosis and histoplasmosis. J Fungi (Basel) 2020;7(1). https://doi.org/10.3390/jof7010012.

46. Di Mango AL, Zanetti G, Penha D, et al. Endemic pulmonary fungal diseases in immunocompetent patients: an emphasis on thoracic imaging. Expert Rev Respir Med 2019;13(3):263–77.

47. Wheat LJ, Azar MM, Bahr NC, et al. Histoplasmosis. Infect Dis Clin North Am 2016;30(1):207–27.

48. Oladele RO, Ayanlowo OO, Richardson MD, et al. Histoplasmosis in Africa: an emerging or a neglected disease? PLoS Negl Trop Dis 2018;12(1):e0006046.

49. Castillo CG, Kauffman CA, Miceli MH. Blastomycosis. Infect Dis Clin North Am 2016;30(1):247–64.

50. Schwartz IS, Munoz JF, Kenyon CR, et al. Blastomycosis in Africa and the middle east: a comprehensive review of reported cases and reanalysis of historical isolates based on molecular data. Clin Infect Dis 2020;73(7):e1560–9.

51. Fang W, Washington L, Kumar N. Imaging manifestations of blastomycosis: a pulmonary infection with potential dissemination. Radiographics 2007;27(3): 641–55. https://doi.org/10.1148/rg.273065122.

52. Orlowski HLP, McWilliams S, Mellnick VM, et al. Imaging Spectrum of invasive fungal and fungal-like infections. Radiographics 2017;37(4):1119–34.

53. Ronald S, Strzelczyk J, Moore S, et al. Computed tomographic scan evaluation of pulmonary

blastomycosis. Winter. Can J Infect Dis Med Microbiol 2009;20(4):112–6.

54. Skolnik K, Huston S, Mody CH. Cryptococcal lung infections. Clin Chest Med 2017;38(3):451–64.

55. Maziarz EK, Perfect JR. Cryptococcosis. Infect Dis Clin North Am 2016;30(1):179–206.

56. Liu K, Ding H, Xu B, et al. Clinical analysis of non-AIDS patients pathologically diagnosed with pulmonary cryptococcosis. J Thorac Dis 2016;8(10):2813–21.

57. Xie LX, Chen YS, Liu SY, et al. Pulmonary cryptococcosis: comparison of CT findings in immunocompetent and immunocompromised patients. Acta Radiol 2015;56(4):447–53.

58. Agrawal R, Yeldandi A, Savas H, et al. Pulmonary mucormycosis: risk factors, radiologic findings, and pathologic correlation. Radiographics 2020; 40(3):656–66.

59. Stemler J, Hamed K, Salmanton-Garcia J, et al. Mucormycosis in the middle east and north africa: analysis of the FungiScope((R)) registry and cases from the literature. Mycoses 2020;63(10):1060–8.

60. Samaddar A, Sharma A. Emergomycosis, an emerging systemic mycosis in immunocompromised patients: current trends and future prospects. Front Med (Lausanne) 2021;8:670731.

61. Schwartz IS, Govender NP, Sigler L, et al. Emergomyces: the global rise of new dimorphic fungal pathogens. PLoS Pathog 2019;15(9):e1007977.

62. Taylor WRJ, Hanson J, Turner GDH, et al. Respiratory manifestations of malaria. Chest 2012;142(2):492–505.

63. Ashley EA, Pyae Phyo A, Woodrow CJ. Malaria. Lancet 2018;391(10130):1608–21.

64. Martinez S, Restrepo CS, Carrillo JA, et al. Thoracic manifestations of tropical parasitic infections: a pictorial review. Radiographics 2005;25(1):135–55.

65. Restrepo CS, Raut AA, Riascos R, et al. Imaging manifestations of tropical parasitic infections. Semin Roentgenol 2007;42(1):37–48.

66. Cheepsattayakorn A, Cheepsattayakorn R. Parasitic pneumonia and lung involvement. Biomed Res Int 2014;2014:874021.

67. Lal C, Huggins JT, Sahn SA. Parasitic diseases of the pleura. Am J Med Sci 2013;345(5):385–9.

68. Shirley DT, Farr L, Watanabe K, et al. A Review of the global burden, new diagnostics, and current therapeutics for amebiasis. Open Forum Infect Dis 2018;5(7):ofy161.

69. Shirley DT, Watanabe K, Moonah S. Significance of amebiasis: 10 reasons why neglecting amebiasis might come back to bite us in the gut. PLoS Negl Trop Dis 2019;13(11):e0007744.

70. Garg MK, Sharma M, Gulati A, et al. Imaging in pulmonary hydatid cysts. World J Radiol 2016;8(6): 581–7.

71. Alvarez Rojas CA, Romig T, Lightowlers MW. Echinococcus granulosus sensu lato genotypes infecting humans–review of current knowledge. Int J Parasitol 2014;44(1):9–18.

72. Gobbi F, Buonfrate D, Angheben A, et al. Pulmonary nodules in African migrants caused by chronic schistosomiasis. Lancet Infect Dis 2017;17(5): e159–65.

73. Aula OP, McManus DP, Jones MK, et al. Schistosomiasis with a focus on Africa. Trop Med Infect Dis 2021; 6(3). https://doi.org/10.3390/tropicalmed6030109.

74. Niemann T, Marti H, Duhnsen S, et al. Pulmonary schistosomiasis - imaging features. J Radiol Case Rep 2010;4(9):37–43.

75. Greaves D, Coggle S, Pollard C, et al. Strongyloides stercoralis infection. BMJ 2013;347:f4610.

76. Lyimo FR, Jusabani AM, Makungu H, et al. Thinking outside malaria: a rare case of disseminated cysticercosis with cardiopulmonary involvement from urban tanzania. Cureus 2021;13(1):e12851.

77. Rabone M, Wiethase J, Clark PF, et al. Endemicity of Paragonimus and paragonimiasis in Sub-Saharan Africa: a systematic review and mapping reveals stability of transmission in endemic foci for a multi-host parasite system. PLoS Negl Trop Dis 2021; 15(2):e0009120.

78. Akgoz A, Mukundan S, Lee TC. Imaging of rickettsial, spirochetal, and parasitic infections. Neuroimaging Clin N Am 2012;22(4):633–57.

79. Lindell RM, Hartman TE, Nadrous HF, et al. Pulmonary cryptococcosis: CT findings in immunocompetent patients. Radiology 2005;236(1):326–31.

Thoracic Infections in Solid Organ Transplants
Radiological Features and Approach to Diagnosis

Michelle Hershman, MD[1], Scott Simpson, DO[1],*

KEYWORDS

- Solid organ transplantation • Lung transplantation • Immunocompromised • Opportunistic infection
- Fungal infection • CMV • Aspergillus • Posttransplant lymphoproliferative disorder

KEY POINTS

- If pulmonary infection is suspected clinically, and a lobar or multifocal pattern of consolidation is present, bacterial and some community-acquired respiratory viruses (CARV) infections should be considered most likely. Failure to respond to antibiotic therapy may indicate a resistant organism, a nonbacterial infection, or a noninfectious pattern of lung injury related to allograft dysfunction or drug toxicity.
- Isolated ground-glass opacity (GGO) is usually acute although nonspecific for infection. Opportunistic infections producing diffuse GGO in solid organ transplantation (SOT) include cytomegalovirus and *Pneumocystis jirovecii* pneumonia. Other opportunistic fungi and mycobacteria do not produce isolated GGO.
- Peripheral opacities may indicate a noninfectious diagnosis. Organizing pneumonia (OP) and infarcts are frequently seen in SOT. A pleuroparenchymal fibrosis pattern on computed tomography (CT) scan is often diagnostic for restrictive allograft syndrome in the setting of lung transplantation and should not be confused with infection.
- Nodules and masses in SOT should prompt testing for opportunistic infections, particularly fungi. Posttransplant lymphoproliferative disorder and OP are often included in the differential diagnosis. Sometimes distinguishing features on CT are present, although definite diagnosis often requires histopathology.
- A bronchiolitis pattern is generally associated with CARV and bacterial infections or aspiration. Noninfectious patterns of lung injury associated with SOT, excepting some forms of chronic lung allograft dysfunction, generally do not produce this CT pattern.

INTRODUCTION

Solid organ transplantations (SOT) continue to increase in number, from 28,000 in 2009 to 39,000 in 2020.[1,2] Infection remains one of the most common complications of SOT,[3–6] the second most common cause of mortality within the first 30 days of lung transplantation (LT) and the primary cause of graft failure after 1 year.

Furthermore, infections are the most common cause of overall morbidity and mortality any time after LT, with two-thirds of infections affecting the respiratory tract.[7] Some infections have been linked to late graft failure.[7] The lungs are the most common site of infection in both heart and lung transplant recipients (LTR) and the second most common site in liver transplantation, only

Cardiothoracic Imaging Division, University of Pennsylvania, 3400 Spruce Street, Philadelphia, PA 19104, USA
[1] Co-first authors.
* Corresponding author.
E-mail address: Scott.Simpson@pennmedicine.upenn.edu

Radiol Clin N Am 60 (2022) 481–495
https://doi.org/10.1016/j.rcl.2022.01.005
0033-8389/22/© 2022 Elsevier Inc. All rights reserved.

preceded by intra-abdominal infections.[8] Pulmonary infections share similarities across solid organ transplant (SOT) recipients[8] and computed tomography (CT) can aid in the diagnosis of a wide array of both infectious and noninfectious complications seen in SOT.[5,7] This article reviews salient clinical and radiological findings of the most common pulmonary infections in SOT recipients. An approach to a differential diagnosis of associated imaging features is also discussed.

TIMELINE OF PULMONARY INFECTIONS AFTER SOLID ORGAN TRANSPLANTATION

Infections in the first postoperative month after SOT are usually caused by nosocomial bacterial infections with antimicrobial-resistant bacteria being of special concern during this time period. Opportunistic infections are uncommon in this time interval because significant therapy-induced immunosuppression has usually not yet been attained.[3] One to 6 months after transplantation, activation of latent infections and opportunistic infections increase in prevalence owing to increasing immunosuppression.[4] After 6 months, immunosuppressive therapy is often tapered, decreasing opportunistic infections, and resulting in a larger proportion of community-acquired pneumonias. Chronic viral infections are commonly seen after 6 months and have been linked to bronchiolitis obliterans (BO) and post-transplant lymphoproliferative disorder (PTLD). Opportunistic infections may still occur despite minimization of immune suppression even in patients with minimal symptoms.[3] A timeline of infections is summarized in **Table 1**.

BACTERIAL INFECTIONS
Overview

Bacteria account for 35% to 66% of total infections and are the most frequent infectious pathogens in lung and heart-lung transplant recipients.[7,9] Bacterial infection has a high incidence in the postoperative setting, with maximum risk during the first 3 weeks after transplantation. During the initial perioperative period, the most frequent organisms causing nosocomial pneumonia are *Staphylococcus aureus*, *Pseudomonas aeruginosa*, and Enterobacteriaceae.[9] Antimicrobial-resistant species are of special concern during this time period, such as methicillin-resistant *S aureus* (MRSA), or vancomycin-resistant enterococcus (VRE), as they are associated with high morbidity and mortality.[3,10] Common community-acquired pathogens seen after the initial postoperative period

Table 1
Timeline of infections after transplantation

Time Since Transplant	Common Infectious Organisms

<1 mo	• Nosocomial organisms (mostly bacteria)
	  ○ S aureus
	  ○ P aeruginosa
	  ○ Enterobacteriae
	• Multi-drug-resistant organisms
	  ○ MRSA
	  ○ VRE
	  ○ Candida
	• Other bacterial: Gram-negative bacteria, legionella
	• Viral: Herpes simplex virus (HSV)

1–6 mo	• Opportunistic organisms
	• With CMV and PJP prophylaxis:
	  ○ Viral: Adenovirus, influenza, RSV
	  ○ Fungal: *Cryptococcus Neoformans*
	  ○ Mycobacteria: MTB, NTM
	• Without CMV and PJP prophylaxis:
	  ○ Bacteria: Nocardia
	  ○ Viruses: Herpesviruses (CMV, EBV, varicella-zoster virus, HSV)
	  ○ Fungal: PJP, Aspergillus
	  ○ Parasites: Toxoplasma, *T cruzi*, Strongyloides

>6 mo	• Community-acquired pathogens • Bacterial: *H influenzae*, *S pneumoniae*, Legionella, *P aeruginosa*, Nocardia • Mycobacterial: MTB, NTM • Viral: Influenza, parainfluenza, adenovirus, RSV, chronic viral infections • Fungal: Aspergillus, atypical molds, mucor

Infections seen <1 mo, 1 to 6 mo, and >6 mo after SOT. At 1 to 6 mo, infections are subdivided between patients with and without prophylaxis.

include *Haemophilus influenzae*, *Streptococcus pneumoniae*, and Legionella.[1] A special consideration in LTR with cystic fibrosis (CF) is *Burkholderia cepacia*. *B cepacia* syndrome is a feared complication that can lead to uncontrollable systemic virulence and lethal postoperative pneumonia, leading to some centers listing infection with this organism as a contraindication to transplantation.[4]

Imaging manifestations of most pulmonary bacterial infections in SOT manifest as a lobar or

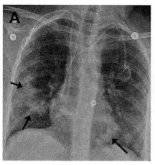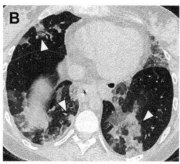

Fig. 1. A 19-year-old woman status post double lung transplant 5 years earlier with *P aeruginosa* pneumonia. (*A*) Frontal chest radiograph shows bilateral multifocal pulmonary opacities (*arrows*). (*B*) CT image shows corresponding multifocal consolidation and associated GGO (*arrowheads*). A pattern of multifocal consolidation is most commonly secondary to a bacterial pneumonia.

bronchopneumonia.[11] Consolidation with or without ground-glass opacities (GGO) predominates and may affect a single lobe or be multifocal. Lobar pneumonias are typical of Streptococcus, Klebsiella, and *H influenzae* (**Fig. 1**). Bronchopneumonia tends to be multifocal and airway centric and typically associated centrilobular nodules, tree-in-bud opacities (TiB), and/or bronchial wall thickening (**Fig. 2**). Common organisms producing a bronchopneumonia pattern include *S aureus*, *P aeruginosa*, *Escherichia coli*, and Klebsiella.[12]

Nocardia

The incidence of Nocardia pneumonia has decreased owing to widespread trimethoprim-sulfamethoxazole prophylaxis for *Pneumocystis jirovecii* pneumonia (PJP).[1] Nocardia is an aerobic bacterial organism found in soil. *Nocardia asteroids* complex species account for the majority of all nocardial infections and mostly affect immunocompromised hosts.[12] Radiological manifestations of pulmonary nocardiosis are usually solid nodules, masses, and consolidation, all of which may cavitate (**Fig. 3**). Nodules and masses may demonstrate a ground-glass halo,[13] an appearance radiologically indistinguishable from more commonly seen angioinvasive fungal infections. On CT, consolidation can demonstrate areas of necrosis predisposing to pulmonary abscess formation. Nocardia can behave locally aggressive, directly involving the pleura and chest wall in advanced infections.[13] Sometimes a solitary nodule or mass is present, which can mimic malignancy.[12,13]

MYCOBACTERIAL INFECTIONS
M tuberculosis

M tuberculosis (MTB) infection is 30 to 100 times higher in SOT than in the general population.[1] The lungs are the most common site of infection, with an overall incidence between 6.4% and 10%. MTB infections usually occur within the first year of LT.[4] Reactivation of occult disease, the most common mechanism of infection, can occur in the native lung after single LT or within the donor lung allograft.[14]

Imaging features of active MTB are conventionally divided into primary or postprimary (reactivation) disease. However, immune status also plays an important role in the imaging manifestation of MTB infection.[15–18] Reactivation MTB demonstrates upper-lobe nodules, masses, and consolidation with frequent cavitation in *immunocompetent* hosts. However, in *immunocompromised* patients, including SOT recipients, reactivation may present with radiological findings classically attributed to primary MTB infection.[19,20] This usually appears as lobar or multifocal consolidation, most often in the middle and lower lobes, mimicking bacterial pneumonias.[14,21,22] The presence of lymphadenopathy (LAD), particularly if necrotic, and failure to respond to conventional antibiotic therapy are important clues.[23] The immunosuppressed, including SOT recipients,

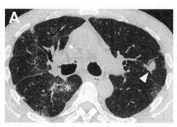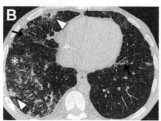

Fig. 2. A 45-year-old male double lung transplant recipient over 20 years ago with *S aureus pneumonia*. CT axial images (*A*, *B*) show GGO (*asterisks*), peribronchial consolidation (*arrowheads*), and airway thickening (*arrows*).

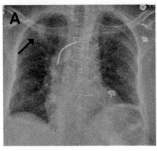
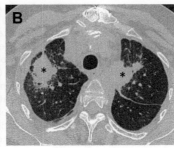

Fig. 3. A 67-year-old female heart transplant recipient with pulmonary nocardiosis identified on repeat biopsy after failing therapy for OP diagnosed on the first biopsy. (*A*) Frontal radiograph shows a masslike opacity (*arrow*) in the right upper lobe. (*B*) HRCT shows bilateral apical masses (*asterisks*) with surrounding GGO on the right depicting a CT halo sign.

are also more susceptible to hematogenous dissemination of MTB, producing a miliary pattern on CT, characterized by 2- to 3-mm well-defined nodules in a random distribution.[20,24] MTB-related pleural effusions can result in empyema, which can extend into the chest wall.[19]

Nontuberculous Mycobacteria

Nontuberculous mycobacteria (NTM) disease rate is higher in LT than in other SOT.[9] The overall incidence of NTM infection is between 3.8% and 22.4% and occurs, on average, 2 years after LT.[4] However, most isolates occur in asymptomatic patients and are transient with the frequent sites of infection being the skin, subcutaneous tissues, and the lungs.[25,26] The most common NTM organisms in LTRs are *Mycobacterium avium complex* (69.8%) followed by *Mycobacterium abscessus* (9.4%) and *Mycobacterium gordonae* (7.5%).[27] Donor lung allografts are a major source of transmission, although infection can also arise from reactivation in the native lung after single LTR and from primary infection.[27,28] *M abscessus* colonization in CF patients has been associated with progressive infection and a poor prognosis despite treatment.[1]

The CT appearance of NTM pulmonary disease is classically divided into apical fibrocavitary, mimicking reactivation MTB, and nodular bronchiectatic (also see article by Hammer and colleagues in this issue). On CT, the nodular bronchiectatic form is characterized by bronchial

wall thickening, mucoid impactions, nodules with or without cavitation, and TiB (**Fig. 4**). Bronchiectasis and scarring commonly develop if the infection is prolonged, sometimes with a characteristic distribution of disease in the paracardiac right middle lobe and lingula.[12] The appearance of NTM infections on CT can be influenced by the species. For instance, *M abscessus* often presents with the nodular bronchiectatic form, whereas *Mycobacterium kansasii* more often causes apical cavitary disease similar to MTB.[29,30] *M abscessus* has also been linked to empyema, sternal wound infections, and dissemination following LT.[29,31,32] Compared with the general population, pulmonary NTM infections in SOT are more likely to have consolidation and cavitary nodules.[12,24,25]

VIRAL INFECTIONS
Overview

Viral infections usually occur after the first postoperative month and are an important cause of morbidity and mortality in SOT.[33] Cytomegalovirus (CMV) infection is the second most common infection in SOT and the most common in LTR without prophylaxis, ranging from 53% to 75%.[34,35] Adenovirus, respiratory syncytial (RSV), parainfluenza, bocavirus, and influenza viruses are common community-acquired respiratory viruses (CARV) affecting SOTs.[33] Viral pneumonias have a wide range of imaging findings, including GGO, consolidation, bronchitis, and bronchiolitis.[8,12]

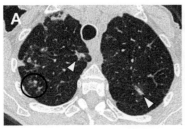
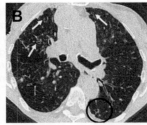

Fig. 4. A 67-year-old male bilateral LTR with the nodular bronchiectatic form of NTM disease. Axial CT images (*A*, *B*) show TiB (*circles*), bronchiectasis (*arrows*), and nodules (*arrowheads*). Cavitary nodules, more common in SOT, were not seen.

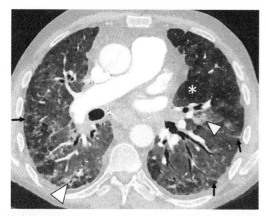

Fig. 5. A 55-year-old male bilateral LTR 1 year earlier with CMV pneumonia and BO. CT shows diffuse GGO, small sites of consolidation (*arrowheads*), and reticular opacities (*arrows*), reflecting CMV pneumonia. Areas of hyperlucent lung (*asterisk*) correspond to air-trapping from coexistent BO.

However, most viral pneumonias rarely if ever produce cavitation and larger nodules and are infrequently lobar in distribution even in SOT recipients.[36–44]

Cytomegalovirus

CMV is the most common viral pathogen seen in SOT.[35] CMV infection is defined as the detection of the virus, whereas CMV disease indicates evidence of infection, such as CMV pneumonia or retinitis.[45] CMV infection can be primary, a result of CMV-seronegative recipients (R−) who receive a CMV-seropositive donor (D+), or secondary, the result of a new exposure or reactivation of latent infection.[8] The incidence of CMV pneumonia is nearly 100% in D+/R− cases.[9] On CT, CMV pneumonia most commonly demonstrates bilateral GGO, often associated with small, poorly defined centrilobular nodules, consolidation, reticulation, and small pleural effusions[11,41,46] (**Fig. 5**). Larger sites of consolidations and nodules with a CT halo sign are atypical and almost always associated with GGO.[8,38] In addition, CMV has an immunomodulatory role that promotes infection with opportunistic infections and has also been linked to BO.[9]

Community-Acquired Respiratory Viruses

LTR have a higher likelihood of CARV compared with other SOT with an incidence of viral infection ranging from 8% to 34%.[36] CARV accounts for nearly 30% of all acute respiratory presentations after LT with a risk of hospitalization of 17% to 50%.[47] Rhinovirus was the most frequently recovered virus in both upper and lower respiratory specimens of LTR followed by endemic coronavirus and influenza viruses[48] (**Fig. 6**A). In the same study, influenza and paramyxoviruses contributed up to 50% of emergency room visits and hospitalizations in SOT. CARV pneumonias also tend to be more severe in SOT. RSV can be associated with respiratory failure and can have a mortality as high as 20%.[1] Adenovirus can present with severe constitutional symptoms and necrotizing pneumonia, intra-alveolar hemorrhage, and diffuse alveolar damage (DAD).[1] CARV, like CMV, have

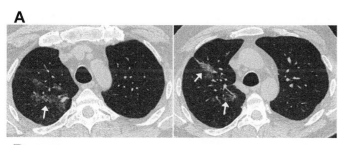

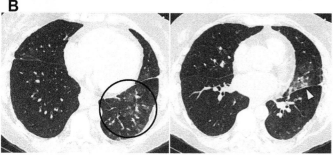

Fig. 6. CT images (*A, B*) in two different LTR patients with CARV infections. (*A*) A 48-year-old male with Rhinovirus pneumonia. CT shows patchy right upper lobe GGO (*arrows*). (*B*) A 47-year-old female with parainfluenza pneumonia. CT axial images show asymmetric left lung patchy GGO (*circle*) and small sites of consolidation (*arrowhead*).

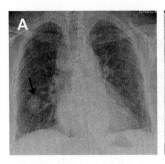
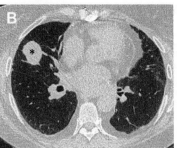

Fig. 7. A 62-year-old female LTR with pulmonary and small bowel PTLD. (*A*) Frontal radiograph shows a mass in the right mid lung zone (*arrow*). (*B*) HRCT shows a solid mass (*asterisk*) in the right middle lobe, which was new from a CT 9 months earlier.

also been associated with an increased risk of bacterial and fungal infections and BO in LTR.[1,49]

Imaging features of CARV are broad, often overlapping with each other as well as some bacterial and opportunistic infections, limiting the use of CT for a specific diagnosis.[8,38,39,41,44,50] Similar to the general population, CARV usually produce one or more of the following CT features in varying severity: bronchial wall thickening, centrilobular nodules, TiB, and GGO[38,44,51] (**Fig. 6B**). Consolidation, if present, is almost always accompanied by other CT findings and is rarely lobar with some exceptions. Pulmonary viral infections in SOT, however, are more likely to result in extensive disease. Widespread consolidation and GGO have been described in immunocompromised patients with RSV, bocavirus, influenza, and parainfluenza viral pneumonias.[33,39,52]

Epstein-Barr Virus

As T-cell immunity wanes with immunosuppression, latently infected B cells with Epstein-Barr virus (EBV) can go unregulated resulting in PTLD. PTLD histologically ranges from a benign polyclonal lymphoid proliferation to an aggressive high-grade lymphoma. PTLD can be seen 1 month to several years after transplantation, peaking at 3 to 4 months, and occurs more commonly in LTR.[4,11] PTLD most commonly affects the transplanted organ. Thus, the lungs are most commonly affected in LTR, compared with other SOT with thoracic monomorphic PTLD ranging from nearly

52% in lung transplants to 4.2% in kidney transplants.[53] Thoracic PTLD usually manifests on imaging as solitary or multiple solid nodules or masses, although it can also affect the pleura and lymph nodes as well[11] (**Fig. 7**). Of note, LAD is a less common feature of thoracic PTLD than pulmonary involvement in LTR.[54]

FUNGAL INFECTIONS
Overview

Invasive fungal infections have a reported mortality of 80% to 100%, with most cases owing to Candida or Aspergillus.[55] Cryptococcus is the third most common fungal infection in SOT recipients, with an incidence of 1.5%.[56] *Scedosporium*, *Fusarium*, and *Mucor* species are other opportunistic fungi of growing concern.[1] *Scedosporium apiospermum* accounts for 25% of invasive fungal infections caused by molds other than *Aspergillus* spp, largely in LTR and patients with CF, and is associated with invasive pulmonary infections and disseminated disease.[4,57] Endemic fungal infections, such as histoplasmosis, are generally rare in SOT.[56,58,59] Fungal infections have a wide variety of imaging manifestations, which can overlap with bacterial and mycobacterial infections. Nodules and masses are the most characteristic presentation in SOT, although nonspecific findings, such as consolidation, may be the only finding.[12,60–64]

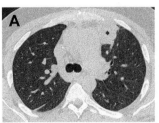
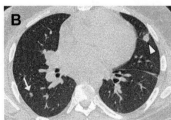

Fig. 8. A 31-year-old male heart transplant recipient with pulmonary aspergillosis. CT images (*A* and *B*) show a solid mass (*asterisk*) and nodules (*arrow*). One nodule demonstrates a small ground-glass halo (*arrowhead*).

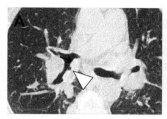
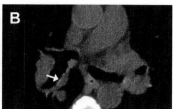

Fig. 9. A 63-year-old female bilateral LTR 1 year earlier with tracheobronchial Aspergillus fumigatus. Axial CT images in lung (A) and soft tissue (B) settings show severe central right-sided airway bronchial wall thickening and nodularity (arrows) and a small site of ulceration (arrowhead).

Aspergillus

Aspergillus is the second most common opportunistic fungal infections in SOT overall, and the most common in LTR.[56] The incidence of pulmonary invasive aspergillosis (IA) in SOT is low, generally less than 10%, although it has a relatively high mortality depending on the SOT. In one study, the incidence of IA in SOT was 1.4%, ranging from 3% in LT to 0.2% in kidney transplantation.[65] Mortalities also range by SOT, being as low as 4% in LT and as high as 88% in liver transplantation.[66] Aspergillus can affect the airways and lungs. Airway colonization and tracheobronchitis can be seen, the latter nearly exclusively occurring in LTR.[67] Tracheobronchitis ranges in severity from mild bronchitis to pseudomembranous and ulcerative disease. If the anastomosis is affected, dehiscence, hemorrhage, or disseminated disease can occur.[9]

Characteristic radiological features of IA include nodules or masses with a ground-glass halo, the latter reflecting alveolar hemorrhage at the periphery of infarcted tissue, and can be seen in up to 95% of patients[68] (Fig. 8). During rebound neutropenia or healing, the "air crescent" sign, caused by contraction of infarcted tissue, may be seen[8] (see article by Godoy and colleagues in this issue). However, in SOT, these characteristic findings are less common, and nonspecific imaging manifestations, such as consolidation, may only be present.[60–62] Tracheobronchial aspergillosis is relatively specific to LT, and severe central tracheobronchial thickening and ulceration should raise suspicion for this infection (Fig. 9).[69] Airway-invasive aspergillosis demonstrates peribronchial consolidation, centrilobular nodules, and TiB and is often poorly distinguished on CT from more common bacterial or viral infections.[8]

Candida

Candida spp are the most common fungal infection in SOT, most often seen in the first few months, however, occur less frequently in the lungs and LTR compared with Aspergillus spp.[56] In one study, pulmonary candidiasis resulted in nodules (88%), TiB (41%), consolidation (65%), and GGO (35%).[64] GGO is almost never an isolated finding, and the CT halo sign is less common compared with IA occurring in 32% of patients.[68] Candidiasis can also cause mediastinitis, empyema, arteritis, bronchial anastomotic infection, or esophagitis.[9]

Pneumocystis jirovecii

P jirovecii is a fungus ubiquitous in nature.[4] Prophylaxis is effective in nearly 100% of patients, dramatically reducing incidence. However, without prophylaxis, prevalence can be as high as 88%.[4,9,70] PJP typically occurs 3 to 6 months after transplantation, and risk significantly decreases after 1 year of SOT except in LTR.[1,71] PJP infects 0.3% to 2.6% of SOT recipients and is higher in lung and heart transplantation owing to more extensive immunosuppressive regimens.[70] On CT, PJP is almost always associated with bilateral GGO,[8] which may be the only finding present. Compared with patients with AIDS, some SOT have been shown to have diffuse GGO and cystic change less often, and patchy GGO and

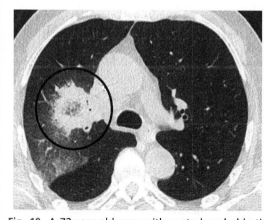

Fig. 10. A 72-year-old man with acute lymphoblastic leukemia undergoing chemotherapy induction with pulmonary mucormycosis. Axial CT image shows a single masslike opacity (circle) with central irregular GGO and thick peripheral consolidation compatible with a reverse halo or bird's nest sign, characteristic of this infection.

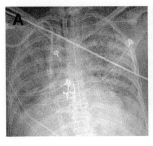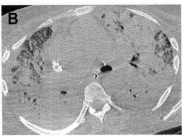

Fig. 11. A 49-year-old female LTR 6 months earlier with *Legionella* pneumonia complicated by ARDS. (*A*) Frontal chest radiograph shows diffuse pulmonary opacities. (*B*) HRCT image shows diffuse consolidation. A pattern of diffuse consolidation is typical of ARDS and pneumonia. Severe bacterial or viral infections could have this appearance.

consolidation more frequently.[72–74] Pleural effusions, LAD, and airway inflammation are uncommonly seen.[8,12,50] CT features of CMV and PJP are similar and often poorly distinguished by CT; however, nodules and consolidation are more often seen in CMV.[8,50]

Mucormycosis

Mucormycosis represents a group of fungal infections in the Mucorales order, including Rhizopus, Mucor, and Rhizomucor.[4] Mucormycosis incidence ranges from 0.2% to 3% in SOT and accounts for 2% of invasive fungal infections.[56,58,75] Mucormycosis is characterized by invasion of vasculature leading to infarction and necrosis in host tissue. Mortality is very high, ranging from 49% to 90%, and management can be difficult.[4] Amphotericin B is the treatment of choice in addition to reduced immunosuppression and possible surgical debridement.[4] The radiological appearance of pulmonary mucormycosis ranges from consolidation to single or multiple masses, the former being associated with a high mortality.[75] The reverse halo, often seen as a single masslike opacity with central irregular GGO and a thick peripheral rim of consolidation, can be characteristic of pulmonary mucormycosis and has been likened to a bird's nest appearance (**Fig. 10**).[4,75,76] The reverse halo is also more commonly seen in Mucor than in Aspergillus infection.[77,78]

APPROACH TO *POTENTIALLY* INFECTIOUS RADIOLOGICAL FINDINGS IN SOLID ORGAN TRANSPLANTATION

The treatment of pulmonary infections is ideally predicated on the identification of the causative organism, although the responsible pathogen may not be isolated.[79] Treatment strategies for presumed infections are usually with broad-spectrum antibiotics and then subsequently narrowed or altered after incorporating additional information.[80] Occasionally, CT findings may direct or redirect management, particularly when the presumed infectious organism does not align with radiological features. Common CT imaging patterns associated with infections in SOT, their differential diagnoses, and helpful imaging clues are subsequently discussed.

Predominant Consolidation

Consolidation in the setting of fever without other explainable cause is suggestive of pneumonia.[38,44,81,82] When consolidation predominates and is multifocal or lobar in distribution, bacterial organisms are most likely. The concurrent presence of TiB greatly increases the likelihood for infection and thus serves as an important biomarker.[51] CARV can produce consolidation, although usually not in isolation and often associated with GGO or TiB. Consolidation can predominate in some viral infections, such

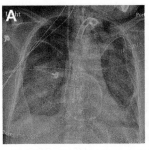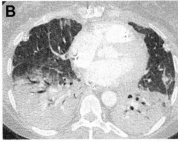

Fig. 12. A 48-year-old woman status post double lung and heart transplantation 1 week earlier with PGD. (*A*) Frontal chest radiograph shows diffuse pulmonary opacities. (*B*) HRCT image obtained shortly thereafter shows diffuse consolidation, noting a dependent distribution typical of early ARDS. Gradual worsening at 72 hours and persistence of opacities without an explainable cause are suggestive of PGD. PGD and ARDS are usually indis-

tinguishable, although PGD should develop within 72 hours of LT.

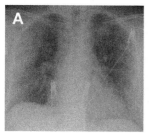
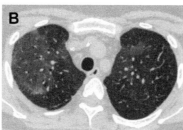

Fig. 13. A 36-year-old female bilateral LTR with OP and acute rejection. (*A*) Frontal chest radiograph (CXR) shows peripheral and upper lobe predominate opacities. (*B*) Axial CT shows bilateral isolated GGO. The differential is broad, although in SOT consideration is also given to some opportunistic infections (PJP, CMV), and acute lung injury patterns related to drug toxicity or allograft dysfunction.

as Adenovirus, RSV, and influenza, particularly in the immunosuppressed, and both bacterial and viral infections are common causes of acute respiratory distress syndrome (ARDS), which can produce diffuse consolidation (**Fig. 11**). Fungal and mycobacterial infections also produce a pattern of consolidation with or without GGO that may be indistinguishable from bacterial infection, although they are much less common.[4,21,34,38,41,81–83]

Noninfectious patterns of lung injury seen in SOT, such as organizing pneumonia (OP), acute fibrinous organizing pneumonia (AFOP), and DAD, also result in consolidation on CT.[84–86] DAD is typically symmetric and diffuse, whereas AFOP and OP can be multifocal or sometimes lobar. A pattern of worsening diffuse consolidation, peaking at 72 hours following LT, is suggestive of primary graft dysfunction (PGD) and is radiographically identical to ARDS[87] (**Fig. 12**).

Isolated Ground-Glass Opacity

Like consolidation, GGO is usually acute and potentially reversible, although is much less specific for infection particularly as an isolated finding.[88,89] Causes for isolated GGO are broad and often discussed in radiology reports categorically. Common acute causes include some infections, particularly viruses, pulmonary edema, alveolar hemorrhage, and diffuse acute lung injury patterns.[44,84,85,88,89] In SOT, CMV, PJP, acute rejection, and drug toxicities should also be included in the differential diagnosis.

Mycobacterial and other fungal infections usually do not produce isolated GGO.[21,41,57,63,82,83] GGO with or without consolidation can be seen with allograft dysfunction in lung transplants, histologically representing DAD and/or OP, may herald the onset of chronic lung allograft dysfunction (CLAD) and are sometimes seen symmetrically in the upper lobes[86,90–92] (**Fig. 13**).

Peripheral Consolidation and/or Ground-Glass Opacity

Peripheral GGO and/or consolidation in the setting of transplants may be noninfectious. OP is a pattern of lung injury seen in SOT, ranging from 10% to 28% of LTR.[92] OP can mimic infections clinically, and thus CT can play an important role in early diagnosis. OP characteristically produces bilateral, lower lobe, peripheral consolidation, and/or GGO.[84] A reverse halo sign may be present, aiding in a more confident radiological diagnosis, although this can also be seen in pulmonary infarcts and mucormycosis.[78,93] An OP pattern can be seen in a small subset of infections, such as influenza A and COVID-19-associated pneumonia.[43,94] SOT also have an increased risk of pulmonary embolism.[95] Infarcts, like OP, are peripheral and can also produce a reverse halo sign. Key distinguishing features on CT include absence of internal air bronchograms, a "bubbly" central opacity, and a wedge-shaped morphology contacting the pleural edge[93] (**Fig. 14**). A pattern of upper lobe subpleural consolidation with features of fibrosis (architectural distortion, traction

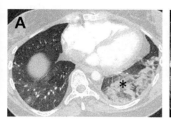
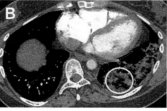

Fig. 14. A 32-year-old male heart transplant recipient with pulmonary infarction from acute pulmonary embolism. (*A*) Axial HRCT in lung window setting shows peripheral left lower lobe consolidation with central GGO (*asterisk*). (*B*) On soft tissue window setting, there is "bubbly" appearance of the central opacity (*circle*). Internal air bronchograms are not seen. These findings are

fairly specific for pulmonary infarction.

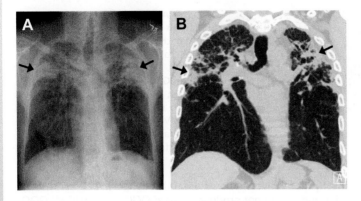

Fig. 15. A 48-year-old male LTR with RAS. (*A*) Frontal CXR and (*B*) coronal CT show upper lobe peripheral consolidation (*arrows*), volume loss, and traction bronchiectasis. This appearance is characteristic of PPFE, a common pattern associated with RAS in LT and should not be confused with infection. Superimposed GGO or consolidation may indicate exacerbation.

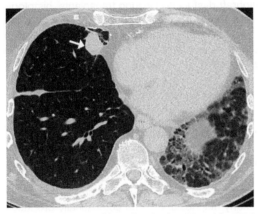

Fig. 16. A 67-year-old male single LTR with PTLD. Axial CT shows a single right middle lobe mass (*arrow*). Differential considerations for a mass in SOT include malignancy such as PTLD, some opportunistic fungal infections, and OP. LAD was not present and is a not reliable distinguishing feature from other causes of pulmonary nodules and masses.

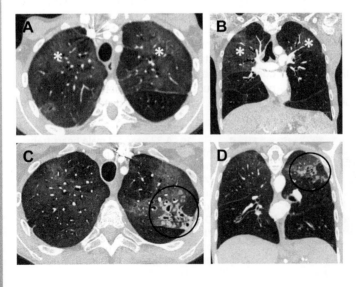

Fig. 17. A 21-year-old male lung and liver transplant recipient for CF with biopsy-proven OP subsequently complicated by *P aeruginosa*. Axial (*A*) and coronal (*B*) CT demonstrate symmetric upper lobe predominant GGO reflecting OP (*asterisks*). Axial (*C*) and coronal (*D*) HRCT 5 months later show persistent GGO and new focal bronchiectasis, centrilobular nodules, and consolidation (*circles*) reflecting superimposed infection and scarring.

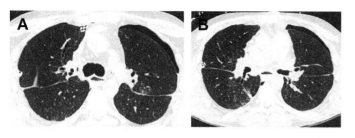

Fig. 18. A 33-year-old male bilateral lung transplant recipient 4 weeks earlier with nontuberculous mycobacterial infection (NTM). (*A, B*) Axial CT images show centrilobular nodules and TiB opacities compatible with bronchiolitis. This is typically related to bacterial and viral infections or aspiration. This patient had a history of CF and was colonized with NTM before transplant.

bronchiectasis) is suggestive of pleuroparenchymal fibrosis (PPFE)[86,91,92,96] (**Fig. 15**). PPFE is a common pattern of fibrosis seen in LT and often characterized clinically as restrictive allograft syndrome (RAS).[96]

Nodules and Masses

The presence of nodules or masses with or without cavitation should raise concern for some opportunistic infections, particularly fungi.[97] *Aspergillus* is a common opportunistic fungal infection seen in SOT and should be included in the initial differential diagnosis. The CT halo and air-crescent signs serve as helpful imaging clues, although are not pathognomonic.[41,57,98,99] Pulmonary candidiasis less often presents with isolated nodules and more frequently with consolidation.[64] Mucormycosis is highly lethal and can demonstrate characteristic findings on CT. The presence of a single masslike opacity with a reverse halo or bird's nest sign may prompt clinicians to potentially alter fungal therapy to include Amphotericin B for presumed pulmonary mucormycosis.[75,77,100,101] Mycobacterial infections result in nodules, although are frequently associated with TiB and consolidation. Rare bacterial causes producing masslike opacities include Nocardia and Actinomycosis.[13,30,102]

Noninfectious causes of nodules and masses in SOT include PTLD and OP, although lung cancers and metastasis are also seen[97,103] (**Fig. 16**). Differentiation between PTLD, OP, and opportunistic fungal infections may not be possible on CT.[97] The presence of chest wall invasion and cavitation is more commonly seen in infections, rarely in PTLD, and almost never in OP.[54,84] Halo and reverse halo signs are uncommon manifestations of PTLD and more commonly seen with fungal infections and OP.[68,104] Significant LAD may suggest PTLD in SOT; however, this is uncommon. Typically, lymph nodes of PTLD are only mild to moderately enlarged and not confidently distinguished from reactive LAD.[54] Furthermore, LAD may not be present even in the setting of pulmonary PTLD.[54]

Bronchiolitis Pattern

A CT bronchiolitis pattern is defined by the presence of TiB and/or centrilobular nodules usually with bronchial wall thickening.[105] A bronchiolitis pattern in SOT, like the general population, is usually related to CARV or bacterial infections, and aspiration[44,51] (**Fig. 17**). Fungal infections, such as airway-invasive aspergillosis and mycobacteria, particularly NTM, can cause a bronchiolitis pattern, although neither is generally given much initial consideration because of the relative higher frequency of other infections (**Fig. 18**). However, the presence of concurrent larger nodules, cavitation, or severe tracheobronchial wall thickening should raise concern for these diagnoses.[67,103] Noninfectious patterns of lung injury seen in SOT generally do not produce bronchiolitis, although obstructive CLAD, such as BO syndrome or azithromycin-reversible allograft dysfunction in LT, can result in bronchiolitis.[86,91,92,96]

SUMMARY

SOT continue to increase in number, and infections remain one of, if not the most important factor affecting patient morbidity and mortality. The number of possible pulmonary infections in SOT is vast, which include community-acquired, nosocomial, and opportunistic pathogens. Incorporating additional information, such as characteristic imaging appearances, time from transplantation, and an approach to imaging features, the radiological differential diagnosis can be narrowed, allowing imaging to remain central in SOT patient management.

CLINICS CARE POINTS

- Understanding the timeline of pulmonary infections after SOT is important in the workup of suspected pneumonia.
- Bacteria are the most common infections after SOT, with some early resistant infections being associated with high morbidity and mortality. Lobar and bronchopneumonia are

the most common findings of bacterial infection on CT.

- Viral infections are a common cause of pneumonia, especially in the outpatient setting and can be associated with severe disease in SOT. Appearance varies on CT and can overlap with bacterial pneumonia.

- Fungal infections should be considered when pulmonary nodules and masses are present, though can also present with consolidation and, in the case of PJP, widespread GGO.

- The appearance of MTB depends on the immune status of the patient and may mimic bacterial pneumonia on CT in SOT. CT appearance of NTM can be species dependent.

- The imaging appearance of pulmonary infections overlaps with noninfectious patterns of lung injury seen in SOT. While CT is a valuable imaging tool to narrow the differential, additional clinical information and occasionally biopsy may be needed to make the diagnosis.

DISCLOSURE

No financial disclosures or conflicts of interest for either author.

REFERENCES

1. Pneumonia infection in organ transplant recipients. ESun Technologies, LLC. Available at: http://www.antimicrobe.org/t35.asp#r30. Accessed August 22, 2021.
2. Organ donation statistics. Health Resources & Services Administration. 2021. Available at: https://www.organdonor.gov/learn/organ-donation-statistics. Accessed September 22, 2021.
3. Fishman JA. Infection in solid-organ transplant recipients. N Engl J Med 2007;357(25):2601–14.
4. Nosotti M, Tarsia P, Morlacchi LC. Infections after lung transplantation. J Thorac Dis 2018;10(6):3849–68.
5. Hemmert C, Ohana M, Jeung MY, et al. Imaging of lung transplant complications. Diagn Interv Imaging 2014;95(4):399–409.
6. Yeung JC, Keshavjee S. Overview of clinical lung transplantation. Cold Spring Harb Perspect Med 2014;4(1):a015628.
7. Speich R, van der Bij W. Epidemiology and management of infections after lung transplantation. Clin Infect Dis 2001;33(Suppl 1):S58–65.
8. Ahuja J, Kanne JP. Thoracic infections in immunocompromised patients. Radiol Clin North Am 2014;52(1):121–36.
9. Len O, Roman A, Gavaldá J. Risks and epidemiology of infections after lung or heart-lung transplantation. Transpl Infections 2016;167–83.
10. Bui KT, Mehta S, Khuu TH, et al. Extended spectrum β-lactamase-producing Enterobacteriaceae infection in heart and lung transplant recipients and in mechanical circulatory support recipients. Transplantation 2014;97(5):590–4.
11. Ng YL, Paul N, Patsios D, et al. Imaging of lung transplantation: review. AJR Am J Roentgenol 2009;192(3 Suppl):S1–13. quiz S14-19.
12. Elicker BM, Webb WR. Pulmonary infections. In: Fundamentals of high-resolution lung CT. Philadelphia: Lippincott Williams and Wilkins; 2013.
13. Kanne JP, Yandow DR, Mohammed TL, et al. CT findings of pulmonary nocardiosis. AJR Am J Roentgenol 2011;197(2):W266–72.
14. Mortensen E, Hellinger W, Keller C, et al. Three cases of donor-derived pulmonary tuberculosis in lung transplant recipients and review of 12 previously reported cases: opportunities for early diagnosis and prevention. Transpl Infect Dis 2014;16(1):67–75.
15. Rozenshtein A, Hao F, Starc MT, et al. Radiographic appearance of pulmonary tuberculosis: dogma disproved. AJR Am J Roentgenol 2015;204(5):974–8.
16. Jones BE, Young SM, Antoniskis D, et al. Relationship of the manifestations of tuberculosis to CD4 cell counts in patients with human immunodeficiency virus infection. Am Rev Respir Dis 1993;148(5):1292–7.
17. Post FA, Wood R, Pillay GP. Pulmonary tuberculosis in HIV infection: radiographic appearance is related to CD4+ T-lymphocyte count. Tuber Lung Dis 1995;76(6):518–21.
18. Geng E, Kreiswirth B, Burzynski J, et al. Clinical and radiographic correlates of primary and reactivation tuberculosis: a molecular epidemiology study. JAMA 2005;293(22):2740–5.
19. Nachiappan AC, Rahbar K, Shi X, et al. Pulmonary tuberculosis: role of radiology in diagnosis and management. Radiographics 2017;37(1):52–72.
20. Horne DJ, Narita M, Spitters CL, et al. Challenging issues in tuberculosis in solid organ transplantation. Clin Infect Dis 2013;57(10):1473–82.
21. Andreu J, Cáceres J, Pallisa E, et al. Radiological manifestations of pulmonary tuberculosis. Eur J Radiol 2004;51(2):139–49.
22. McAdams HP, Erasmus J, Winter JA. Radiologic manifestations of pulmonary tuberculosis. Radiol Clin North Am 1995;33(4):655–78.
23. Burrill J, Williams CJ, Bain G, et al. Tuberculosis: a radiologic review. Radiographics 2007;27(5):1255–73.
24. Washington L, Miller WT. Mycobacterial infection in immunocompromised patients. J Thorac Imaging 1998;13(4):271–81.
25. Lee Y, Song JW, Chae EJ, et al. CT findings of pulmonary non-tuberculous mycobacterial infection in non-AIDS immunocompromised patients: a case-

controlled comparison with immunocompetent patients. Br J Radiol 2013;86(1024):20120209.

26. Piersimoni C. Nontuberculous mycobacteria infection in solid organ transplant recipients. Eur J Clin Microbiol Infect Dis 2012;31(4):397–403.

27. Kesten S, Chaparro C. Mycobacterial infections in lung transplant recipients. Chest 1999;115(3):741–5.

28. Knoll BM, Kappagoda S, Gill RR, et al. Non-tuberculous mycobacterial infection among lung transplant recipients: a 15-year cohort study. Transpl Infect Dis 2012;14(5):452–60.

29. Chernenko SM, Humar A, Hutcheon M, et al. Mycobacterium abscessus infections in lung transplant recipients: the international experience. J Heart Lung Transplant 2006;25(12):1447–55.

30. Doucette K, Fishman JA. Nontuberculous mycobacterial infection in hematopoietic stem cell and solid organ transplant recipients. Clin Infect Dis 2004;38(10):1428–39.

31. Fairhurst RM, Kubak BM, Shpiner RB, et al. Mycobacterium abscessus empyema in a lung transplant recipient. J Heart Lung Transpl 2002;21(3):391–4.

32. Smibert O, Snell GI, Bills H, et al. Mycobacterium abscessus complex - a particular challenge in the setting of lung transplantation. Expert Rev Anti Infect Ther 2016;14(3):325–33.

33. Matar LD, McAdams HP, Palmer SM, et al. Respiratory viral infections in lung transplant recipients: radiologic findings with clinical correlation. Radiology 1999;213(3):735–42.

34. Maurer JR, Tullis DE, Grossman RF, et al. Infectious complications following isolated lung transplantation. Chest 1992;101(4):1056–9.

35. Zamora MR. Cytomegalovirus and lung transplantation. Am J Transplant 2004;4(8):1219–26.

36. Gottlieb J, Schulz TF, Welte T, et al. Community-acquired respiratory viral infections in lung transplant recipients: a single season cohort study. Transplantation 2009;87(10):1530–7.

37. Shalhoub S, Husain S. Community-acquired respiratory viral infections in lung transplant recipients. Curr Opin Infect Dis 2013;26(4):302–8.

38. Koo HJ, Lim S, Choe J, et al. Radiographic and CT features of viral pneumonia. Radiographics 2018;38(3):719–39.

39. Anderson DJ, Jordan MC. Viral pneumonia in recipients of solid organ transplants. Semin Respir Infect 1990;5(1):38–49.

40. Brooks RG, Hofflin JM, Jamieson SW, et al. Infectious complications in heart-lung transplant recipients. Am J Med 1985;79(4):412–22.

41. Collins J, Müller NL, Kazerooni EA, et al. CT findings of pneumonia after lung transplantation. AJR Am J Roentgenol 2000;175(3):811–8.

42. Kang EY, Patz EF, Müller NL. Cytomegalovirus pneumonia in transplant patients: CT findings. J Comput Assist Tomogr 1996;20(2):295–9.

43. Marchiori E, Zanetti G, Fontes CA, et al. Influenza A (H1N1) virus-associated pneumonia: high-resolution computed tomography-pathologic correlation. Eur J Radiol 2011;80(3):e500–4.

44. Miller WT, Mickus TJ, Barbosa E, et al. CT of viral lower respiratory tract infections in adults: comparison among viral organisms and between viral and bacterial infections. AJR Am J Roentgenol 2011;197(5):1088–95.

45. Ljungman P, Boeckh M, Hirsch HH, et al. Definitions of cytomegalovirus infection and disease in transplant patients for use in clinical trials. Clin Infect Dis 2017;64(1):87–91.

46. Erasmus JJ, McAdams HP, Tapson VF, et al. Radiologic issues in lung transplantation for end-stage pulmonary disease. AJR Am J Roentgenol 1997;169(1):69–78.

47. Glanville AR. Community-acquired respiratory viruses after lung transplantation: common, sometimes silent, potentially lethal. Thorax 2014;69(1):1–2.

48. Bridevaux PO, Aubert JD, Soccal PM, et al. Incidence and outcomes of respiratory viral infections in lung transplant recipients: a prospective study. Thorax 2014;69(1):32–8.

49. Garcia-Vidal C, Royo-Cebrecos C, Peghin M, et al. Environmental variables associated with an increased risk of invasive aspergillosis. Clin Microbiol Infect 2014;20(11):O939–45.

50. Kunihiro Y, Tanaka N, Kawano R, et al. Differential diagnosis of pulmonary infections in immunocompromised patients using high-resolution computed tomography. Eur Radiol 2019;29(11):6089–99.

51. Miller WT, Panosian JS. Causes and imaging patterns of tree-in-bud opacities. Chest 2013;144(6):1883–92.

52. Yang E, Rubin BK. Childhood" viruses as a cause of pneumonia in adults. Semin Respir Infect 1995;10(4):232–43.

53. Opelz G, Dohler B. Lymphomas after solid organ transplantation: a collaborative transplant study report. Am J Transplant 2004;4(2):222–30.

54. Borhani AA, Hosseinzadeh K, Almusa O, et al. Imaging of posttransplantation lymphoproliferative disorder after solid organ transplantation. Radiographics 2009;29(4):981–1000.

55. Singh N, Aguado JM, Bonatti H, et al. Zygomycosis in solid organ transplant recipients: a prospective, matched case-control study to assess risks for disease and outcome. J Infect Dis 2009;200(6):1002–11.

56. Pappas PG, Alexander BD, Andes DR, et al. Invasive fungal infections among organ transplant recipients: results of the Transplant-Associated Infection Surveillance Network (TRANSNET). Clin Infect Dis 2010;50(8):1101–11.

57. Solé A, Salavert M. Fungal infections after lung transplantation. Curr Opin Pulm Med 2009;15(3):243–53.

58. Kauffman CA, Freifeld AG, Andes DR, et al. Endemic fungal infections in solid organ and hematopoietic cell transplant recipients enrolled in the Transplant-Associated Infection Surveillance Network (TRANSNET). Transpl Infect Dis 2014; 16(2):213–24.

59. Assi M, Martin S, Wheat LJ, et al. Histoplasmosis after solid organ transplant. Clin Infect Dis 2013; 57(11):1542–9.

60. Park SY, Kim SH, Choi SH, et al. Clinical and radiological features of invasive pulmonary aspergillosis in transplant recipients and neutropenic patients. Transpl Infect Dis 2010;12(4):309–15.

61. Park SY, Lim C, Lee SO, et al. Computed tomography findings in invasive pulmonary aspergillosis in non-neutropenic transplant recipients and neutropenic patients, and their prognostic value. J Infect 2011;63(6):447–56.

62. Qin J, Fang Y, Dong Y, et al. Radiological and clinical findings of 25 patients with invasive pulmonary aspergillosis: retrospective analysis of 2150 liver transplantation cases. Br J Radiol 2012;85(1016): e429–35.

63. Althoff Souza C, Müller NL, Marchiori E, et al. Pulmonary invasive aspergillosis and candidiasis in immunocompromised patients: a comparative study of the high-resolution CT findings. J Thorac Imaging 2006;21(3):184–9.

64. Franquet T, Müller NL, Lee KS, et al. Pulmonary candidiasis after hematopoietic stem cell transplantation: thin-section CT findings. Radiology 2005;236(1):332–7.

65. Gavalda J, Len O, San Juan R, et al. Risk factors for invasive aspergillosis in solid-organ transplant recipients: a case-control study. Clin Infect Dis 2005;41(1):52–9.

66. Neofytos D, Garcia-Vidal C, Lamoth F, et al. Invasive aspergillosis in solid organ transplant patients: diagnosis, prophylaxis, treatment, and assessment of response. BMC Infect Dis 2021;21(1):296.

67. Kramer MR, Denning DW, Marshall SE, et al. Ulcerative tracheobronchitis after lung transplantation. A new form of invasive aspergillosis. Am Rev Respir Dis 1991;144(3 Pt 1):552–6.

68. Georgiadou SP, Sipsas NV, Marom EM, et al. The diagnostic value of halo and reversed halo signs for invasive mold infections in compromised hosts. Clin Infect Dis 2011;52(9):1144–55.

69. Isnard J, Trogrlic S, Haloun A, et al. [Heart and heart-lung transplants thorax complications: major radiologic forms]. J Radiol 2007;88(3 Pt 1):339–48.

70. Iriart X, Challan Belval T, Fillaux J, et al. Risk factors of Pneumocystis pneumonia in solid organ recipients in the era of the common use of posttransplantation prophylaxis. Am J Transplant 2015;15(1):190–9.

71. Gordon SM, LaRosa SP, Kalmadi S, et al. Should prophylaxis for Pneumocystis carinii pneumonia in solid organ transplant recipients ever be discontinued? Clin Infect Dis 1999;28(2):240–6.

72. Vogel MN, Vatlach M, Weissgerber P, et al. HRCT-features of Pneumocystis jiroveci pneumonia and their evolution before and after treatment in non-HIV immunocompromised patients. Eur J Radiol 2012;81(6):1315–20.

73. Christe A, Walti L, Charimo J, et al. Imaging patterns of Pneumocystis jirovecii pneumonia in HIV-positive and renal transplant patients - a multicentre study. Swiss Med Wkly 2019;149:w20130.

74. Ebner L, Walti LN, Rauch A, et al. Clinical course, radiological manifestations, and outcome of Pneumocystis jirovecii pneumonia in HIV patients and renal transplant recipients. PLoS One 2016; 11(11):e0164320.

75. Agrawal R, Yeldandi A, Savas H, et al. Pulmonary mucormycosis: risk factors, radiologic findings, and pathologic correlation. Radiographics 2020; 40(3):656–66.

76. Walker CM, Abbott GF, Greene RE, et al. Imaging pulmonary infection: classic signs and patterns. AJR Am J Roentgenol 2014;202(3):479–92.

77. Jung J, Kim MY, Lee HJ, et al. Comparison of computed tomographic findings in pulmonary mucormycosis and invasive pulmonary aspergillosis. Clin Microbiol Infect 2015;21(7):684.e1-8.

78. Wahba H, Truong MT, Lei X, et al. Reversed halo sign in invasive pulmonary fungal infections. Clin Infect Dis 2008;46(11):1733–7.

79. Ogawa H, Kitsios GD, Iwata M, et al. Sputum gram stain for bacterial pathogen diagnosis in community-acquired pneumonia: a systematic review and Bayesian meta-analysis of diagnostic accuracy and yield. Clin Infect Dis 2020;71(3):499–513.

80. Dulek DE, Mueller NJ, Practice AIDCo. Pneumonia in solid organ transplantation: guidelines from the American Society of Transplantation Infectious Diseases Community of Practice. Clin Transplant 2019;33(9):e13545.

81. Kjeldsberg KM, Oh K, Murray KA, et al. Radiographic approach to multifocal consolidation. Semin Ultrasound CT MR 2002;23(4):288–301.

82. Franquet T. Imaging of pneumonia: trends and algorithms. Eur Respir J 2001;18(1):196–208.

83. Brown MJ, Miller RR, Müller NL. Acute lung disease in the immunocompromised host: CT and pathologic examination findings. Radiology 1994; 190(1):247–54.

84. Kligerman SJ, Franks TJ, Galvin JR. From the radiologic pathology archives: organization and fibrosis as a response to lung injury in diffuse alveolar damage, organizing pneumonia, and acute fibrinous and organizing pneumonia. Radiographics 2013;33(7):1951–75.

85. Obadina ET, Torrealba JM, Kanne JP. Acute pulmonary injury: high-resolution CT and

histopathological spectrum. Br J Radiol 2013; 86(1027):20120614.

86. Brun AL, Chabi ML, Picard C, et al. Lung transplantation: CT assessment of chronic lung allograft dysfunction (CLAD). Diagnostics (Basel) 2021; 11(5).

87. Belmaati EO, Steffensen I, Jensen C, et al. Radiological patterns of primary graft dysfunction after lung transplantation evaluated by 64-multi-slice computed tomography: a descriptive study. Interact Cardiovasc Thorac Surg 2012;14(6): 785–91.

88. Miller WT, Shah RM. Isolated diffuse ground-glass opacity in thoracic CT: causes and clinical presentations. AJR Am J Roentgenol 2005;184(2):613–22.

89. Parekh M, Donuru A, Balasubramanya R, et al. Review of the chest CT differential diagnosis of ground-glass opacities in the COVID era. Radiology 2020;297(3):E289–302.

90. Dettmer S, Shin HO, Vogel-Claussen J, et al. CT at onset of chronic lung allograft dysfunction in lung transplant patients predicts development of the restrictive phenotype and survival. Eur J Radiol 2017;94:78–84.

91. Byrne D, Nador RG, English JC, et al. Chronic lung allograft dysfunction: review of CT and pathologic findings. Radiol Cardiothorac Imaging 2021;3(1): e200314.

92. Hota P, Dass C, Kumaran M, et al. High-resolution CT findings of obstructive and restrictive phenotypes of chronic lung allograft dysfunction: more than just bronchiolitis obliterans syndrome. AJR Am J Roentgenol 2018;211(1):W13–21.

93. Revel MP, Triki R, Chatellier G, et al. Is it possible to recognize pulmonary infarction on multisection CT images? Radiology 2007;244(3):875–82.

94. Kwee TC, Kwee RM. Chest CT in COVID-19: what the radiologist needs to know. Radiographics 2020;40(7).1848–65.

95. Evans CF, Iacono AT, Sanchez PG, et al. Venous thromboembolic complications of lung transplantation: a contemporary single-institution review. Ann Thorac Surg 2015;100(6):2033–9.

96. Verleden GM, Glanville AR, Lease ED, et al. Chronic lung allograft dysfunction: definition, diagnostic criteria, and approaches to treatment-a consensus report from the Pulmonary Council of the ISHLT. J Heart Lung Transpl 2019;38(5): 493–503.

97. Copp DH, Godwin JD, Kirby KA, et al. Clinical and radiologic factors associated with pulmonary nodule etiology in organ transplant recipients. Am J Transplant 2006;6(11):2759–64.

98. Franquet T, Müller NL, Giménez A, et al. Spectrum of pulmonary aspergillosis: histologic, clinical, and radiologic findings. Radiographics 2001;21(4): 825–37.

99. Mehrad B, Paciocco G, Martinez FJ, et al. Spectrum of Aspergillus infection in lung transplant recipients: case series and review of the literature. Chest 2001;119(1):169–75.

100. Legouge C, Caillot D, Chrétien ML, et al. The reversed halo sign: pathognomonic pattern of pulmonary mucormycosis in leukemic patients with neutropenia? Clin Infect Dis 2014;58(5):672–8.

101. Connolly JE, McAdams HP, Erasmus JJ, et al. Opportunistic fungal pneumonia. J Thorac Imaging 1999;14(1):51–62.

102. Kramer MR, Marshall SE, Starnes VA, et al. Infectious complications in heart-lung transplantation. Analysis of 200 episodes. Arch Intern Med 1993; 153(17):2010–6.

103. Lee P, Minai OA, Mehta AC, et al. Pulmonary nodules in lung transplant recipients: etiology and outcome. Chest 2004;125(1):165–72.

104. Thomas R, Madan R, Gooptu M, et al. Significance of the reverse halo sign in immunocompromised patients. AJR Am J Roentgenol 2019;213(3): 549–54.

105. Hwang JH, Kim TS, Lee KS, et al. Bronchiolitis in adults: pathology and imaging. J Comput Assist Tomogr 1997;21(6):913–9.

Invasive Fungal Pneumonia in Immunocompromised Patients

Myrna C.B. Godoy, MD, PhD[a],*, Hanna R. Ferreira Dalla Pria, MD[a],
Mylene T. Truong, MD[a], Girish S. Shroff, MD[a], Edith M. Marom, MD[b]

KEYWORDS

- Hematopoietic stem cell transplantation • Adverse effects • Pulmonary aspergillosis
- Pulmonary mucormycosis • Pulmonary candidiasis • Fungal pneumonia
- Computed X- ray tomography

KEY POINTS

- In the setting of hematopoietic stem cell transplantation (HSCT) most invasive fungal infections occur in the neutropenic or preengraftment phase (up to 2–3 weeks after HSCT) and are most commonly caused by *Aspergillus, Mucor, Fusarium,* and *Candida* species.
- The typical CT findings of angioinvasive aspergillosis include nodules (>1 cm) or masses surrounded by a halo of ground-glass attenuation ("CT halo sign") and pleural-based, wedge-shaped areas of consolidation, the latter representing hemorrhagic infarction.
- The reversed halo sign (RHS) on CT is characterized by a central ground-glass opacity surrounded by a complete or incomplete ring of consolidation and is suspicious for pulmonary mucormycosis in immunosuppressed patients, especially in the context of concomitant sinusitis and prior voriconazole prophylaxis.
- The noninfectious complications seen in the neutropenic phase of HSCT (pulmonary edema, diffuse alveolar hemorrhage, drug toxicity, idiopathic pneumonia syndrome, and engraftment syndrome), in contrast to fungal infection, tend to present with a diffuse pattern of disease.

INTRODUCTION

Immunocompetent individuals are estimated to inhale hundreds of fungal conidia daily without developing a clinical infection. By contrast, many patients with hematologic malignancies (HM) or hematopoietic stem cell transplantation (HSCT) recipients have impaired antifungal defenses, which lead to a disproportionate number of fungal pneumonias in these hosts.[1]

HSCT is a well-established treatment of various oncologic and hematologic diseases. Pulmonary complications, including infectious and noninfectious conditions, are common in HSCT recipients. Invasive fungal infections (IFIs) remain a leading cause of morbidity in patients with HM/HSCT, associated with a high mortality rate, despite widespread use of antifungal prophylaxis in the last 30 years.

Imaging, particularly CT, plays an important role in the diagnosis of these potentially life-threatening complications. Appropriate image interpretation of the posttransplant patient requires a combination of pattern recognition and knowledge of the clinical setting. A specific pattern of involvement can help suggest a likely diagnosis

The authors have nothing to disclose.
[a] Department of Thoracic Imaging, The University of Texas MD Anderson Cancer Center, 1515 Holcombe Boulevard, Unit 371, Houston, TX 77030, USA; [b] Department of Diagnostic Radiology, The Chaim Sheba Medical Center, Affiliated with the Tel Aviv University, 2 Derech Sheba St, Ramat Gan 5265601, Israel
* Corresponding author. Department of Thoracic Imaging, The University of Texas MD Anderson Cancer Center, 1515 Holcombe Boulevard, Unit 371, Houston, TX 77030.
E-mail address: mgodoy@mdanderson.org

radiologic.theclinics.com

in some specific cases. Polymerase chain reaction analysis and serologic tests, used in combination with imaging findings, have improved the timeliness and accuracy of diagnosis of IFIs. This review describes the CT imaging features of the most common invasive fungal pneumonias (IFPs) in patients with HM/HSCT.

Basic Principles of Hematopoietic Stem Cell Transplantation

HSCT is a widely used treatment that involves the ablation of bone marrow with either high-dose chemotherapy and/or total body radiation therapy and transfusion of pluripotent stem cells to repopulate the bone marrow and restore hematopoiesis.[2,3] It is used not only in the treatment of HM, such as leukemia, lymphoma, and multiple myeloma but also in some solid organ malignancies, such as breast, germ cell tumors, renal, and ovarian tumors; aplastic anemia; congenital immunodeficiency syndromes; thalassemia; sickle cell anemia; and amyloidosis.[4] Additionally, more recently, this treatment has been increasingly used in immunologic conditions, such as multiple sclerosis, immune cytopenia, systemic sclerosis, systemic lupus erythematosus, rheumatoid arthritis, and Crohn's disease.[4]

The term HSCT is currently favored over bone marrow transplantation because a variety of potential sources of stem cells can be used, including bone marrow, peripheral blood, and fetal cord blood.[5] Types of HSCT include autologous stem cell transplantation (patient's own stem cells are used), allogeneic stem cell transplantation (stem cells used are typically from a relative or nonrelative leukocyte antigen (HLA) matched donor) or syngeneic (donated by the patient's identical twin).[5] Engraftment usually occurs over a period of 2 to 4 weeks, during which time the patient is wholly dependent on blood products and antibiotic, antifungal and antiviral therapy. This is followed by the slow reconstitution of the immune system, which takes at least 1 year to completely recover.[6]

Timeline of Pulmonary Complications

A wide variety of pulmonary complications including both infectious and noninfectious etiologies can occur following HSCT. Different complications tend to predominate at specific phases following transplantation, as a reflection of changes in patients' immune status. Most IFIs occur in the first phase after HSCT, the neutropenic or preengraftment phase (up to 2–3 weeks after HSCT), when patients are profoundly neutropenic and at severe risk for bacterial and fungal infections. Fungal infections occur in up to 10% of patients undergoing HSCT and have a reported mortality rate of 80% to 90%.[1] It has been shown that survival can be improved with the early administration of antifungal therapy.[7] The fungal pneumonias are most commonly caused by *Aspergillus, Mucor, Fusarium,* and *Candida* species.[1,8] Noninfectious complications that occur during the neutropenic phase include pulmonary edema, diffuse alveolar hemorrhage (DAH), idiopathic pneumonia syndrome (IPS), and engraftment syndrome (also known as periengraftment respiratory distress syndrome or PERDS).[3]

During the second phase post-HSCT, the early posttransplantation phase (2–3 weeks to 100 days after HSCT), the focus of risk shifts to viral disease, particularly cytomegalovirus (CMV) pneumonia, as well as other opportunistic infections, such as *Pneumocystis jiroveci* pneumonia (PJP). In the late posttransplantation phase (beyond 100 days after HSCT), the main pulmonary complications include bronchiolitis obliterans (BO) and cryptogenic organizing pneumonia (COP), which can be related to chronic graft-versus-host disease.[9]

Clinical Manifestations of Invasive Fungal Pneumonia

Due to immunosuppression, HSCT recipients presenting with pulmonary complications may not necessarily have signs of infection, such as fever and leukocytosis. A detailed clinical history including knowledge of the underlying condition requiring HSCT, type of HSCT, time frame since HSCT, exposures, and adherence to posttransplant prophylaxis medications can aid in narrowing the broad differential.[10] Persistent fevers, cough, chest pain, progressive dyspnea, and hemoptysis are among the clinical features that can be encountered in cases of fungal pneumonia, which may require further investigation.[11]

Invasive and noninvasive tests are used in the diagnosis of fungal pneumonia. Historically, the challenging diagnosis of pulmonary disease after HSCT required lung biopsy. However, recent advancements in diagnosis and therapy for respiratory infections have changed how clinicians approach pulmonary abnormalities, with a marked decline in lung biopsies during the last 2 decades.[12] The standard clinical workup for suspected fungal pneumonia can include serum galactomannan (GM), respiratory viral panel, other bloodwork, and imaging, including chest radiographs and/or computed tomography (CT) (See Brixey and colleagues' article, "Non-Imaging Diagnostic Tests For Pneumonia,"in this issue).

The diagnostic yield of sputum culture and bronchoalveolar lavage (BAL) is often low.[10]

Chest CT and radiography play crucial roles in establishing the likelihood of pneumonia during the infectious workup of HSCT recipients. Chest radiographs are often the first-line imaging obtained during an infectious workup in patients with HSCT given their wide availability and low cost. Radiographs may demonstrate features of pneumonia, as well as provide information about the overall extent of disease/severity; however, in cases whereby the radiographs are normal or when only minimal/subtle features of potential infection are demonstrated, a chest CT should be obtained. CT has higher sensitivity than radiographs in detecting pneumonia and high negative predictive value in excluding pneumonia.[10] Therefore, a normal CT study would suggest an extrapulmonary source of infection. Moreover, specific CT patterns can help narrow the differential diagnosis and, in some instances, suggest a specific etiology.

Computed Tomography Findings of Invasive Fungal Infection

Invasive fungal pneumonias (IFPs) predominate the neutropenic phase when patients are at severe risk for bacterial and fungal infections. The typical CT findings of IFIs include lung nodules of 1 cm or more, lung masses, segmental or subsegmental consolidation—often as a result of pulmonary infarction, and several associated signs: the CT halo sign, reversed halo sign (RHS), hypodense sign, and the air-crescent sign, which are discussed later in discussion.[5,13] These CT findings are the major clinical criteria for diagnosing probable IFP.[8]

Other infections can mimic fungal pneumonia in patients with HSCT including bacterial, viral, or less commonly mycobacterial infections. Large nodules, larger than 1 cm, and the presence of the CT halo sign or the RHS are more suggestive of fungal rather than bacterial or viral etiologies.[14]

Invasive Pulmonary Aspergillosis

Pulmonary aspergillosis consists of a clinical spectrum of lung diseases caused by *Aspergillus* organisms. *Aspergillus* is a genus of ubiquitous soil fungi. Organisms usually enter the body after the inhalation of spores. The manifestations of pulmonary aspergillosis are determined by the number and virulence of the organisms and the patient's immune response. The spectrum can be subdivided into five categories: saprophytic aspergillosis (aspergilloma), hypersensitivity reaction (allergic bronchopulmonary aspergillosis), semi-invasive (chronic necrotizing) aspergillosis, airway-invasive aspergillosis, and angioinvasive aspergillosis (AIA).[15,16]

Whereas the other forms can occur in immunocompetent and mildly immunocompromised patients, invasive pulmonary aspergillosis (IPA), including airway-invasive aspergillosis and angioinvasive aspergillosis (AIA), occurs almost exclusively in immunocompromised patients with severe neutropenia due to acquired immune deficiency syndrome (AIDS) or HM/HSCT. Angioinvasive infection is the more common of the 2 types.

Aspergillus organisms account for a substantial majority of the documented IFIs in patients with HM/HSCT, with *A. fumigatus* identified more than *A. flavus*, while *A. terreus* and *A. ustus* are increasingly noted in severely immunocompromised populations.[1,10,17]

Airway-invasive aspergillosis

Airway-invasive aspergillosis occurs in up to 10% of cases of invasive aspergillosis and is characterized histologically by the presence of organisms deep to the basement membrane of the airway. Clinical manifestations include acute tracheobronchitis, bronchiolitis, and bronchopneumonia.[5,16] Patients with acute tracheobronchitis usually have normal radiologic findings, but occasionally, tracheal or bronchial wall thickening may be seen on CT (**Fig. 1**). Bronchiolitis is characterized by the presence of centrilobular nodules and branching linear or nodular opacities ("tree-in-bud" appearance). The centrilobular nodules have a patchy distribution in the lung. *Aspergillus* bronchopneumonia results in predominantly peribronchial areas of consolidation indistinguishable from bronchopneumonia caused by other micro-organisms.[5,16,18] Less frequently, lobar consolidation may occur. At pathology, the peribronchial infiltrates represent bronchopneumonia and the nodules represent *Aspergillus* bronchiolitis with a variable degree of peribronchiolar organizing pneumonia and hemorrhage.[18]

Angioinvasive aspergillosis

AIA is the most common form of IPA, histologically characterized by the invasion and occlusion of small to medium-sized pulmonary arteries by fungal hyphae. This leads to the formation of necrotic, hemorrhagic nodules or pleural-based, wedge-shaped hemorrhagic infarcts.[19] The clinical diagnosis is difficult; patients may present with cough, fever, and chest pain. Hemoptysis and pneumothorax may occur, but are rarely a presenting feature and actually can occur during or after recovery from the infection. AIA has a mortality rate of 50% to 85%.[20]

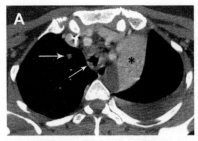
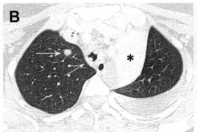
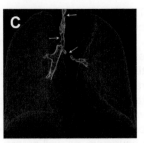

Fig. 1. Airway-invasive Aspergillosis. *Aspergillus* tracheitis in a 41-year-old woman with acute lymphocytic leukemia. (*A, B*) CT images, mediastinal (*A*) and lung (*B*) window settings show extensive circumferential nodular thickening of the wall of the trachea (diagonal *arrows*) and left main bronchus (not shown) with luminal narrowing and obstruction of the left upper lobe bronchus resulting in LUL collapse (*asterisks*). A right upper lobe nodule (horizontal *arrow*) relates to the infectious process. (*C*) 3-D Volume Rendering image better illustrates the craniocaudal extension of disease and the severity of stenosis of the tracheal (horizontal *arrows*) and left main bronchus with obstruction left upper lobe bronchus (diagonal *arrow*). Tracheal biopsy showed extensive necrosis with extensive deposition of fungal-hyphae organisms, compatible with *Aspergillus* species.

The typical CT findings of AIA include nodules (>1 cm) or masses surrounded by a halo of ground-glass attenuation ("CT halo sign") (**Fig. 2**) and pleural-based, wedge-shaped areas of consolidation. The solid central component was shown to correspond to a central fungal nodule/mass surrounded by a halo/rim of hemorrhage and coagulative necrosis, whereas the peripheral wedge-shaped areas of consolidation correspond to hemorrhagic infarcts.[16,21] In severely neutropenic oncologic patients, the halo sign is highly suggestive of AIA. However, the differential diagnosis includes several other conditions, including mucormycosis and candidiasis. The halo sign is considered an early finding of AIA, seen in more than 90% of patients at initial presentation. However, if imaging is performed 1 week later, only approximately 20% of patients will still demonstrate this sign.[5,22]

Occlusion of a vessel leading to a parenchymal lesion (due to fungal invasion) on multi-detector CT pulmonary angiography (CTPA), the so-called CT vessel occlusion sign, has been described as a potentially more sensitive and specific early sign in AIA that may be identified even earlier than the CT halo sign (**Fig. 3**).[23,24] Pseudoaneurysm formation secondary to the vascular damage has also been reported.[25] Although the use of intravenous contrast with a CT angiogram protocol has been shown to add value in the diagnosis and

follow-up of patients with IFPs, the clinical treating team may wish to avoid intravenous contrast in patients with renal dysfunction or those on antifungal therapy at risk for nephrotoxicity.

Additional signs seen in AIA include the hypodense sign (central hypodensity in a lung nodule or mass), the air-crescent sign (collection of air in a crescent shape that separates the wall of a cavity from an inner mass), and the RHS (central area of ground-glass opacity surrounded by a ring of consolidation), all of them representing lung necrosis.[13,26]

The hypodense sign is a highly specific feature of fungal infection and represents a relative hypodensity/low attenuation within the pulmonary nodule.[27] The hypodense sign is a precursor to cavitation and the air crescent sign (**Fig. 4**), which is a late finding, specific for IPA, often occurring 2 to 3 weeks after the initiation of treatment and improvement in neutropenia. It indicates air occupying the space between retracted necrotic lung tissue and the surrounding healthy lung parenchyma.[10] This sign is also not pathognomonic of aspergillosis, but in the setting of severe immunosuppression, it is highly suggestive of invasive fungal disease.[5,13] The RHS is more frequently seen in pulmonary zygomycosis (PZ), although also present in AIA, and will be described subsequently.

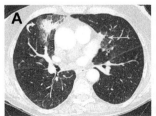
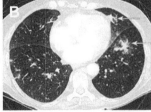

Fig. 2. Angioinvasive aspergillosis in a 27-year-old woman with acute myelocytic leukemia. CT images (*A, B*) show multiple pulmonary nodules (*arrows*) and an area of mass-like consolidation in the right middle lobe (curved *arrow*), with surrounding ground-glass opacities, consistent with the CT halo sign. The bronchoalveolar lavage showed a highly positive *Aspergillus* antigen (Galactomannan test).

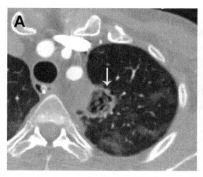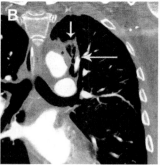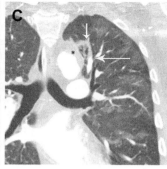

Fig. 3. Angioinvasive aspergillosis in a 46-year-old man with acute myelocytic leukemia following hematopoietic stem cell transplant. Axial CT (*A*) shows the left upper lobe cavitary nodule (vertical *arrow*). Coronal reformations with soft tissue (*B*) and lung windows (*C*) show the vessel occlusion sign with an irregular cutoff of the left upper lobe apicoposterior segmental pulmonary artery (horizontal *arrows*). Note direct involvement of the abutting transverse aorta (*asterisks*).

The most important factor in the management of aspergillosis is a timely and accurate diagnosis. It is important to identify the fungus because of the spectrum of sensitivity to available drugs. For instance, voriconazole, the drug of choice for aspergillosis, does not cover zygomycetes.[28] An early diagnosis of IPA with timely intravenous antimycotic therapy has been shown to significantly impact the survival rate. In a study by Von Eiff and colleagues,[29] delayed the initiation of antifungal treatment later than 10 days after the onset of pulmonary aspergillosis resulted in a mortality rate of 90%, as compared with 41% with an earlier start of antimycotics.

Pulmonary zygomycosis (mucormycosis)

Pulmonary zygomycosis (PZ), also known as mucormycosis, is an increasingly common and often fatal, opportunistic invasive infection caused by fungi belonging to the class Zygomycetes, order Mucorales, which includes the genera *Rhizopus*, *Mucor*, *Lichtheimia* and *Cunninghamella*.[15,30] Six distinct clinical syndromes are recognized: rhinocerebral, pulmonary, gastrointestinal, cutaneous, disseminated and miscellaneous mucormycosis. Pulmonary infection is the second most common form of presentation, after rhinocerebral mucormycosis.[15] The hallmark of

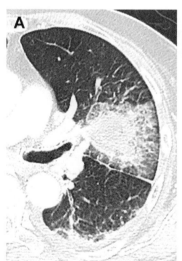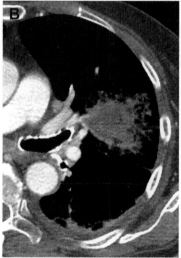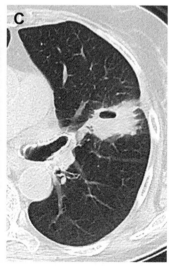

Fig. 4. Angioinvasive aspergillosis in a 75-year-old woman with myelodysplastic syndrome. The patient developed productive cough while undergoing chemotherapy. Initial CT image, lung window settings, shows a left upper lobe mass with the CT halo sign (*A*). Mediastinal window settings image shows the hypodense sign, due to central necrosis, and a small left pleural effusion (*B*). Bronchoalveolar lavage was positive for galactomannan. These findings are consistent with the diagnosis of probable invasive aspergillosis. Follow-up CT imaging (*C*) obtained 3 weeks later shows the interval development of cavitation and decrease in size of the lesion following antifungal therapy. Because cavitation is dependent on leukocyte function, it occurs during bone marrow recovery, and therefore, cavitation usually indicates that the infection is improving.

PZ is rapidly progressive pneumonia that occurs in neutropenic patients, with angioinvasion and tissue necrosis, advancement across tissue planes, and propensity for dissemination. On histopathology, Zygomycetes hyphae are broad and irregular with right-angled branching, as opposed to *Aspergillus* hyphae, which are thinner with more acute-angled branching.[15] Symptoms include fever, cough, chest pain, and dyspnea.[31] Patients with uncontrolled diabetes or ketoacidosis are also at risk for infection, but tend to present a more indolent clinical course with a better outcome than oncologic patients.[15,30,31] In patients with HM and HSCT, reported mortality rates exceed 65% and 90%, respectively, despite aggressive antifungal therapy.[31]

The CT findings of PZ are nonspecific and include progressive lobar or multilobar consolidation (seen in 66% of cases), pulmonary masses (either solitary or multiple, present in 25% of cases), pulmonary nodules (solitary or multiple, present in 16%), the halo sign and the RHS (**Fig. 5**).[13,32,33]

The RHS is characterized by a central ground-glass opacity surrounded by a complete or incomplete ring of consolidation on CT.[33–35] It has also been described as the "atoll sign," because of its resemblance to a coral atoll, and the "bird's nest sign."[35] First reported in COP, it was initially thought to be specific for this disease,[36] but was subsequently described in a variety of pulmonary diseases.[33,37,38] Despite being no longer considered specific, its presence in association with ancillary CT findings and the clinical history can be useful in narrowing the differential diagnosis. High suspicion for pulmonary mucormycosis should be raised in immunosuppressed patients when the CT scan shows the RHS, especially in the context of concomitant sinusitis and voriconazole prophylaxis (**Fig. 6**).[39] RHS can also be seen in patients with IPA, but would be more likely in the absence of prophylaxis.

Cavitation is seen in as many as 40% of cases, with the air-crescent sign reported in approximately 13% of cases.[32] The upper lobes are most commonly involved.[32] It may be associated with mediastinal or hilar lymphadenopathy, vascular invasion with possible development of pulmonary artery pseudoaneurysm, and invasion of contiguous structures such as the chest wall, spine, aorta, pericardium, and diaphragm.[32] Although the invasion of adjacent structures is more frequently seen with PZ, other entities can present similar findings, including AIA (**Fig. 7**) and the so-called "fungal-like" bacterial pneumonias, such as Nocardia and Actinomycosis infections, which can present with nodules or consolidations that cavitate and may involve the pleura or chest wall.[40]

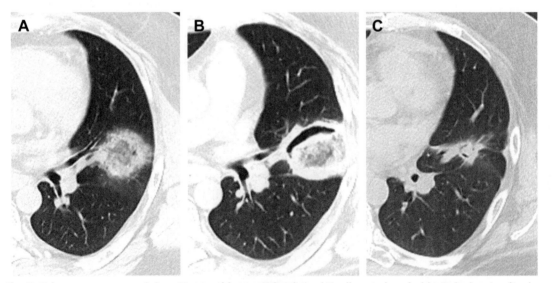

Fig. 5. Pulmonary zygomycosis in a 40-year-old man with relapsed T-cell acute lymphoblastic leukemia after hematopoietic stem cell transplantation undergoing chemotherapy. The patient presented with fever. Initial chest CT scan (*A*) shows a left upper lobe mass with central ground-glass attenuation (RHS). Similar lesions are seen in the lower lobe (not shown). Bronchioloalveolar lavage (BAL) was negative. Subsequent imaging obtained 40 days later (after the improvement of patient's neutropenia) (*B*) shows the development of cavitation with an air crescent sign. There was an increase in size and attenuation of the lower lobe lesions. Biopsy showed branched fungal hyphae compatible with Mucor/Rhizopus and infarcted and hemorrhagic tissue. Silver stain showed positive fungal structures. Progressive improvement was seen after antifungal therapy covering mucormycosis, as demonstrated in a CT obtained 8 months later (*C*).

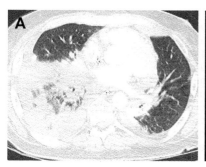 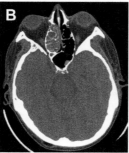

Fig. 6. Pulmonary zygomycosis in a 53-year-old man with chronic myelocytic leukemia. (A) Chest CT image shows a large mass-like consolidation involving the right lower lobe with a central ground-glass opacity, consistent with the reversed halo sign (RHS). The bronchoalveolar lavage showed numerous broad, aseptate fungal hyphae, consistent with zygomycetes. (B) Maxillofacial CT image shows sinonasal opacification primarily on the right side which included the ethmoid, frontal (not shown), and maxillary (not shown) sinuses. Biopsy of the ethmoid sinus showed fungal hyphae and necrosis, consistent with invasive fungal sinusitis. Although the RHS can also be seen in patients with invasive pulmonary aspergillosis its presence in immunosuppressed patients is, by itself, highly suspicious for pulmonary mucormycosis. Mucormycosis is still more likely in the context of concomitant sinusitis and voriconazole prophylaxis.

Distinguishing between the AIA and PZ based on CT findings alone is difficult. Features that favor mucormycosis over aspergillosis include the presence of multiple nodules (≥10) and, to a lesser degree, the presence of pleural effusions at initial CT.[39] The RHS is more commonly encountered with mucormycosis than aspergillosis (54% vs 6%, respectively).[25,41] Similarly, invasion of contiguous structures is more often seen with PZ.

Pulmonary candidiasis

Candidiasis is an infection caused by *Candida* species, most commonly *Candida albicans*. Candida, such as *Aspergillus* and *Mucoraceae*, are ubiquitous fungi. Risk factors for the development of *Candida* pneumonia include AIDS, chemotherapy-induced neutropenia, and HM/HSCT.[42] The prophylactic use of "azole" medications (such as fluconazole) has significantly decreased the rate of candidiasis in immunosuppressed patients.[10] Two main mechanisms of

pulmonary infection include the aspiration of contaminated oropharyngeal secretions and hematogenous dissemination.[5]

The CT finding in *Candida* pneumonia can overlap significantly with those discussed previously, including the presence of pulmonary nodules, reported in 88% to 95% of cases, and areas of consolidation in 50% to 65%.[42,43] Nodules range from 3 to 30 mm in diameter and may present as the only finding (24%) or as the predominant finding (65%). They can be centrilobular or random distribution (**Fig. 8**). Centrilobular nodules are more common in aspergillosis than candidiasis (96% vs 52%) while random nodules are more common in candidiasis than aspergillosis (48% vs 4%), probably representing hematogenous spread in reported cases of candidiasis.[43] Other findings frequently associated with nodules in *Candida* pneumonia include ground-glass opacities (35%), airspace consolidation, tree-in-bud opacities and the CT halo sign (33%).[42,43] Cavitation is less common (4%).[43]

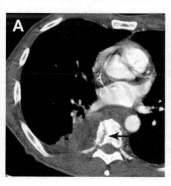 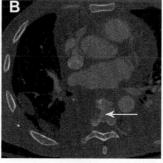

Fig. 7. Pulmonary angioinvasive aspergillosis in 78-year-old man with acute myelocytic leukemia. (A) CT image, mediastinal window settings, shows a right lower lobe mass with the hypodense sign, consistent with necrosis, which involves the right paraspinal region and is associated with lytic changes in the adjacent vertebral body (arrow), suspicious for invasive fungal pneumonia, with associated osteomyelitis. (B) CT image obtained 10 days later, bone window settings show an increase in size of the mass with progressive destruction of the right lateral aspect of the abutting vertebral body (arrow). Bilateral moderate-sized pleural and pericardial effusions are present. The patient underwent right lower lobectomy. Pathology showed extensive necrosis with granulomatous inflammation and numerous fungal organisms consistent with *Aspergillus* species with prominent vascular permeation. Although the invasion of adjacent structures is more frequently seen in cases of mucormycosis, other invasive pneumonias can present with similar findings, as illustrated here in a patient with AIA.

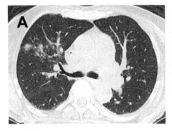
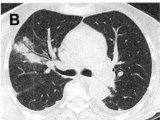

Fig. 8. Pulmonary Candidiasis in a 75-year-old woman with acute myelocytic leukemia undergoing chemotherapy. The patient presented with hypotension and no fever. CT image (*A*) shows poorly marginated clustered pulmonary nodules in the right upper lobe with predominant centrilobular distribution. She then presented with fever and dry cough. A repeat CT 6 days later (*B*) shows the development of consolidation in the right upper lobe. Bronchoalveolar lavage was positive for *Candida glabrata*.

Pulmonary fusariosis

Fusarium species have been increasingly recognized as lethal pathogens in patients with HM. The *Fusarium* species are soil saprophytes and plant and bacterial pathogens. Only a few of the 50 different species have been reported as pathogenic in humans. Among these, *Fusarium solani* has the highest virulence, causing half of the reported human fusariosis cases. This infection is typically acquired through the inhalation of airborne conidia that germinate and invade lung blood vessels in the setting of profound, sustained immunosuppression.[44,45]

The clinical symptoms of pulmonary fusariosis are nonspecific and may include fever and sinopulmonary symptoms. *Fusarium* has a worse outcome and fewer therapeutic options than the much more common aspergillosis.[44,45]

Nodules or masses are the most common findings at CT, seen in 82% of patients (**Fig. 9**). Nodules have been reported in the range of 3 to 27 mm and masses 3 to 6.7 cm. The halo sign and tree-in-bud opacities are not commonly seen. Additional findings include pleural effusions, pericardial effusion, and mild (<1.5 cm) mediastinal or hilar adenopathy.[44]

Differential Diagnosis

Noninfectious complications seen in the neutropenic phase include pulmonary edema, DAH, drug toxicity, IPS, and engraftment syndrome.[3] In contrast to fungal infection, noninfectious complications in this phase tend to present with a diffuse pattern of disease. Pulmonary edema manifests as prominent pulmonary vessels, interlobular septal thickening, ground-glass opacities, and pleural effusions. DAH and drug reactions manifest as bilateral areas of ground-glass attenuation or consolidation, with the development of reticulation at a later stage.[3,46] Among infectious complications, several diseases can cause nonspecific findings, such as nodules and consolidations. In particular, bacterial pneumonias are also frequently seen in the neutropenic phase. However, more specific findings such as the halo sign, RHS, and hypodense sign can aid in the diagnosis.

In conclusion, imaging plays an important role in the early detection and management of immunosuppressed patients with IFIs. Appropriate image interpretation requires a combination of pattern recognition, knowledge of the clinical setting, and awareness of the main differential diagnosis when imaging patients with HM or following HSCT. Details regarding the underlying condition requiring stem cell transplantation, type of stem cell transplantation, time frame since stem cell transplantation, exposures, and adherence to posttransplant prophylaxis medications help support the radiologic interpretation of potential complications. Radiologists should be familiar with the subtle features that may help to differentiate these various fungal infections.

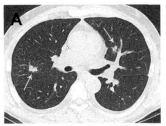
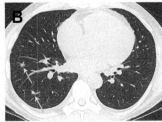

Fig. 9. Pulmonary Fusariosis in a 53-year-old man with acute myelocytic leukemia, after hematopoietic stem cell transplantation presenting with disseminated *Fusarium* infection. CT images (*A, B*) show multiple bilateral irregular pulmonary nodules measuring up to 1.6 cm (*arrows*) and small bilateral pleural effusions. Note lack of the CT halo sign, which is not usually seen in pulmonary fusariosis, as opposed to the other invasive fungal pneumonias.

CLINICS CARE POINTS

- Pulmonary complications, including infectious and non-infectious conditions, are common in HSCT recipients. Invasive fungal infections (IFIs) remain a leading cause of morbidity in HM/HSCT patients, associated with a high mortality rate, despite widespread use of antifungal prophylaxis in the last 30 years. Fungal infections occur in up to 10% of patients undergoing HSCT and have a reported mortality rate of 80 to 90%.[1] It has been shown that survival can be improved with early administration of antifungal therapy.[7]

- Most IFIs occur in the first phase after HSCT, the neutropenic or pre-engraftment phase (up to 2-3 weeks after HSCT), when patients are profoundly neutropenic and at severe risk for bacterial and fungal infections. The fungal pneumonias are most commonly caused by *Aspergillus, Mucor, Fusarium and Candida* species.[1,8]

- Due to immunosuppression, HSCT recipients presenting with pulmonary complications may not necessarily have signs of infection, such as fever and leukocytosis. A detailed clinical history including knowledge of the underlying condition requiring HSCT, type of HSCT, time frame since HSCT, exposures, and adherence to post-transplant prophylaxis medications can aid in narrowing the broad differential.[10] Persistent fevers, cough, chest pain, progressive dyspnea and hemoptysis are among the clinical features that can be encountered in cases of fungal pneumonia, which may require further investigation.[11]

- Noninfectious complications that occur during the neutropenic phase include pulmonary edema, diffuse alveolar hemorrhage (DAH), idiopathic pneumonia syndrome (IPS), and engraftment syndrome (also known as peri-engraftment respiratory distress syndrome or PERDS).[3]

REFERENCES

1. Young AY, Leiva Juarez MM, Evans SE. Fungal pneumonia in patients with hematologic malignancy and hematopoietic stem cell transplantation. Clin Chest Med 2017;38(3):479–91.

2. Coy DL, Ormazabal A, Godwin JD, et al. Imaging evaluation of pulmonary and abdominal complications following hematopoietic stem cell transplantation. Radiographics 2005;25(2):305–17 [discussion: 318].

3. Peña E, Souza CA, Escuissato DL, et al. Noninfectious pulmonary complications after hematopoietic stem cell transplantation: practical approach to imaging diagnosis. Radiographics 2014;34(3): 663–83.

4. Ljungman P, Urbano-Ispizua A, Cavazzana-Calvo M, et al. Allogeneic and autologous transplantation for haematological diseases, solid tumours and immune disorders: definitions and current practice in Europe. Bone Marrow Transpl 2006;37(5):439–49.

5. Shroff GS, Marom EM, Wu CC, et al. Imaging of pneumonias and other thoracic complications after hematopoietic stem cell transplantation. Curr Probl Diagn Radiol 2019;48(4):393–401.

6. Evans A, Steward CG, Lyburn ID, et al. Imaging in haematopoietic stem cell transplantation. Clin Radiol 2003;58(3):201–14.

7. Caillot D, Casasnovas O, Bernard A, et al. Improved management of invasive pulmonary aspergillosis in neutropenic patients using early thoracic computed tomographic scan and surgery. J Clin Oncol 1997; 15(1):139–47.

8. Ascioglu S, Rex JH, de Pauw B, et al. Defining opportunistic invasive fungal infections in immunocompromised patients with cancer and hematopoietic stem cell transplants: an international consensus. Clin Infect Dis 2002;34(1):7–14.

9. Patriarca F, Poletti V, Costabel U, et al. Clinical presentation, outcome and risk factors of late-onset non-infectious pulmonary complications after allogeneic stem cell transplantation. Curr Stem Cell Res Ther 2009;4(2):161–7.

10. Revels J W, Fadl S A, Wang S S, et al. Imaging features of fungal pneumonia in haematopoietic stem cell transplant patients. Pol J Radiol 2021;86(1): 335–43.

11. Hussien A, Lin CT. CT findings of fungal pneumonia with emphasis on aspergillosis. Emerg Radiol 2018; 25(6):685–9.

12. Cheng GS, Stednick ZJ, Madtes DK, et al. Decline in the use of surgical biopsy for diagnosis of pulmonary disease in hematopoietic cell transplantation recipients in an Era of improved diagnostics and empirical therapy. Biol Blood Marrow Transplant 2016;22(12):2243–9.

13. Godoy MC, Marom EM, Carter BW, et al. Computed tomography imaging of lung infection in the oncologic setting: typical features and potential pitfalls. Semin Roentgenol 2015;50(3):192–6.

14. Escuissato DL, Gasparetto EL, Marchiori E, et al. Pulmonary infections after bone marrow transplantation: high-resolution CT findings in 111 patients. AJR Am J Roentgenol 2005;185(3):608–15.

15. Gazzoni FF, Severo LC, Marchiori E, et al. Fungal diseases mimicking primary lung cancer:

radiologic-pathologic correlation. Mycoses 2014; 57(4):197–208.

16. Franquet T, Müller NL, Giménez A, et al. Spectrum of pulmonary aspergillosis: histologic, clinical, and radiologic findings. Radiographics 2001;21(4): 825–37.

17. Smith JA, Kauffman CA. Pulmonary fungal infections. Respirology 2012;17(6):913–26.

18. Logan PM, Primack SL, Miller RR, et al. Invasive aspergillosis of the airways: radiographic, CT, and pathologic findings. Radiology 1994;193(2):383–8.

19. Denning DW. Invasive aspergillosis. Clin Infect Dis 1998;26(4):781–803.

20. Kousha M, Tadi R, Soubani AO. Pulmonary aspergillosis: a clinical review. Eur Respir Rev 2011;20(121): 156–74.

21. Hruban RH, Meziane MA, Zerhouni EA, et al. Radiologic-pathologic correlation of the CT halo sign in invasive pulmonary aspergillosis. J Comput Assist Tomogr 1987;11(3):534–6.

22. Caillot D, Couaillier JF, Bernard A, et al. Increasing volume and changing characteristics of invasive pulmonary aspergillosis on sequential thoracic computed tomography scans in patients with neutropenia. J Clin Oncol 2001;19(1):253–9.

23. Sonnet S, Buitrago-Téllez CH, Tamm M, et al. Direct detection of angioinvasive pulmonary aspergillosis in immunosuppressed patients: preliminary results with high-resolution 16-MDCT angiography. AJR Am J Roentgenology 2005;184(3):746–51.

24. Stanzani M, Sassi C, Lewis RE, et al. High resolution computed tomography angiography improves the radiographic diagnosis of invasive mold disease in patients with hematological malignancies. Clin Infect Dis 2015;60(11):1603–10.

25. Wahba H, Truong MT, Lei X, et al. Reversed halo sign in invasive pulmonary fungal infections. Clin Infect Dis 2008;46(11):1733–7.

26. Potente G. Computed tomography in invasive pulmonary aspergillosis. Acta Radiologica 1989;30(6):587–90.

27. Horger M, Einsele H, Schumacher U, et al. Invasive pulmonary aspergillosis: frequency and meaning of the "hypodense sign" on unenhanced CT. Br J Radiol 2005;78(932):697–703.

28. Livio P, Luana F, Morena C. Pulmonary aspergillosis in hematologic malignancies: lights and shadows. Haematologica 2008;93(11):1611–6.

29. von Eiff M, Roos N, Schulten R, et al. Pulmonary aspergillosis: early diagnosis improves survival. Respiration 1995;62(6):341–7.

30. McAdams HP, Rosado-de-Christenson ML, Templeton PA, et al. Thoracic mycoses from opportunistic fungi: radiologic-pathologic correlation. Radiographics 1995;15(2):271–86.

31. Ibrahim AS, Kontoyiannis DP. Update on mucormycosis pathogenesis. Curr Opin Infect Dis 2013; 26(6):508–15.

32. McAdams HP, Rosado de Christenson M, Strollo DC, et al. Pulmonary mucormycosis: radiologic findings in 32 cases. AJR Am J Roentgenology 1997;168(6):1541–8.

33. Godoy MC, Viswanathan C, Marchiori E, et al. The reversed halo sign: update and differential diagnosis. Br J Radiol 2012;85(1017):1226–35.

34. Hansell DM, Bankier AA, MacMahon H, et al. Fleischner society: glossary of terms for thoracic imaging. Radiology 2008;246(3):697–722.

35. Zompatori M, Poletti V, Battista G, et al. Bronchiolitis obliterans with organizing pneumonia (BOOP), presenting as a ring-shaped opacity at HRCT (the atoll sign). A case report. Radiol Med 1999;97(4):308–10.

36. Voloudaki AE, Bouros DE, Froudarakis ME, et al. Crescentic and ring-shaped opacities. CT features in two cases of bronchiolitis obliterans organizing pneumonia (BOOP). Acta Radiologica 1996;37(6): 889–92.

37. Marchiori E, Zanetti G, Escuissato DL, et al. Reversed halo sign: high-resolution CT scan findings in 79 patients. Chest 2012;141(5):1260–6.

38. Marchiori E, Zanetti G, Hochhegger B, et al. Reversed halo sign on computed tomography: state-of-the-art review. Lung 2012;190(4):389–94.

39. Chamilos G, Marom EM, Lewis RE, et al. Predictors of pulmonary zygomycosis versus invasive pulmonary aspergillosis in patients with cancer. Clin Infect Dis 2005;41(1):60–6.

40. Orlowski HLP, McWilliams S, Mellnick VM, et al. Imaging spectrum of invasive fungal and fungal-like infections. Radiographics 2017;37(4):1119–34.

41. Jung J, Kim MY, Lee HJ, et al. Comparison of computed tomographic findings in pulmonary mucormycosis and invasive pulmonary aspergillosis. Clin Microbiol Infect 2015;21(7):684.e1-8.

42. Franquet T, Müller NL, Lee KS, et al. Pulmonary candidiasis after hematopoietic stem cell transplantation: thin-section CT findings. Radiology 2005; 236(1):332–7.

43. Althoff Souza C, Müller NL, Marchiori E, et al. Pulmonary invasive aspergillosis and candidiasis in immunocompromised patients: a comparative study of the high-resolution CT findings. J Thorac Imaging 2006;21(3):184–9.

44. Marom EM, Holmes AM, Bruzzi JF, et al. Imaging of pulmonary fusariosis in patients with hematologic malignancies. AJR Am J Roentgenology 2008; 190(6):1605–9.

45. Lionakis MS, Kontoyiannis DP. Fusarium infections in critically ill patients. Semin Respir Crit Care Med 2004;25(2):159–69.

46. Worthy SA, Flint JD, Muller NL. Pulmonary complications after bone marrow transplantation: high-resolution CT and pathologic findings. Radiographics 1997;17(6):1359–71.

Pulmonary Infections in People Living with HIV

Tomás Franquet, MD, PhD[a],*, Pere Domingo, MD, PhD[b,c]

KEYWORDS

- Thoracic imaging • Infection • Chest radiography • Computed tomography • People living with HIV

KEY POINTS

- Infection of the lungs and airways by bacterial, viral, fungal, and protozoal agents is common in people living with HIV (PLWH).
- Among PLWH, the combination of clinical and radiographic findings performs better than radiographic findings alone in the detection and follow-up of pneumonia.
- Despite the declining incidence of *Pneumocystis jiroveci* among patients with HIV, *P jiroveci* pneumonia (PJP) may be the presenting illness in PLWH.

INTRODUCTION

The landscape of HIV infection has forever changed since the introduction and massive implementation of combination antiretroviral therapy (cART) in 1996.[1] Before this date, natural history of HIV infection was dominated by a chain of opportunistic infections and cancers uncommon outside the HIV field, the so-called AIDS-defining conditions.[2] The relentless sequence of infections and cancer significantly impacted patients' quality of life, leading to patients' health deterioration and eventually death.[2] In fact, in 1981 the AIDS epidemic was heralded by the appearance of rare cases of pneumonia (*Pneumocystis jiroveci* pneumonia [PJP]) and uncommon skin cancer (Kaposi sarcoma), predominantly in men who had sex with men.[3]

The widespread adoption of cART, initially in high-resource countries, has changed the natural history of the disease, causing unprecedented declines in HIV-associated morbidity and mortality in people living with HIV (PLWH).[4] Immune reconstitution secondary to gaining control of viral replication led to sweeping decreases in AIDS-defining conditions.[5] However, it was noticed that PLWH had an excess of age-associated comorbidities, which

soon became the most common cause of death in otherwise virologically controlled patients.[5] The success of cART caused an unparalleled increase in PLWH life expectancy with better quality of life and a shift in PLWH-associated comorbidities from infectious to noninfectious ones. Such a shift greatly diminished pulmonary infections, which had been a leading cause of morbidity and mortality in the pre-cART era.[6,7]

Since the introduction of cART, life expectancy of PLWH has substantially increased. The number of PLWH is increasing worldwide because of continued spread of disease and improved survival.[8] Three patient scenarios are relevant to pulmonary infections in PLWH.

1. PLWH having unrestricted access to medical care who adhere to modern cART and immunization schedules, and can achieve adequate immune reconstitution levels.
2. PLWH who have discontinued effective cART, who decline to seek medical care or adhere to cART, or who do not respond to cART.
3. PLWH who are unaware of their condition whose infection progresses to advanced stages of immunosuppression.

[a] Department of Diagnostic Radiology, Hospital de la Santa Creu i Sant Pau, Universidad Autónoma de Barcelona, Carrer Sant Quintí, 89, Barcelona 08041, Spain; [b] Department of Infectious Diseases, Hospital de la Santa Creu i Sant Pau, Barcelona, Universidad Autónoma de Barcelona, Carrer Sant Quintí, 89, Barcelona 08041, Spain; [c] Institut de Recerca Biomèdica del Hospital de Sant Pau, Carrer Sant Quintí, 77, Barcelona 08041, Spain
* Corresponding author.
E-mail address: tfranquet@santpau.cat

Scenarios two and three are similar, both characterized by severe CD4 lymphopenia and the appearance of opportunistic infections reminiscent of those seen in the pre-cART era. In scenario one, the incidence of lung infection is superimposable to that of patients not infected by HIV; however, as the patient ages chronic lung disease can contribute to morbidity and mortality. Additional factors may modulate these scenarios including lung damage from host-dependent factors, such as exposure to toxins, smoking, and illicit or recreative drugs. Local ecology may influence the cause of infectious lung diseases, such as the prevalence of tuberculosis (TB) in the community. Finally, chemoprophylaxis or vaccination may modify the incidence of infectious lung disease in PLWH. These include *P jiroveci* primary and secondary prophylaxis, *Mycobacterium tuberculosis* chemoprophylaxis, pneumococcal, meningococcal, influenza, and (more recently) COVID-19 vaccines. All of them are included in the vaccination schedule for PLWH.[9]

Despite these advances, AIDS-related infections (particularly TB) and bacterial infections (particularly pneumonia and bacteremia) continue to be leading causes of hospital admission and in-hospital mortality in PLWH worldwide.[10] In this article, we review the epidemiologic, pathophysiologic, and imaging features of pulmonary infections in PLWH. Conventional chest radiography and chest computed tomography (CT) remain the most useful imaging modalities for evaluation of the immunocompromised patient presenting with a suspected pulmonary infection.

THE SPECTRUM OF INFECTIOUS LUNG DISEASES IN THE MODERN COMBINATION ANTIRETROVIRAL THERAPY ERA

Because of the reasons outlined previously the epidemiology of lung disease, particularly lung infections, has changed remarkably in PLWH over the last decades. Although the incidence of opportunistic infection has declined substantially, respiratory infection caused by opportunistic pathogens remains a significant cause of morbidity and mortality in PLWH.[11]

Currently, bacterial pneumonia ranks first among the causes of pulmonary infectious disease in PLWH, followed by PJP and TB. Endemic fungi, parasites, and viruses may contribute to the burden of infectious pulmonary disease worldwide; however, striking differences in the relative incidence of some pathogens depend on the geographic location.[12]

HIV infection is associated with a greater than 10-fold increase in the incidence of bacterial pneumonia.[13] Additional risk factors are intravenous drug use and smoking.[14] Although bacterial pneumonia can occur throughout the course of HIV infection, its incidence increases as CD4 cell counts decrease.[15] Recurrent bacterial pneumonia was included as an AIDS-defining condition by the Centers for Disease Control and Prevention in 1992. Controlling viral replication is protective against the development of bacterial pneumonia.[15] Data from randomized clinical trials have demonstrated that the risk of bacterial pneumonia is reduced by cART even when the CD4 count is greater than 500 cells/mm^3.[15]

IMAGING APPROACH

The evaluation of respiratory symptoms and suspected pneumonia in PLWH is challenging. Imaging plays a crucial role in the detection and management of PLWH with a suspected respiratory infection. Although some chest radiographic findings are pathognomonic for specific conditions, in most cases, the diagnostic process depends on correlating the chest radiographic findings with the clinical scenario. In some situations, the diagnosis may only be confirmed on follow-up radiologic study and clinical features.[16]

Focal airspace consolidation has been shown to be the most common manifestation of bacterial infection. However, chest radiograph has limited sensitivity for the detection of early infection, being normal in up to 10% of patients with proven pulmonary disease.[17–19] Serial chest roentgenograms can aid detection of pulmonary disease, but faint opacities may be difficult to detect. Furthermore, neutrophil counts are often low, and this may result in a poor inflammatory response, which may further decrease the sensitivity of the chest radiographs.[18]

Although CT is not recommended for the initial evaluation of PLWH with suspected pulmonary infection, it is especially useful in the assessment of patients with respiratory symptoms, a clinical suspicion for pneumonia or bacterial airway infections, and normal or nonspecific chest radiographs.[17,20] In addition, CT is an important adjunct to the physical examination, allowing evaluation for lymphadenopathy in regions that are not externally accessible (eg, mediastinum, intra-abdominal sites), and assessment of internal organs for evidence of infection.

The most common CT patterns in acute pulmonary infections are nodules, tree-in-bud appearance, ground-glass attenuation, consolidation, or a combination. Ground-glass attenuation is a common but nonspecific CT finding that may result from pyogenic, fungal, or viral pneumonia.[20,21] Proof of the cause of pneumonia is not obtained in most cases.

BACTERIAL INFECTIONS

Bacterial infections, including pyogenic airway disease and bacterial pneumonia, are the most common pulmonary infections diagnosed in PLWH. Like persons without HIV infection, the most common bacterial cause of community-acquired pneumonia among PLWH is *Streptococcus pneumoniae*. Other bacteria causing pneumonia include *Haemophilus influenzae*, *Staphylococcus aureus*, and *Pseudomonas aeruginosa*. Less common pathogens include *Legionella*, *Rhodococcus*, and *Nocardia*.

Airway diseases caused by bacterial agents, such as *H influenzae*, *P aeruginosa*, *Streptococcus viridans*, and *S pneumoniae*, also occur with increased frequency in PLWH. These abnormalities are typically absent or subtle on chest radiographs. CT findings consist of bronchial dilatation and wall thickening, tree-in-bud appearance of centrilobular nodules, and branching opacities (**Fig. 1**). Recurrent bacterial bronchitis may lead to bronchiectasis.

Streptococcus pneumoniae

S pneumoniae is the most common causative agent of bacterial pneumonia in PLWH (40% of those for an etiologic diagnosis) and carries a high rate of bacteremia and recurrence.[22] Despite controversies, the introduction of pneumococcal conjugate vaccine together with the classical polysaccharide vaccine has led to recommended immunization schedule with pneumococcal conjugate vaccine 13/polysaccharide vaccine 23. The combination has been demonstrated immunogenic in PLWH; however, the durability of protection remains unknown.[15]

The radiographic presentation of PLWH-associated bacterial pneumonia is like that in persons without HIV infection. Radiographically, acute pneumococcal pneumonia consist of a homogeneous consolidation that crosses segmental boundaries (nonsegmental) but involves only one lobe (lobar pneumonia) (**Fig. 2**). Because the consolidation begins in the peripheral airspaces of the lung, it almost invariably abuts against a visceral pleural surface, either interlobar or over the convexity of the lung.[11] Cavitation and pneumatocele formation are unusual, but when present suggest a polymicrobial infection. Pleural effusion is common and is seen in up to half of patients.

Occasionally, infection may manifest as a spherical focus of consolidation without visible air bronchograms that simulates a mass (round pneumonia) and is commonly located posteriorly and in the lower lobes (**Fig. 3**). Round pneumonia is a rare manifestation of lower respiratory tract infection in adults. It is primarily seen in children because they have poorly developed pathways of collateral ventilation and smaller alveoli. Although round pneumonias are usually caused by *S pneumoniae* or *H influenzae*, the work-up should also include evaluation for Q fever and *Legionella micdadei*.[23] In immunocompromised patients, round pneumonia may be the initial manifestation of a rapidly progressive, life-threatening lung infection.[24]

Haemophilus influenzae

H influenzae ranks second among the causes of bacterial pneumonia with etiologic diagnosis in PLWH.[25] It most often affects PLWH with advanced infection and with a subacute presentation.[25] Other factors that predispose to *Haemophilus* pneumonia include chronic obstructive lung disease (COPD), malignancy, and alcoholism. Pneumonia is often associated with a previous history of upper respiratory tract infection followed by onset of high fever, cough, dyspnea, purulent sputum, and pleuritic chest pain.[26]

The typical radiographic appearance of *H influenza* pneumonia consists of multilobar involvement with lobar or segmental consolidation and pleural effusion (**Figs. 4** and **5**). In 30% to 50% of patients, the pattern is that of lobar consolidation like that of *S pneumoniae*.[27,28]

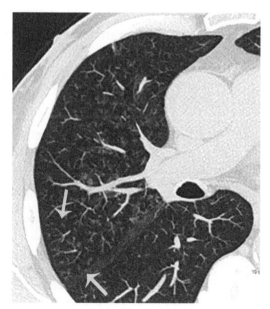

Fig. 1. Pyogenic airway disease. Thin maximum intensity projection reformatted CT image shows diffuse centrilobular branching nodular and linear opacities resulting in a tree-in-bud appearance (*arrows*).

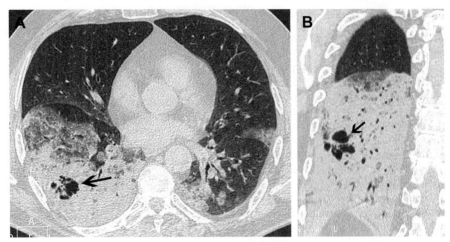

Fig. 2. Pneumococcal pneumonia. (*A*) Axial and (*B*) coronal CT images show heterogenous lobar consolidation with irregular air lucencies caused by necrosis (*arrows*).

Staphylococcus aureus

S aureus is the third most frequent cause of pneumonia in PLWH and is frequently community-acquired.[29] It is usually seen in intravenous drug users who develop tricuspid endocarditis with secondary pulmonary emboli.[30] PLWH have also been disproportionally affected by methicillin-resistant *S aureus* colonization even when on antiretroviral therapy.[31] Risk factors for the development of staphylococcal pneumonia in PLWH include underlying pulmonary disease (eg, COPD, carcinoma), chronic illnesses (eg, diabetes mellitus, renal failure), or viral infection.

The characteristic CT manifestation of *S aureus* is as a bronchopneumonia (lobular pneumonia) with or without cavitation or pneumatocele formation (**Fig. 6**). It is bilateral in approximately 40% of patients.[32] Pyogenic airway infections involving the walls of the bronchi and bronchioles result in airway wall thickening and dilation.[33] Pleural effusions occur in 30% to 50% of patients.

Pseudomonas aeruginosa

P aeruginosa was a common cause of bacterial pneumonia in the pre-cART era.[34] Difficult-to-treat chronic bronchopulmonary infections were described in PLWH with advanced

Fig. 3. Round pneumonia. Chest radiograph shows a masslike area of consolidation in the left upper lobe (*arrow*). Gram stains of sputum demonstrated *Streptococcus pneumoniae*.

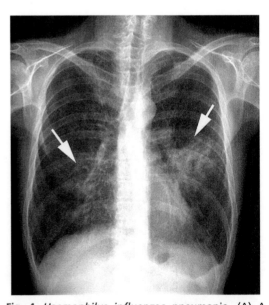

Fig. 4. *Haemophilus influenzae* pneumonia. (A) A 49-year-old man with fever. Posteroanterior chest radiograph shows bilateral areas of consolidation with ill-defined margins (*arrows*). A community-acquired *H influenzae* pneumonia was diagnosed.

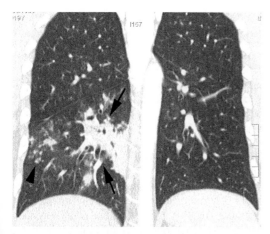

Fig. 5. Bronchopneumonia caused by *Haemophilus influenzae*. Coronal reformatted CT shows a focal area of consolidation in the right lower lobe with visible air bronchogram and poorly defined margins (*arrows*). Also evident are small nodular opacities and a few tree-in-bud opacities (*arrowhead*).

immunosuppression.[35] *P aeruginosa* causes confluent bronchopneumonia that is often extensive and frequently cavitates.

The radiologic manifestations are nonspecific and consist most commonly of patchy areas of consolidation and widespread poorly defined nodular opacities.[36] CT findings consist of multifocal, predominantly upper lobe, airspace consolidation, random large nodules, tree-in-bud opacities, ground-glass opacity, necrosis, and pleural effusion (**Fig. 7**).[37,38]

Other less common pathogens that can cause bacterial pneumonia in PLWH are *Legionella pneumophila*, *Rhodococcus equi*, and *Nocardia*, the two latter appearing in profoundly immunosuppressed patients.

Legionella sp

Legionella pneumonia is an infrequent cause of bacterial pneumonia in PLWH on antiretroviral therapy.[8] Other risk factors for *L pneumophila* pneumonia include posttransplantation, cigarette smoking, renal disease, and exposure to contaminated water.[39]

Imaging findings include consolidation that is initially peripheral, similar to *S pneumoniae* pneumonia. In many cases focal consolidation with a lower lobe predilection enlarges to occupy all or a large portion of a lobe (lobar pneumonia), to involve contiguous lobes, or to become bilateral.[40,41] Rapid progression of multilobar opacities with asymmetric distribution may occur despite an appropriate antibiotic therapy (**Fig. 8**). Occasionally legionella infections may result in a round pneumonia. Unilateral pleural effusions are common.[41]

Rhodococcus equi

R equi is a gram-positive, weak acid-fast coccobacilli that is isolated from the stools of foals. Rhodococcosis is a rare zoonotic infection that occurs in immunocompromised patients, such as transplant recipients and PLWH with a CD4 cell count less than 50 cells/μL. *R equi* pulmonary infection may mimic reactivated TB. Imaging manifestations consists of homogeneous nonsegmental airspace consolidation with or without cavitation, mediastinal or hilar lymphadenopathy, and/or multiple pulmonary nodules (**Fig. 9**).[42]

Nocardia

Nocardiosis is caused by members of the family Nocardiaceae, of which the most important genus is *Nocardia asteroides*. Nocardiosis is a rare cause of pulmonary infection in PLWH. The radiologic appearance of pulmonary nocardiosis is like that seen in immunocompetent patients. The most frequent imaging manifestations consists of homogeneous nonsegmental airspace consolidation that is usually peripheral, abuts the adjacent pleura, and is often extensive. Cavitation is common, seen in one-third or more of patients, and

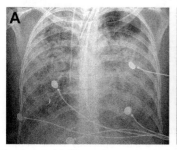
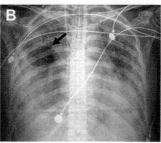
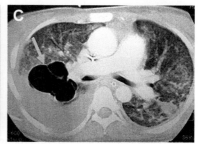

Fig. 6. Methicillin-resistant *Staphylococcus aureus*. (*A*) Portable chest radiograph shows extensive bilateral dense consolidations in upper lobes. (*B*) Follow-up radiograph shows a well-defined air-collection in the upper right lung (*arrow*). (*C*) CT shows a pneumatocele in the upper right lobe (*arrow*). A right pleural effusion is also demonstrated. Community-acquired methicillin-resistant *S aureus* pneumonia was diagnosed.

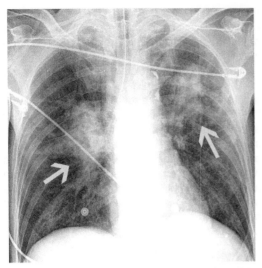

Fig. 7. *Pseudomonas* pneumonia. Portable chest radiograph shows extensive bilateral poorly defined areas of consolidation in the upper lobes (*arrows*).

may occur in areas of consolidation, within nodular opacities, or within masses (**Fig. 10**). Occasionally a halo of ground-glass opacity surrounds the nodule or mass.[43,44] Endobronchial spread can occur and infection can also extend directly to the pleura and chest wall, resulting in pleural effusion and chest wall abscess.[43]

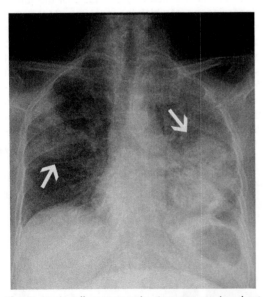

Fig. 8. *Legionella* pneumonia. Anteroposterior chest radiograph shows bilateral dense and poorly defined "rounded" consolidations in the right upper and left lower lobes (*arrows*). Community-acquired *Legionella pneumophila* pneumonia was diagnosed.

Mycobacterium tuberculosis and Nontuberculous Mycobacteria

Although cART reduces the incidence of opportunistic infections its initiation can also trigger a pathologic hyperinflammatory response to viable or dead *M tuberculosis*, known as TB immune reconstitution inflammatory syndrome.[45] Immune reconstitution inflammatory syndrome associated with TB is well recognized among HIV-infected patients initiating cART.

TB and nontuberculous mycobacteria (NTM) have killed more PLWH than any other group of infections. Although its incidence in HIV-infected patients has decreased with the use of antiretroviral therapy, at least one-third of patients infected with HIV worldwide are infected with *M tuberculosis*, and TB is the leading cause of death in PLWH residing in low-income and middle-income countries.[46] TB can occur at any stage of HIV-related disease but, with CD4 cell counts less than 200 cells/mm^3, disseminated infection occurs more frequently.[47]

Overall, the most common NTM resulting in pulmonary disease is the *Mycobacterium avium* complex (MAC).[48,49] NTM infections can appear as a classic form that mimics reactivation TB, in a bronchiectatic form, or as hypersensitivity pneumonitis.[50] Typical radiographic findings of MAC pulmonary infection include upper lobe involvement with or without cavitation (**Fig. 11**).[46,51] The cavities are usually thin-walled and frequently associated with apical pleural thickening. Endobronchial spread of disease is common and manifests as unilateral or bilateral small ill-defined nodules on chest radiograph. CT scan shows the nodules to be centrilobular and frequently

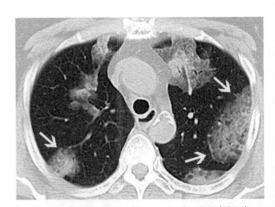

Fig. 9. *Rhodococcus equi* pneumonia. Axial CT shows large, rounded, ground-glass opacities in the periphery of both lungs (*arrows*). A geographic ground-glass pattern is observed in the anterior upper lobes. Patient presented with advanced AIDS and a CD4 cell count less than 100 cells/μL.

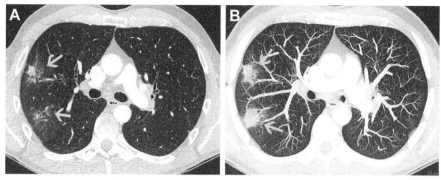

Fig. 10. Nocardial pneumonia. (*A*) CT at the level of the carina shows peripheral subpleural ill-defined nodules with surrounding ground-glass opacity (*arrows*). (*B*) On the thin maximum intensity projection reformatted image an associated halo sign is clearly demonstrated (*arrows*).

associated with branching opacities (tree-in-bud pattern) (**Fig. 12**).[52,53] Multifocal bronchiectasis is the most common radiographic feature of MAC in HIV populations.[48,49]

FUNGAL INFECTIONS

Fungal lung infections can occur in immune-competent and immune-compromised individuals. Their increasing incidence is likely multifactorial but caused in part by a growing population of immunocompromised individuals, including those living in resource-poor settings with a high incidence of HIV infections.

PLWH are at risk of developing fungal infections, which require intact T-cell function for containment. Fungal pneumonias other than PJP have been reported in PLWH, most commonly *Cryptococcus* and *Aspergillus*.[54–56] Other fungal infections are caused by *Histoplasma capsulatum* and *Coccidioides immitis*.[56] Incidence of invasive

pulmonary aspergillosis (IPA) ranging from 3.5 to 19 cases of per 1000 person-years was observed in the 1990s but has substantially decreased with improvement in antiretroviral therapy.[57] Despite antiretroviral therapy, fungal opportunistic pneumonias are an important cause of mortality and morbidity among PLWH.[58]

Pneumocystis jiroveci

Pneumocystis is an opportunistic fungus associated with the AIDS-defining illness PJP. Formerly known as *Pneumocystis carinii*, the species infecting humans has been renamed *P jiroveci*.[54]

PJP was rare in the era before HIV/AIDS but its incidence increased dramatically during the early phases of the AIDS epidemic. PJP also develops in HIV-uninfected patients who are immunocompromised secondary to hematologic or malignant neoplasms, or caused by immunosuppressive therapy for stem cell or solid organ transplantation

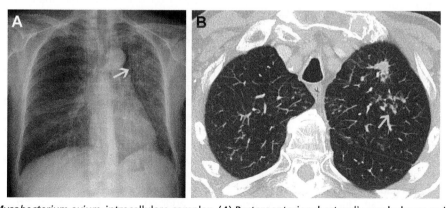

Fig. 11. *Mycobacterium avium*–intracellulare complex. (*A*) Posteroanterior chest radiograph shows an ill-defined left upper lobe opacity (*arrow*) with associated minimal collapse of the left upper lobe. (*B*) Axial CT image at the level of the left upper lobe shows a spiculated nodular opacity. Note the presence of a few tree-in-bud opacities nearby the nodule (*arrow*) representing NTM infection. The differential diagnosis and clinical concern were of a primary lung carcinoma.

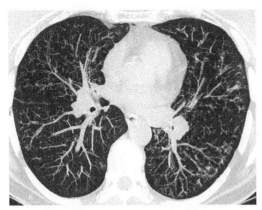

Fig. 12. *Mycobacterium avium*–intracellulare bronchiolitis. CT shows diffuse tree-in-bud opacities by NTM infection.

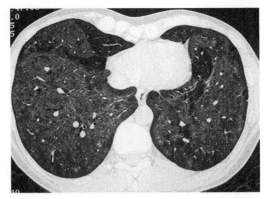

Fig. 13. *Pneumocystis jiroveci* pneumonia. CT shows extensive bilateral and homogeneous ground-glass opacities. Bronchoalveolar lavage showed *P jiroveci*.

or for autoimmune disorders.[55] *Pneumocystis* organisms can colonize the airways of children and adults with acute or chronic syndromes, such as COPD.[14,54]

The widespread implementation of cART and primary and secondary prophylaxis since 1987 dramatically reduced its incidence.[56] Currently, PLWH who fit in scenarios two and three are the most frequently affected, usually when the CD4 count falls to less than 200 cells/mm^3.[59]

Abnormal chest radiographs have been reported in up to 90% of patients with suspected PJP. Imaging findings consist of bilateral perihilar or diffuse symmetric interstitial pattern, which may be finely granular, reticular, or ground-glass in appearance (**Fig. 13**). As the disease progresses, alveolar infiltrates may also develop.

The widespread use of *P jiroveci* prophylaxis has led to a larger proportion of patients presenting with normal radiographs, such that a normal radiograph does not exclude the diagnosis. The most common CT manifestation of PJP consists of patchy or confluent, symmetric, bilateral ground-glass opacities. Less common manifestations include bilateral areas of consolidation, interlobular septal thickening, intralobular linear opacities, cystic lesions, and nodules.[60]

Cryptococcal Disease

Because most symptomatic cryptococcal disease is associated with CD4 counts less than 100/mm^3 its incidence has declined in the cART era. It remains a significant cause of opportunistic infection in PLWH in sub-Saharan Africa and in low- and middle-income countries.[61] The lung is the portal of entry, and cryptococcal pneumonia may present concomitantly or in the absence of cryptococcal meningoencephalitis, which is the most frequent and serious manifestation of cryptococcal infection.[62] HIV-negative patients have atypical presentations and worse outcomes with cryptococcal infection compared with PLWH.[63]

Radiographic features in pulmonary infection are varied and may reveal single or multiple nodular lesions (with or without cavitation), mass lesions, patchy airspace consolidations, interstitial infiltrates, mediastinal or hilar adenopathy, or pleural effusions (**Fig. 14**).[64–66] The most common CT findings consist of reticulonodular opacities, focal or widespread airspace consolidation, and ground-glass opacities.[64]

Invasive Pulmonary Aspergillosis

IPA is usually diagnosed in individuals with impaired immune function; those with neutropenia; solid organ transplant recipients; and patients on multiple drug therapies that suppress granulocyte function, such as high-dose corticosteroids.[11,67] In PLWH, major risk factors for IPA include CD4 cell counts less than 50 cells/mm^3 and neutropenia.[68]

Imaging findings are characterized by multiple, ill-defined, 1- to 3-cm-diameter nodules mainly involving the peripheral lung regions and the lower lobes.[69] Nodules may gradually coalesce into larger masses or areas of consolidation (**Fig. 15**). The classic radiologic finding associated with IPA is the halo sign, which is a rim of ground-glass opacity surrounding a pulmonary nodule.[70,71] The halo sign has also been observed in TB and mucormycosis. Cavitation in the nodules or masses occurs in 40% of affected patients and often results in an air-crescent sign.[34]

In addition, as with bacterial bronchopneumonia, imaging may also show segmental, lobar, or diffuse pulmonary consolidation; pleural-based densities; cavitary lesions; and/or less commonly pleural effusions.[69,71–73]

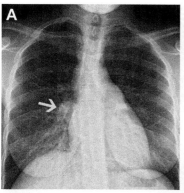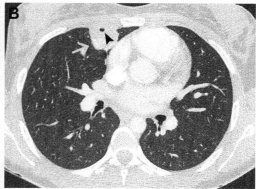

Fig. 14. Cryptococcosis. (*A*) Posteroanterior chest radiograph shows a nodular opacity adjacent to the right heart border (*arrow*). (*B*) Nonenhanced CT shows a cavitated mass in the middle lobe (*arrow*).

Endemic Fungi

Endemic fungi, such as *H capsulatum*, *C immitis*, and *Blastomyces dermatitidis*, may cause infection in PLWH in endemic areas (Southwest United States, northern Mexico, and parts of Central and South America). Latent infections can reactivate in individuals whose immune responses have been compromised, such as by corticosteroid therapy, immune-modulating agents, chemotherapy, or HIV.[74,75] Most cases of histoplasmosis or coccidioidomycosis are disseminated in PLWH with less than 100 CD4 cells/mm^3 (**Figs. 16** and **17**).[76] However, when the CD4 cell count is more than 250 cells/mm^3, focal pneumonia is most common.

Penicillium marneffei, a fungus endemic in Thailand and other countries in Southeast Asia, affects PLWH with greater than 100 cells/mm^3, causing disseminated disease with significant

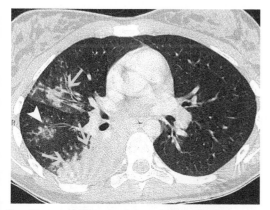

Fig. 15. Aspergillosis. CT image shows a homogeneous consolidation of the apical segment of the right lower lobe (*arrow*). Note the presence of a few tree-in-bud opacities nearby the consolidation (*arrowhead*). A focal consolidation is also visible in the middle lobe (*arrow*).

respiratory involvement.[77] Pulmonary disease can present with a wide range of imaging findings, including reticular opacities, consolidation, single or multiple nodules (including miliary nodules), lymphadenopathy, and pleural effusions.[50,78]

VIRAL INFECTIONS

Influenza is a common cause of respiratory illness in PLWH, although its incidence is reduced in the cART era.[28] During the influenza virus A/h1N1 pandemic, the prognosis of patients on well-controlled cART was similar to uninfected population.[29] International guidelines recommend annual influenza vaccination for PLWH.[8,22]

PLWH are particularly susceptible to pneumonias caused by cytomegalovirus (CMV) and herpesviruses. The presumptive role of CMV as a cause of pneumonia is uncertain until the CD4 cell count falls to less than 50 cells/mm^3. CMV pneumonia incidence in patients with AIDS has decreased dramatically since the introduction of cART.[79] CMV pneumonia, however, continues to be diagnosed in PLWH who fall into scenarios two and three in the introduction.

The CT scan manifestations of CMV pneumonia include multiple small nodular opacities, areas of consolidation, and ground-glass opacities.[80,81] The nodules tend to have a centrilobular distribution reflecting the presence of bronchiolitis. Small nodular opacities have also been reported in patients with adenovirus, influenza virus, herpes simplex virus, and herpes varicella-zoster virus pulmonary infections (**Fig. 18**).[82]

PARASITIC INFECTIONS
Toxoplasma gondii

Toxoplasma gondii is a well-recognized cause of parasitic opportunistic infection of central nervous system in patients with AIDS.[83] Pulmonary

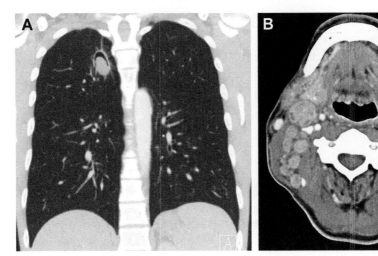

Fig. 16. A 34-year-old man living with HIV with disseminated coccidioidomycosis. (*A*) Necrotic cavity right upper lobe. (*B*) Extensive neck lymphadenopathy. Node biopsy positive for coccidioidomycosis.

toxoplasmosis is an infrequent manifestation of this infection. It can still be seen in the cART era but occurs mainly in patients with advanced immunodeficiency (CD4 cell counts <50 cells/mm³).[84] The clinical and radiologic appearance of *T gondii* pneumonia are indistinguishable from those of PJP.[85]

COVID-19 IN PEOPLE LIVING WITH HIV

Several factors suggest that PLWH could be at increased risk of developing severe COVID-19.[86] Even on cART many PLWH have incomplete immune reconstitution and persistent immune activation. In addition, HIV infection is an independent risk factor for COPD, diffusing capacity impairment, asthma, and pulmonary hypertension. These noninfectious conditions, and the prevalence in PLWH of other risk factors for respiratory infections, such as smoking, are associated with increased COVID-19 severity.[86]

The prevalence of SARS-CoV-2 infection in PLWH ranges from 0.3% to 0.8%, similar to that in the general population. PLWH are reported to make up 0.8% to 2% of those patients hospitalized with COVID-19, which does not suggest increased hospitalization rates among PLWH.[86] Matched cohorts found no significant differences in adverse outcomes in PLWH hospitalized for COVID-19 compared with patients not infected with HIV.[87] A large prospective cohort in Spain, however, found greater age- and sex-standardized mortality from COVID-19 in PLWH than in the general population.[88] Recently, three population studies from the United Kingdom and South Africa concluded that living with HIV raises

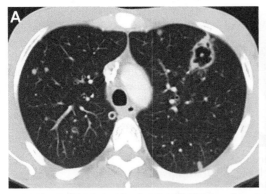
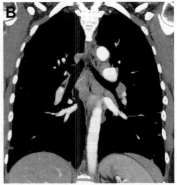

Fig. 17. Man living with HIV with disseminated histoplasmosis. (*A*) Dominant cavity left upper lobe with numerous other nodules, some cavitary. (*B*) Coronal mediastinal window demonstrates modest enlargement of mediastinal and hilar nodes.

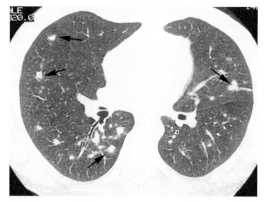

Fig. 18. Cytomegalovirus pneumonia. CT shows multiple scattered, poorly defined nodules (*arrows*) some of them surrounded by a halo of ground-glass opacity.

- Tuberculous and non-tuberculous pulmonary mycobacterial infections are a leading cause of morbidity and mortality in low- and medium-income countries.
- PJP is the most common AIDS-defining pulmonary infection in the era of modern antiretroviral therapy.
- HIV infection does not carry an excess risk of infection by SARS-CoV-2, but it carries a worse prognosis, especially in PLWH with uncontrolled HIV infection.
- Conventional chest radiography and computed tomography remain the most helpful imaging modalities for assessing suspected pulmonary infection in PLWH.

the risk of dying from COVID-19 (from 1.63- to 2.3-fold increased risk), after adjusting for age and other factors.[89,90]

SUMMARY

Although the wide availability of cART in high-income countries has shifted the burden of disease among PLWH toward chronic, age-related morbidities, infection remains a major cause of death and hospitalization worldwide. Infections with pyogenic bacteria, mycobacteria, and fungal pathogens remain more common than in the general population. Differential diagnosis in PLWH who have discontinued cART or were only recently aware of HIV infection and present with profound immunosuppression, differs considerably from PLWH successfully treated with cART. Although imaging manifestations of these infections are pleomorphic and may overlap with one another, knowledge of cART treatment status can help radiologists create a more tailored differential diagnosis and assist clinicians at the bedside.

CLINICS CARE POINTS

- Knowledge of antiretroviral therapy status is of paramount importance in assessing pulmonary infections in PLWH.
- AIDS-related and bacterial infections are the leading causes of pulmonary infection-related morbidity and mortality in PLWH.
- Streptococcus pneumoniae is the most common causative agent of microbiologically-proven bacterial pneumonia.

DISCLOSURE

This work was partially supported by grants PI16/0503, PI17/0420; PI17/0498; PI20/0106; PI20/0137, and COV20/00070, Instituto de Salud Carlos III, Madrid, Spain. PD is supported by a grant from the Programa de Intensificación de Investigadores (INT19/00036)-ISCIII.

REFERENCES

1. Gazzard B. Antiretroviral therapy for HIV: medical miracles do happen. Lancet 2005;366(9483):346–7.
2. Moore RD, Chaisson RE. Natural history of opportunistic disease in an HIV-infected urban clinical cohort. Ann Intern Med 1996;124(7):633–42.
3. Centers for Disease C. Kaposi's sarcoma and *Pneumocystis pneumonia* among homosexual men–New York City and California. MMWR Morb Mortal Wkly Rep 1981;30(25):305–8.
4. Buchacz K, Baker RK, Moorman AC, et al. Rates of hospitalizations and associated diagnoses in a large multisite cohort of HIV patients in the United States, 1994-2005. AIDS 2008;22(11):1345–54.
5. Llibre JM, Falco V, Tural C, et al. The changing face of HIV/AIDS in treated patients. Curr HIV Res 2009; 7(4):365–77.
6. Maitre T, Cottenet J, Beltramo G, et al. Increasing burden of noninfectious lung disease in persons living with HIV: a 7-year study using the French nationwide hospital administrative database. Eur Respir J 2018;52(3):1800359.
7. Wallace JM, Hansen NI, Lavange L, et al. Respiratory disease trends in the Pulmonary Complications of HIV Infection Study cohort. Pulmonary Complications of HIV Infection Study Group. Am J Respir Crit Care Med 1997;155(1):72–80.
8. Benito N, Moreno A, Miro JM, et al. Pulmonary infections in HIV-infected patients: an update in the 21st century. Eur Respir J 2012;39(3):730–45.

9. Iribarren JA, Rubio R, Aguirrebengoa K, et al. Executive summary: prevention and treatment of opportunistic infections and other coinfections in HIV-infected patients: May 2015. Enferm Infecc Microbiol Clin 2016;34(8):517–23.

10. Ford N, Shubber Z, Meintjes G, et al. Causes of hospital admission among people living with HIV worldwide: a systematic review and meta-analysis. Lancet HIV 2015;2(10):e438–44.

11. Skalski JH, Limper AH. Fungal, viral, and parasitic pneumonias associated with human immunodeficiency virus. Semin Respir Crit Care Med 2016; 37(2):257–66.

12. Benito N, Rano A, Moreno A, et al. Pulmonary infiltrates in HIV-infected patients in the highly active antiretroviral therapy era in Spain. J Acquir Immune Defic Syndr 2001;27(1):35–43.

13. Feikin DR, Feldman C, Schuchat A, et al. Global strategies to prevent bacterial pneumonia in adults with HIV disease. Lancet Infect Dis 2004;4(7): 445–55.

14. Gordin FM, Roediger MP, Girard PM, et al. Pneumonia in HIV-infected persons: increased risk with cigarette smoking and treatment interruption. Am J Respir Crit Care Med 2008;178(6):630–6.

15. Garrido HMG, Schnyder JL, Tanck MWT, et al. Immunogenicity of pneumococcal vaccination in HIV infected individuals: a systematic review and meta-analysis. EClinicalMedicine 2020;29-30: 100576.

16. Franquet T. Imaging of pneumonia: trends and algorithms. Eur Respir J 2001;18(1):196–208.

17. Primack SL, Muller NL. High-resolution computed tomography in acute diffuse lung disease in the immunocompromised patient. Radiol Clin North Am 1994; 32(4):731–44.

18. Boersma WG, Daniels JM, Lowenberg A, et al. Reliability of radiographic findings and the relation to etiologic agents in community-acquired pneumonia. Respir Med 2006;100(5):926–32.

19. Basi SK, Marrie TJ, Huang JQ, et al. Patients admitted to hospital with suspected pneumonia and normal chest radiographs: epidemiology, microbiology, and outcomes. Am J Med 2004;117(5): 305–11.

20. Tanaka N, Matsumoto T, Kuramitsu T, et al. High resolution CT findings in community-acquired pneumonia. J Comput Assist Tomogr 1996;20(4):600–8.

21. Primack SL, Hartman TE, Lee KS, et al. Pulmonary nodules and the CT halo sign. Radiology 1994; 190(2):513–5.

22. Saindou M, Chidiac C, Miailhes P, et al. Pneumococcal pneumonia in HIV-infected patients by antiretroviral therapy periods. HIV Med 2008;9(4):203–7.

23. Wagner AL, Szabunio M, Hazlett KS, et al. Radiologic manifestations of round pneumonia in adults. AJR Am J Roentgenol 1998;170(3):723–6.

24. Soubani AO, Epstein SK. Life-threatening "round pneumonia. Am J Emerg Med 1996;14(2):189–91.

25. Cordero E, Pachon J, Rivero A, et al. Haemophilus influenzae pneumonia in human immunodeficiency virus-infected patients. The Grupo Andaluz para el Estudio de las Enfermedades Infecciosas. Clin Infect Dis 2000;30(3):461–5.

26. Johnson SR, Thompson RC, Humphreys H, et al. Clinical features of patients with beta-lactamase producing Haemophilus influenzae isolated from sputum. J Antimicrob Chemother 1996;38(5):881–4.

27. Pearlberg J, Haggar AM, Saravolatz L, et al. Hemophilus influenzae pneumonia in the adult. Radiographic appearance with clinical correlation. Radiology 1984;151(1):23–6.

28. Okada F, Ando Y, Tanoue S, et al. Radiological findings in acute Haemophilus influenzae pulmonary infection. Br J Radiol 2012;85(1010):121–6.

29. Afessa B, Green B. Bacterial pneumonia in hospitalized patients with HIV infection: the pulmonary complications, ICU support, and prognostic factors of hospitalized patients with HIV (PIP) Study. Chest 2000;117(4):1017–22.

30. Kaye MG, Fox MJ, Bartlett JG, et al. The clinical spectrum of Staphylococcus aureus pulmonary infection. Chest 1990;97(4):788–92.

31. Shadyab AH, Crum-Cianflone NF. Methicillin-resistant Staphylococcus aureus (MRSA) infections among HIV-infected persons in the era of highly active antiretroviral therapy: a review of the literature. HIV Med 2012;13(6):319–32.

32. Flaherty RA, Keegan JM, Sturtevant HN. Post-pneumonic pulmonary pneumatoceles. Radiology 1960; 74:50–3.

33. Aviram G, Fishman JE, Boiselle PM. Thoracic infections in human immunodeficiency virus/acquired immune deficiency syndrome. Semin Roentgenol 2007;42(1):23–36.

34. Hirschtick RE, Glassroth J, Jordan MC, et al. Bacterial pneumonia in persons infected with the human immunodeficiency virus. Pulmonary Complications of HIV Infection Study Group. N Engl J Med 1995; 333(13):845–51.

35. Domingo P, Ferre A, Baraldes MA, et al. Pseudomonas aeruginosa bronchopulmonary infection in patients with AIDS, with emphasis on relapsing infection. Eur Respir J 1998;12(1):107–12.

36. Winer-Muram HT, Jennings SG, Wunderink RG, et al. Ventilator-associated Pseudomonas aeruginosa pneumonia: radiographic findings. Radiology 1995; 195(1):247–52.

37. Shah RM, Wechsler R, Salazar AM, et al. Spectrum of CT findings in nosocomial Pseudomonas aeruginosa pneumonia. J Thorac Imaging 2002;17(1):53–7.

38. Okada F, Ono A, Ando Y, et al. Thin-section CT findings in Pseudomonas aeruginosa pulmonary infection. Br J Radiol 2012;85(1020):1533–8.

39. Davis GS, Winn WC Jr. Legionnaires' disease: respiratory infections caused by *Legionella* bacteria. Clin Chest Med 1987;8(3):419–39.

40. Dietrich PA, Johnson RD, Fairbank JT, et al. The chest radiograph in Legionnaires' disease. Radiology 1978;127(3):577–82.

41. Kroboth FJ, Yu VL, Reddy SC, et al. Clinicoradiographic correlation with the extent of Legionnaire disease. AJR Am J Roentgenology 1983;141(2):263–8.

42. Wicky S, Cartei F, Mayor B, et al. Radiological findings in nine AIDS patients with *Rhodococcus equi* pneumonia. Eur Radiol 1996;6(6):826–30.

43. Ahuja J, Kanne JP. Thoracic infections in immunocompromised patients. Radiol Clin North Am 2014; 52(1):121–36.

44. Yoon HK, Im JG, Ahn JM, et al. Pulmonary nocardiosis: CT findings. J Computer Assisted Tomogr 1995; 19(1):52–5.

45. Cevaal PM, Bekker LG, Hermans S. TB-IRIS pathogenesis and new strategies for intervention: insights from related inflammatory disorders. Tuberculosis (Edinb). 2019;118:101863.

46. Henkle E, Winthrop KL. Nontuberculous mycobacteria infections in immunosuppressed hosts. Clin Chest Med 2015;36(1):91–9.

47. Haas MK, Daley CL. Mycobacterial lung disease complicating HIV infection. Semin Respir Crit Care Med 2016;37(2):230–42.

48. Hartman TE, Swensen SJ, Williams DE. *Mycobacterium avium*-intracellulare complex: evaluation with CT. Radiology 1993;187(1):23–6.

49. Pupaibool J, Limper AH. Other HIV-associated pneumonias. Clin Chest Med 2013;34(2):243–54.

50. Ketai L, Jordan K, Busby KH. Imaging infection. Clin Chest Med 2015;36(2):197–217, viii.

51. Restrepo CS, Katre R, Mumbower A. Imaging manifestations of thoracic tuberculosis. Radiol Clin North Am 2016;54(3):453–73.

52. Erasmus JJ, McAdams HP, Farrell MA, et al. Pulmonary nontuberculous mycobacterial infection: radiologic manifestations. Radiographics 1999;19(6): 1487–505.

53. Martinez S, McAdams HP, Batchu CS. The many faces of pulmonary nontuberculous mycobacterial infection. AJR Am J Roentgenology 2007;189(1):177–86.

54. Bienvenu AL, Traore K, Plekhanova I, et al. *Pneumocystis* pneumonia suspected cases in 604 non-HIV and HIV patients. Int J Infect Dis 2016;46:11–7.

55. Cilloniz C, Dominedo C, Alvarez-Martinez MJ, et al. *Pneumocystis* pneumonia in the twenty-first century: HIV-infected versus HIV-uninfected patients. Expert Rev Anti Infect Ther 2019;17(10):787–801.

56. Furrer H, Egger M, Opravil M, et al. Discontinuation of primary prophylaxis against *Pneumocystis carinii* pneumonia in HIV-1-infected adults treated with combination antiretroviral therapy. Swiss HIV Cohort Study. New Engl J Med 1999;340(17):1301–6.

57. Denis B, Guiguet M, de Castro N, et al. Relevance of EORTC criteria for the diagnosis of invasive *Aspergillosis* in HIV-infected patients, and survival trends over a 20-year period in France. Clin Infect Dis 2015;61(8):1273–80.

58. Huang L, Crothers K. HIV-associated opportunistic pneumonias. Respirology 2009;14(4):474–85.

59. Tominski D, Katchanov J, Driesch D, et al. The late-presenting HIV-infected patient 30 years after the introduction of HIV testing: spectrum of opportunistic diseases and missed opportunities for early diagnosis. HIV Med 2017;18(2):125–32.

60. Obmann VC, Bickel F, Hosek N, et al. Radiological CT patterns and distribution of invasive pulmonary *Aspergillus*, non-*Aspergillus*, cryptococcus and *Pneumocystis jirovecii* mold infections: a multicenter study. Rofo 2021;193(11):1304–14.

61. Zavala S, Baddley JW. Cryptococcosis. Semin Respir Crit Care Med 2020;41(1):69–79.

62. Meyohas MC, Roux P, Bollens D, et al. Pulmonary cryptococcosis: localized and disseminated infections in 27 patients with AIDS. Clin Infect Dis 1995; 21(3):628–33.

63. George IA, Spec A, Powderly WG, et al. Comparative epidemiology and outcomes of human immunodeficiency virus (HIV), non-HIV non-transplant, and solid organ transplant associated cryptococcosis: a population-based study. Clin Infect Dis 2018; 66(4):608–11.

64. Friedman EP, Miller RF, Severn A, et al. Cryptococcal pneumonia in patients with the acquired immunodeficiency syndrome. Clin Radiol 1995;50(11):756–60.

65. Zinck SE, Leung AN, Frost M, et al. Pulmonary cryptococcosis: CT and pathologic findings. J Computer Assisted Tomogr 2002;26(3):330–4.

66. Xie LX, Chen YS, Liu SY, et al. Pulmonary cryptococcosis: comparison of CT findings in immunocompetent and immunocompromised patients. Acta Radiol 2015;56(4):447–53.

67. Holding KJ, Dworkin MS, Wan PC, et al. Aspergillosis among people infected with human immunodeficiency virus: incidence and survival. Adult and Adolescent Spectrum of HIV Disease Project. Clin Infect Dis 2000;31(5):1253–7.

68. Mylonakis E, Barlam TF, Flanigan T, et al. Pulmonary aspergillosis and invasive disease in AIDS: review of 342 cases. Chest 1998;114(1):251–62.

69. Franquet T, Muller NL, Gimenez A, et al. Spectrum of pulmonary aspergillosis: histologic, clinical, and radiologic findings. Radiographics 2001;21(4): 825–37.

70. Kuhlman JE, Fishman EK, Burch PA, et al. CT of invasive pulmonary aspergillosis. AJR Am J Roentgenology 1988;150(5):1015–20.

71. Miller WT Jr, Sais GJ, Frank I, et al. Pulmonary aspergillosis in patients with AIDS. Clinical and radiographic correlations. Chest 1994;105(1):37–44.

72. Kuhlman JE. Imaging pulmonary disease in AIDS: state of the art. Eur Radiol 1999;9(3):395–408.

73. Marom EM, Kontoyiannis DP. Imaging studies for diagnosing invasive fungal pneumonia in immunocompromised patients. Curr Opin Infect Dis 2011;24(4):309–14.

74. Lortholary O, Denning DW, Dupont B. Endemic mycoses: a treatment update. J Antimicrob Chemother 1999;43(3):321–31.

75. Sarosi GA, DAvies SF. Endemic mycosis complicating human immunodeficiency virus infection. West J Med 1996;164(4):335–40.

76. Kaplan JE, Benson C, Holmes KK, et al. Guidelines for prevention and treatment of opportunistic infections in HIV-infected adults and adolescents: recommendations from CDC, the National Institutes of Health, and the HIV Medicine Association of the Infectious Diseases Society of America. MMWR Recomm Rep 2009;58(RR-4):1–207.

77. Kawila R, Chaiwarith R, Supparatpinyo K. Clinical and laboratory characteristics of penicilliosis marneffei among patients with and without HIV infection in Northern Thailand: a retrospective study. BMC Infect Dis 2013;13:464.

78. Ketai L, Jordan K, Marom EM. Imaging infection. Clin Chest Med 2008;29(1):77–105, vi.

79. Drew WL. Cytomegalovirus disease in the highly active antiretroviral therapy era. Curr Infect Dis Rep 2003;5(3):257–65.

80. Franquet T. Respiratory infection in the AIDS and immunocompromised patient. Eur Radiol 2004;14(Suppl 3):E21–33.

81. Franquet T, Lee KS, Muller NL. Thin-section CT findings in 32 immunocompromised patients with cytomegalovirus pneumonia who do not have AIDS. AJR Am J Roentgenology 2003;181(4):1059–63.

82. Franquet T. Imaging of pulmonary viral pneumonia. Radiology 2011;260(1):18–39.

83. Porter SB, Sande MA. Toxoplasmosis of the central nervous system in the acquired immunodeficiency syndrome. New Engl J Med 1992;327(23):1643–8.

84. Rabaud C, May T, Lucet JC, et al. Pulmonary toxoplasmosis in patients infected with human immunodeficiency virus: a French National Survey. Clin Infect Dis 1996;23(6):1249–54.

85. Goodman PC, Schnapp LM. Pulmonary toxoplasmosis in AIDS. Radiology 1992;184(3):791–3.

86. Gutierrez MDM, Mur I, Mateo MG, et al. Pharmacological considerations for the treatment of COVID-19 in people living with HIV (PLWH). Expert Opin Pharmacother 2021;22(9):1127–41.

87. Karmen-Tuohy S, Carlucci PM, Zervou FN, et al. Outcomes among HIV-positive patients hospitalized with COVID-19. J Acquir Immune Defic Syndr 2020;85(1):6–10.

88. Del Amo J, Polo R, Moreno S, et al. Incidence and severity of COVID-19 in HIV-positive persons receiving antiretroviral therapy: a cohort study. Ann Intern Med 2020;173(7):536–41.

89. Geretti AM, Stockdale AJ, Kelly SH, et al. Outcomes of COVID-19 related hospitalization among people with HIV in the ISARIC WHO Clinical Characterization Protocol (UK): a prospective observational study. Clin Infect Dis 2020;73(7):e2095–106.

90. Boulle A, Davies MA, Hussey H, et al. Risk factors for COVID-19 death in a population cohort study from the Western Cape Province, South Africa. Clin Infect Dis 2020;73(7):e2005–15.

Nonimaging Diagnostic Tests for Pneumonia

Anupama Gupta Brixey, MD[a],*, Raju Reddy, MD[b], Shewit P. Giovanni, MD, MS[b]

KEYWORDS

- Pneumonia • Diagnosis • Laboratory tests • Bacterial • Fungal • Viral • Culture • Antigen

KEY POINTS

- Interpreting radiologists can narrow the differential diagnosis for suspected pneumonia by combining imaging findings with knowledge of nonimaging diagnostic tests for lung pathogens.
- Results from the recently developed urine pneumococcal antigen (for *Streptococcus pneumoniae*) and urine *Legionella* antigen tests, both of which demonstrate sensitivities of at least 70%, return rapidly and are often available at the time of image interpretation.
- The use of molecular testing and multiplex diagnostic platforms for viral detection in respiratory secretions allow clinicians to identify pathogens with extraordinary high speed and accuracy; however, these results should be correlated with the imaging presentation.
- Bronchoalveolar lavage galactomannan and serum 1 to 3 beta-D-glucan have high specificity and may facilitate a rapid diagnosis of invasive aspergillus in the appropriate clinical setting.

INTRODUCTION

Lower respiratory tract infections that progress to pneumonia are extremely common and account for greater morbidity and mortality than any other type of infection.[1] Of the greater than 5 million cases of community-acquired pneumonias (CAPs) that are diagnosed per year in the United States, approximately 20% require hospitalization with mortality ranging from 12% to 40%.[2]

Broad categories of infection (such as bacterial, fungal, and viral) can occasionally be suggested by characteristic imaging features, but determination of a specific organism by imaging alone is nearly impossible. Although, clinicians usually rely on the radiologist to detect thoracic infections and occasionally to hypothesize the category of the pathogen, further diagnostic testing such as sputum, blood, pleural fluid, and so forth, is usually used. These nonimaging diagnostic tests are often obtained quickly and available to the radiologist when images are interpreted. Understanding these test results can help the radiologist add value by narrowing the differential diagnosis and offering suggestions for further workup.

This article reviews the methodology of available nonimaging diagnostic tests, as well as the commonly used diagnostic tests for the major categories of organisms (bacterial, fungal, viral, and parasitic/protozoan).

METHODS FOR DIAGNOSTIC TESTING— TRADITIONAL

The role of sputum evaluation as a diagnostic tool in directing antimicrobial treatment in CAP is limited. Current guidelines only recommend acquiring pretreatment expectorated sputum Gram stain and culture in adult patients with severe CAP or when risk factors for methicillin-resistant *Staphylococcus aureus* (MRSA) or *Pseudomonas aeruginosa* are present.[3] Blood cultures should not be routinely collected from patients with CAP in the outpatient setting but are recommended before initiation of

[a] Department of Diagnostic Radiology, Section of Cardiothoracic Imaging, Oregon Health and Science University, 3181 SW Sam Jackson Park Road Mail Code L340, Portland, OR 97239, USA; [b] Department of Pulmonary and Critical Care, Oregon Health and Science University, 3181 SW Sam Jackson Park Road, Portland, OR 97239, USA
* Corresponding author.
E-mail address: brixey@ohsu.edu

Radiol Clin N Am 60 (2022) 521–534
https://doi.org/10.1016/j.rcl.2022.01.009

antibiotics in adults with severe CAP or risk factors for MRSA or *P aeruginosa*.[4,5]

Bronchoscopy with bronchoalveolar lavage (BAL) may be required to obtain more definitive samples in immunocompromised patients and can detect a pathogen causing pneumonia in up to 70% to 80% of these patients.[6] Bronchoscopy may also be performed in patients with persistent symptoms and radiologic findings despite antibiotic treatment. Data are scarce on optimal timing of bronchoscopy, but retrospective studies suggest the yield is best if performed within 4 days of initial presentation and before 7 days of completion of antimicrobial therapy.[5]

In the setting of suspected pneumonia diagnostic thoracentesis is often performed when the effusion is greater than 10 or 20 mm in depth on a decubitus radiograph.[5,7] Percutaneous computed tomography (CT)-guided transthoracic needle lung biopsy and surgical lung biopsy are occasionally considered in patients with suspected nonresolving pulmonary infections when less invasive methods are nondiagnostic. Studies have shown that CT-guided lung biopsies revealed the causative organism and changed antibiotic therapy in up to 30% to 40% of cases in which they were performed.[8]

METHODS FOR DIAGNOSTIC TESTING—NEWER METHODS

Respiratory viruses may be detected by viral culture; however, this approach can be too slow to effectively guide acute patient management. Rapid antigen detection kits have turnaround in minutes and are widely available but with low sensitivity.[9] Molecular diagnostic approaches and antigen detection in respiratory secretions through the use of nucleic acid amplification testing (NAAT) have emerged as modern technologies in identifying viruses.[10] NAAT using polymerase chain reaction (PCR), reverse-transcriptase PCR (RT-PCR), and quantitative real-time PCR provide rapid results with sensitivity and specificity approaching 100% and are considered the diagnostic standard for detection of viruses.[9] Samples are most commonly collected from a nasopharyngeal swab.[4]

Urine antigen testing can be used to diagnose significant etiologies of respiratory infections such as *Legionella pneumophilia*, *Streptococcus pneumoniae*, and *Histoplasma capsulatum*, particularly in patients with severe CAP, relevant clinical history, or immunocompromised patients.[5,11]

BACTERIAL PNEUMONIA

Bacterial pneumonias can be classified by mechanism of development (CAP, healthcare-associated [HCAP], hospital-acquired [HAP], or ventilator-associated [VAP]) or by organism ("typical" vs "atypical"). Typical organisms can be Gram stained and cultured on a standard medium and include *S pneumoniae, methicillin-sensitive Staphylococcus aureus,* and *Haemophilus influenzae,* Group A streptococci, gram-negative rods, and anaerobes, among others. Typical organisms often cause CAP but can also cause HCAP and HAP (such as MRSA and *P aeruginosa*), as well as VAP (such as *Acinetobacter* spp, *P aeruginosa,* and multidrug-resistant organisms). Atypical organisms require special media to be cultured and include organisms such as *Legionella* spp, *Mycoplasma pneumoniae,* and *Chlamydia* spp).

C-reactive protein (CRP) is a nonspecific acute-phase protein. Although not specific for pneumonia, in the setting of clinical symptoms, it can be useful in establishing the diagnosis of CAP. High plasma levels of CRP are more common with *S pneumoniae* and *Legionella pneumophila*, as well as with patients with more severe CAP.[12] A threshold of 106 mg/L in men and 110 mg/L in women (normal value <10 mg/L) has been suggested as a determinant of inpatient versus outpatient care for the treatment of CAP (sensitivity 81% and specificity 81%). Furthermore, patients with extremely high levels should be ensured to have antibiotic coverage against both *S pneumoniae* and *L pneumophila*.

For patients with suspected pneumonia, the most common nonimaging test obtained is a complete blood count with differential. In the setting of bacterial pneumonia, leukocytosis is often present (typically with a white blood cell count in the range of 15,000–30,000 cells per mm^3) accompanied by a leftward shift (increased neutrophil count). Leukopenia with a white blood cell count of less than 5000 cells per mm^3 is less common but indicates a poorer prognosis, particularly in pneumococcal pneumonia.[13]

S pneumoniae (eg, pneumococcal pneumonia) is the most commonly identified bacterial organism in CAP.[14] Sputum Gram stain and culture sensitivity have been shown to be as low as 31% and 44%, respectively,[15] and yield drops dramatically when cultures are obtained after administration of antibiotics. Urine pneumococcal antigen test, introduced in 2003, has a sensitivity of 70.4% and a specificity of 89.7%, with results available quickly (**Fig. 1**). Blood cultures are positive in up to 24.8% of patients with pneumococcal pneumonia.[16]

MRSA is an important cause of HAP, HCAP, as well as CAP and VAP, often causing a necrotic pneumonia. If MRSA is suspected, treatment with vancomycin is often instituted but can be

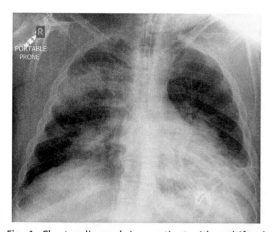

Fig. 1. Chest radiograph in a patient with multifocal consolidation and small left parapneumonic effusion secondary to pneumococcal (*Streptococcus pneumoniae*) pneumonia. Parapneumonic effusions are present in up to one-third of patients with pneumococcal pneumonia.

discontinued if MRSA infection is excluded. Therefore, use of a screening nasal swab for the detection of MRSA colonization has become routine.[17] In a recent meta-analysis, screening the nares for MRSA had a high specificity of 90.3% for ruling out MRSA pneumonia, allowing for de-escalation of antibiotics.[18] Radiologists can exclude MRSA from the differential diagnosis if the nares screening test is negative at the time of dictation.

Legionella species resulting in pneumonia are one of the organisms classified as "atypical" infections as they require a special medium to be cultured. Although there are numerous *Legionella* species, *L pneumophila* (most commonly serotype 1) is the most virulent and is responsible for greater than 95% of infections. Consideration of *Legionella* is important because antibiotic treatment for typical CAP may not cover this organism. In patients with *L pneumophila* serotype 1, antigen test on a urine sample can be performed. In a meta-analysis, the pooled sensitivity of the urine antigen was 74% and the specificity was 99%[19] (Fig. 2). Urine antigen tests and sputum cultures are commonly obtained for diagnosis but PCR testing on sputum or lavage fluid is considered the gold standard.[20]

Nontuberculous mycobacteria (NTM) encompass a large number (greater than 160) of acid-fast positive staining bacteria[21] but a much smaller number of these organisms are associated with pneumonia, typically causing chronic symptoms. Treatment decisions for NTM are complex and are partially based on the presence of cavitary disease, smear-positivity of sputum, as well as the species of NTM (see Faisal Jamal and Mark M Hammer's article, "Nontuberculous Mycobacterial Infections," in this issue).

Given that NTM can demonstrate cavitary lesions by imaging, differentiation of NTM from tuberculous infections is crucial (Fig. 3). Sputum specimens for acid-fast bacteria smear and culture are the mainstay of diagnosis, with at least 3 specimens obtained 24 hours apart in the morning. Smear results will return quickly but cultures can

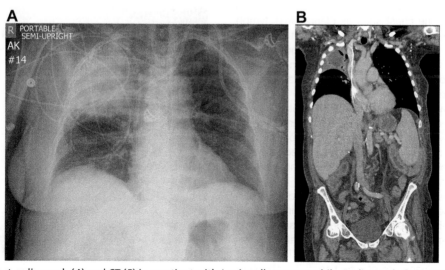

Fig. 2. Chest radiograph (A) and CT (B) in a patient with *Legionella pneumophila*. Radiograph demonstrates focal right upper lobe consolidation. Follow-up chest CT demonstrates hypoattenuating consolidation with internal gas compatible with necrosis. Urine *Legionella* antigen was positive at the time of radiographic imaging, allowing the radiologist to corroborate the imaging findings with test results.

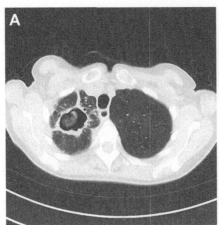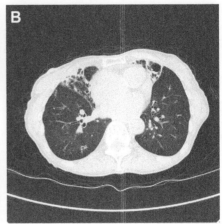

Fig. 3. (*A*) Chest CT in a man with COPD and evidence of fibrocavitary NTM involving the right upper lobe containing a mycetoma, and with surrounding bronchiectasis and tree-in-bud nodularity. (*B*) Chest CT in an elderly woman with noncavitary NTM involving the middle lobe and lingula (a common distribution).

take weeks; in one study, 20% of cultures become positive after 2 weeks and 10% of cultures after 3 weeks.[22] BAL is reserved for cases where sputum specimens cannot be obtained, or when specimens are negative but there is high clinical concern. Nucleic acid probes can be used within 1 day after recognizable culture growth and are available for several NTM species including MAC. More recently, real-time PCR tests have become available and can detect the presence of NTM directly on the sputum sample, not just the culture, with some assays reporting both excellent sensitivity and specificity of 99%.[23]

Imaging findings of mycobacterium tuberculosis (TB), can appear similar to NTM (**Fig. 4**). The same techniques used for NTM can also be used for TB sources in the chest such as pleural fluid, lymph nodes, abscesses, and so forth. Culture specimens for TB turn positive in the range of 17 to 25 days.[22] Given the long culture time and the ramifications of untreated TB, additional methods such as real-time PCR have become integral to timely diagnosis. Quantiferon TB Gold In-Tube (QFT-IT) can be ordered by clinicians, more commonly for detection of latent TB, but also for evaluation of active TB. However, its negative predictive value is only 79%, so it should not be used alone to exclude active TB.

Nocardia spp are ubiquitous gram-positive bacteria found in soil that causes disease in immunocompromised hosts in two-thirds of cases and in immunocompetent hosts in the remaining one-third.[24] In most cases, intrapulmonary infection is the predominant site of infection.[25] Timely diagnosis of *Nocardia* spp is important, given its tendency to relapse off of treatment, progress on treatment, and ability to disseminate, particularly

to the brain. Unfortunately, diagnosis can be impeded by accidental destruction of *Nocardia* in the laboratory from sputum decontamination solutions. If there is a high radiological suspicion for Nocardiosis, this should be made clear to the clinician and the laboratory (**Fig. 5**). Given that *Nocardia* spp are not colonizers, a positive sputum culture for *Nocardia* should always be considered an active infection. An invasive procedure such as BAL was required 44% of the time to establish the diagnosis of Nocardiosis.[26] Given its rapidity, PCR testing is the preferred method of diagnosis, combining sensitivity and specificity of 100% with a rapid turnaround time.

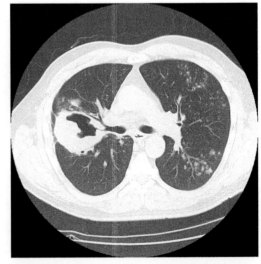

Fig. 4. Chest CT in a patient with active pulmonary tuberculosis. Appearance similar to **Fig. 3**, fibrocavitary NTM, exemplifying the importance of microbiologic evaluation.

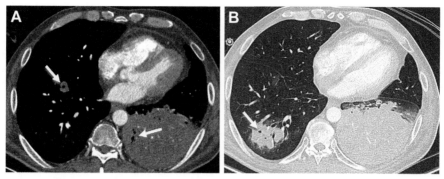

Fig. 5. Chest CT of pulmonary nocardia infection in a 55-year-old man receiving systemic chemotherapy. (A) Low attenuation consolidation in the left lower lobe and middle lobe nodule both containing bubbles of air at sites of necrosis (arrows). (B) More inferior CT section shows a consolidative mass in the right lower lobe which also contains a focus of necrosis.

FUNGAL PNEUMONIA

Fungal pneumonias are divided into endemic and opportunistic infections. Endemic fungal infections include organisms such as *Coccidioides immitis*, *Cryptococcus gattii*, *H capsulatum*, and *Blastomyces dermatitidis* and affect immunocompetent individuals in geographic regions where the fungi are present in the environment (see Jeffrey P. Kanne's article, "North American Endemic Fungal Infections," in this issue). Opportunistic fungal infections include pathogens such as *Aspergillus fumigatus*, *Candida albicans*, and *Mucor* spp, which are ubiquitous environmental fungi that typically do not cause disease unless the host is immunocompromised.

Coccidioidomycosis is caused by the endemic fungi *C immitis* and *Coccidioides posadasii*. It is found in the desert regions of the southwestern United States and northwestern Mexico, accounting for 29% of cases of CAP in these areas[27,28] (Fig. 6).

Diagnosis of coccidioidomycosis relies on serologic testing including immunoglobulin (Ig) antibodies subtype M (indicating acute infection) via enzyme-linked immunoassays (EIAs) and immunodiffusion and IgG antibodies (indicating prior infection) by complement fixation.[29] The sensitivity of EIAs for detection of acute infection ranges from 21% to 100% depending on immune status and symptom burden.[29,30] Up to 20% of patients seroconvert after an initial negative test, therefore, an initial negative test should not deter the radiologist from this diagnosis if the imaging findings are suspicious.[31]

Sensitivity of cytology and histology is low (33%) and these tests are rarely used alone.[32,33] In contrast, urine coccidioidomycosis antigen is positive in approximately 70% of patients.[34,35] Specimen culture remains the gold standard, but is insensitive with one study demonstrating a 54% rate of positivity. Owing to the overall low sensitivity of testing for *Coccidioides*, the American

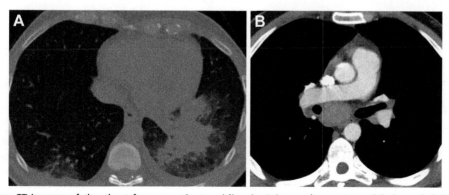

Fig. 6. Two CT images of the chest from a patient residing in Arizona demonstrate (A) dense left lower lobe consolidation with surrounding ground glass and septal thickening, as well as (B) presence of multifocal mediastinal lymphadenopathy on soft tissue images. Coccidioidomycosis was diagnosed via positive serologies.

Thoracic Society (ATS) recommends using more than one test for diagnosis.[36] Specificity for both antigen testing and IgM is high in symptomatic patients (>96%), so a positive result should be regarded as indicative of active disease.[29,30,35,37]

Cryptococcus spp are unique in that they can be considered both opportunistic and endemic fungi, affecting both immunocompromised and immunocompetent hosts.[38,39] *Cryptococcus neoformans* is the most common pathogen but *C gattii* is endemic to several parts of the world, recently recognized in the Pacific Northwest. In addition to pneumonia, Cryptococcal organisms can also exist in a latent stage as a granuloma presenting as a chronic pulmonary nodule[40] (**Fig. 7**).

Options for laboratory detection of *Cryptococcus* spp are similar to *Coccidioides* spp and include antigen detection tests, molecular PCR tests, direct microscopic examination of a cytologic or histopathologic specimen, and specimen culture. The classic method of serum cryptococcal antigen detection using EIA has a sensitivity of 83% to 100% with higher sensitivities in immunocompromised patients.[41,42] A newer method of antigen testing using lateral flow assay allows detection of antigen in as soon as 5 minutes[43] and may often be available at the time of radiologic interpretation. Sensitivity of urine antigen testing is also high at 94%.[44]

Histoplasmosis fumigatus is a fungus endemic to the Ohio and Mississippi river valleys and is found in soil containing bird and bat droppings. It most commonly occurs in immunocompetent hosts and can result in either subclinical/minimal symptoms, or disseminated disease.

Testing for histoplasmosis is similar to the endemic fungi above. Although fungal culture is the gold standard, testing begins with urine antigen (sensitivity 79.5% and specificity 99%) and serum antigen (sensitivity 83.9% and specificity 97%) detection.[45] Combining antigen and serologic testing increases the diagnostic yield to 93.3% for pulmonary histoplasmosis.[46] Unfortunately, serologies may be of low utility in patients with solid organ transplants.[47] Sensitivities and specificities for laboratory tests tend to be higher in patients with disseminated histoplasmosis in which antigen levels may correlate with severity of illness.[47,48]

Blastomycosis is an endemic fungal infection caused by *B dermatitidis*, found primarily in the central and southeastern United States. The most common site of infection is the lungs although it can disseminate to skin, bones, and the central nervous system[36] (**Fig. 8**). No one test has sufficient sensitivity to be used alone for the diagnosis of Blastomycosis.[36] Use of multiple simultaneous tests to increase diagnostic yield and improve accuracy is recommended by the ATS. Antigen testing is the usual first step and can be detected in urine (sensitivity 55%–93%), serum (sensitivity 55.6%), or BAL (sensitivity 62.5%) specimens.[49,50] Combining antigen and serology testing increases the diagnostic yield to 97.6%.[51] Although fungal culture or direct visualization remain the gold standards, diagnostic yield

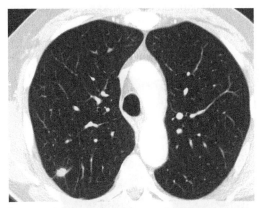

Fig. 7. Axial chest CT demonstrates presence of a rounded soft tissue density solitary pulmonary nodule in the posterior aspect of the right upper lobe. A serum cryptococcal antigen was positive in a 1:20 dilution. Diagnosis of *Cryptococcus* spp was confirmed with surgical wedge resection.

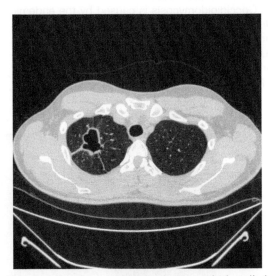

Fig. 8. Axial chest CT demonstrates a thick-walled right upper lobe cavitary lesion in a 38-year-old man residing in Nashville, Tennessee. The patient underwent bronchoscopy with transbronchial biopsies with tissue cultures confirming the diagnosis of Blastomycosis.

is low, requires an experienced microbiologist, and cultures may take 5 weeks to grow.[52]

Pneumocystis pneumonia is caused by *Pneumocystis jirovecii*, formerly *Pneumocystis carinii*. It occurs in immunocompromised patients, particularly those with defects in cell-mediated immunity such as AIDS and glucocorticoid use.[53] The most common radiographic finding is centrally predominant ground-glass opacities without pleural effusions and with occasional presence of cysts or pneumothorax[54] (**Fig. 9**). Laboratory findings that suggest pneumocystis infection include elevated lactate dehydrogenase and elevated serum beta-D-glucan levels but these are not specific to pneumocystis pneumonia.[55,56] Other diagnostic options include PCR testing or direct visualization on a respiratory specimen.[57,58]

The diagnostic yield of sputum for direct visualization of PJP ranges from 4% to 58%,[59–61] is higher in patients with human immunodeficiency virus (HIV) compared with non-HIV patients.[60,61] Diagnostic yield of BAL fluid is also higher in patients with HIV.[59] As sensitivity for direct visualization can be low, serum beta-D-glucan may be useful. The sensitivity and specificity of serum beta-D-glucan depend on the threshold used to define positivity.[62] High levels of beta-D-glucan (>200 pg/mL) increase specificity to 100%. Nucleic acid amplification of a respiratory specimen has a higher sensitivity of 82%. Although not widely available,[58] it does have a negative predictive value at 98.7%.

Invasive aspergillosis (IA) is caused by *A fumigatus*, *Aspergillus flavus*, and *Aspergillus terreus*, which are ubiquitous and are frequent colonizers of the respiratory tract. Therefore, it is not uncommon to culture aspergillus in a sputum or BAL specimen. However, tissue invasion is rare and primarily occurs in immunocompromised patients.[63] Radiologic findings are discussed in detail elsewhere in this issue (see Godoy and colleagues' article, "Invasive Fungal Pneumonia in Immunocompromised Patients"). Presence of a halo sign manifest by a solid lesion with surrounding ground glass can suggest the diagnosis in an immunocompromised patient (**Fig. 10**). As aspergillus is a frequent colonizer, diagnosis of IA requires clinical evidence of active infection in addition to fungal invasion into tissue, elevation of serum or BAL galactomannan (GM), or beta-D-glucan or culture of aspergillus within a sterile site.[36]

Galactomannan is a component of the fungal cell wall and can be detected by EIA. Using positivity as an optical index greater than 0.5, sensitivity and specificity for serum galactomannan are 79% and 88%, respectively.[64] BAL galactomannan greater than 1.0 has a much higher sensitivity and specificity of 90% and 94%, respectively.[64] As galactomannan is also present on fungi other than *Aspergillus* such as *Candida*, *Histoplasma*, *Blastomyces*, and *Penicillium*, serum galactomannan can yield false positives.[65]

Beta-D-glucan is also a component of the fungal cell wall and aside from aspergillus is also present on *Candida* spp. and *P jiroveci*. Its utility is similar to serum galactomannan. In a meta-analysis of 1771 patients, sensitivity was low at 50% but specificity was outstanding at 99% for detection of invasive aspergillus.[66] False-positive results may occur with infection with *P aeruginosa*.[67] Newer methods to diagnose pulmonary aspergillosis and IA include serum and BAL PCR (sensitivity 79.2%, specificity 79.6%, and sensitivity

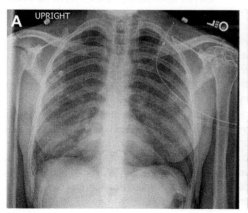
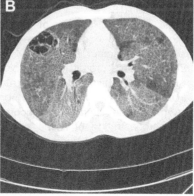

Fig. 9. (*A*) Front radiograph demonstrates the presence of bilateral perihilar ground-glass opacities without pleural effusions. (*B*) Axial high-resolution CT demonstrates a middle lobe cyst in conjunction with "crazy paving," septal thickening on a background of ground-glass opacities. Pneumocystis stain demonstrating organisms on induced sputum sample.

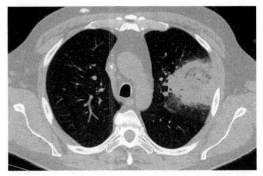

Fig. 11. CT from a febrile neutropenic patient demonstrates focal subpleural consolidation with central ground glass (reversed halo sign) shown to be caused by Mucormycosis by BAL PCR. A single subpleural lesion is a common imaging appearance for this disease.

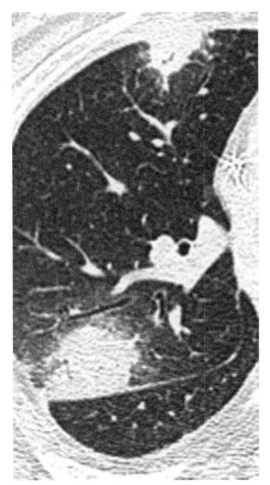

Fig. 10. Axial CT of the right lung of an immunocompromised patient demonstrates 2 solid pulmonary masses with surrounding ground glass, a halo sign. The patient was diagnosed with angioinvasive aspergillus by bronchoscopy.

90.2%, specificity 96.4%, respectively), which are recommended by the ATS.[36,68,69]

Mucormycosis accounts for 8% of invasive fungal infections in immunocompromised patients[70] usually from the genera *Rhizopus*, *Mucor*, and *Rhizomucor*.[71] These organisms are ubiquitous and are frequent colonizers of the respiratory tract, but can result in disease in immunocompromised hosts (**Fig. 11**). The diagnosis of mucormycosis requires demonstration of tissue invasion and clinical symptoms of pneumonia. On microscopic examination, the hyphae have an irregular branching pattern, unlike aspergillus which tends to branch at 90°.[72,73] PCR testing has also been used although is not widely available.[74,75] In one study of 27 patients with confirmed mucormycosis, 22 patients had a positive PCR.[75] Equally important, PCR positivity occurred in 12 of 15 cases that were negative by culture, indicating the utility of PCR.

VIRAL PNEUMONIA

Respiratory viruses are a major cause of pneumonia in immunocompetent and immunocompromised populations (see Febbo and colleagues' article, "Viral Pneumonias," in this issue). Over the last several decades, NAAT PCR-based testing has emerged as a technique that can simultaneously detect multiple respiratory virus nucleic acids. These assays can detect multiple previously unrecognized respiratory viruses on a single sample[76] with a quick turnaround time while maintaining high sensitivity and specificity of greater than 90%.[10]

Influenza virus (**Fig. 12**) is the most significant cause of viral pneumonia. Rapid antigen testing can be specific (up to 94.5%) at detecting the virus from respiratory secretions, although sensitivity is low (40.5%) so cannot be used to exclude infection. Rapid influenza molecular assays based on PCR detection are recommended to identify different subtypes of influenza viruses with a reported sensitivity and specificity of up to 100%.[10,76]

CAP caused by the currently pandemic (SARS-CoV-2) (**Fig. 13**) can be detected by rapid antigen tests but has low sensitivity due to variable viral loads, which has limited their use. NAAT (RT-PCR) remains the currently recommended test[77] (see Sing and colleagues' article, "Review of Thoracic Imaging Manifestations of COVID-19 & Other Pathologic Coronaviruses," in this issue). Diagnostic testing is recommended on an upper respiratory specimen, preferably a nasopharyngeal sample, with acceptable alternative

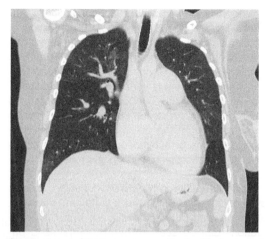

Fig. 12. Coronal CT image in a patient with fever and cough demonstrates bilateral upper lobe ground-glass opacities, which was later confirmed to be influenza A positive by PCR nasopharyngeal swab.

specimens obtained from the anterior nares, nasal midturbinate, oropharyngeal tract, or BAL fluid. Viral load is greatest in throat swabs at the time of viral onset and rapid specimen collection is recommended as soon as the decision to evaluate for the virus is made.[78]

VZV infection—which is associated with chickenpox and shingles—can lead to severe pneumonia in the elderly, pregnant, and immunocompromised patients although the incidence has decreased due to efficacy of the varicella vaccine.[76] Acute VZV infection can be diagnosed by PCR testing or isolating the virus/growth on cell culture, such as from vesicle fluid.[79]

Patients who have undergone a solid organ/hematopoietic stem cell transplant or have active hematologic malignancies are at risk for CMV pneumonia. Diagnosis can be made by PCR assay, CMV viral load quantification, or cytologic examination of the BAL fluid or lung biopsy samples.[76] PCR testing is the most sensitive method of detecting CMV. Quantitative real-time PCR

can be helpful in monitoring viral loads in the blood although has a low specificity and positive predictive value in BAL fluid.[80]

Herpes simplex virus (HSV)—more commonly HSV-1 rather than HSV-2—can be a rare cause of pneumonia in immunocompromised patients and those who are critically ill or mechanically ventilated (Fig. 14). It has been reported in approximately 3% of patients with hematologic malignancies and 1% of hematopoietic stem cell transplant recipients.[81] When detected in BAL samples of ventilated patients, it is unclear whether it represents viral shedding or a true pathogen.[76] The virus can be detected through rapid antigen testing detection (sensitivity of 80% and specificity of 100%) or shell-vial culture (sensitivity of 57% and specificity of 100%) from respiratory secretions, BAL fluid, or lung tissue.[81] Although PCR testing is more rapid and sensitive, it is unable to distinguish between active disease and contamination from the oral cavity. Finally, histopathologic inspection of BAL fluid or lung tissue can demonstrate characteristic findings of multinucleated giant cells "owl-eyes."[81]

PNEUMONIA SECONDARY TO PARASITES/PROTOZOA

Parasitic infections are increasingly encountered in western countries in both immunocompromised and immunocompetent individuals. In the United States, most cases occur with travel to endemic regions.[82,83] (See Restrepo and colleagues' article, "Endemic Thoracic Infections in Latin America and the Caribbean," in this issue; Ching Ching and Lynette LS Teo's article, "Endemic Thoracic Infections in Southeast Asia," in this issue; Rydzak and colleagues' article, "Endemic Thoracic Infections in sub-Saharan Africa," in this issue)

Pulmonary amebiasis is rare but is the second most common site of this infection outside the abdomen[83] and often extends from the liver

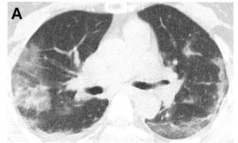
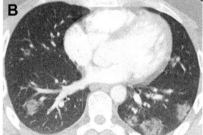

Fig. 13. Two axial CT images of the chest demonstrate basilar and peripheral predominant mixed ground glass and consolidative opacities in a distribution typical for SARS-CoV-2 viral pneumonia.

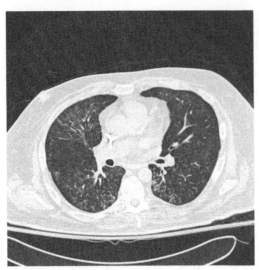

Fig. 14. Axial chest CT demonstrates extensive bilateral ground-glass opacities and centrilobular nodules in an immunocompromised patient diagnosed with HSV pneumonia by BAL culture.

(Fig. 15). Diagnostic options include serology, antigen detection, and trophozoite visualization on aspirated fluid. Antibody detection is positive in greater than 90% of patients and is the most widely available test.[83,84] Often, patients in endemic areas have antibodies from remote prior exposure[83] so clinical history is important.

Acute pulmonary schistosomiasis (Katayama syndrome) is caused by *Schistosoma mansoni* (Africa and South America) and *Schistosoma haematobium* (Africa and the Middle East). Peripheral

eosinophilia can occur but is nonspecific. Diagnostic tools include microscopic visualization of eggs in stool or urine (the gold standard), antigen detection in serum, serum and urine PCR testing, serologic testing. Uncommonly, biopsy can be performed if testing is negative and clinical suspicion remains high. Antibodies develop 6 to 12 weeks after exposure, so PCR testing may be more useful in[85] the acute setting.[86] Pulmonary manifestations of schistosomiasis often occur in chronic infection where diagnosis relies on serologic testing.[87]

Pulmonary strongyloidiasis usually causes symptoms of cough, throat irritation, dyspnea, and wheezing but severe disease from "hyperinfection" can be seen in immunosuppressed patients (see articles by Ryzdak, Teo, and Restreppo).[88] Serology is the main diagnostic tool. Most serologic tests measure IgG response and a specificity of 81% has been reported in patients with proven disease.[89] Limitations of serologic testing include reduced sensitivity in immunocompromised patients and inability to distinguish current from prior infection.[89] Other options include direct microscopic visualization of a stool specimen, but sensitivity is low at 21% due to intermittent larval excretion.[90]

SUMMARY

The differential diagnosis of organisms causing pneumonia can often be narrowed by a combination of imaging patterns and nonimaging diagnostic tests. The breadth and speed with which these nonimaging tests can be obtained has markedly increased in this century. Knowledge of the accuracy of diagnostic tests that have been performed as well familiarity with the utility of additional diagnostic tests can allow the radiologists to assist clinicians in suggesting the optimal course of action.

DISCLOSURE

The authors have nothing to disclose.

REFERENCES

1. Mizgerd JP. Acute lower respiratory tract infection. N Engl J Med 2008;358(7):716–27.
2. Armstrong GL, Conn LA, Pinner RW. Trends in infectious disease mortality in the United States during the 20th century. JAMA 1999;281(1):61–6.
3. Metlay JP, Waterer GW, Long AC, et al. Diagnosis and treatment of adults with community-acquired pneumonia. An official clinical practice guideline of the american thoracic society and infectious

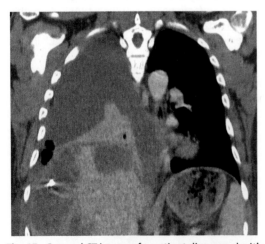

Fig. 15. Coronal CT image of a patient diagnosed with *Entamoeba histolytica* by elevated *E histolytica* serum antibodies demonstrates multiple intrahepatic abscesses and a large loculated right pleural effusion with intrapleural gas secondary to empyema.

diseases society of America. Am J Respir Crit Care Med 2019;200(7):e45–67.

4. Evans SE, Jennerich AL, Azar MM, et al. Nucleic acid-based testing for noninfluenza viral pathogens in adults with suspected community-acquired pneumonia. An official american thoracic society clinical practice guideline. Am J Respir Crit Care Med 2021;203(9):1070–87.

5. Miller JM, Binnicker MJ, Campbell S, et al. A guide to utilization of the microbiology laboratory for diagnosis of infectious diseases: 2018 update by the infectious diseases society of america and the american society for microbiology. Clin Infect Dis 2018;67(6):813–6.

6. Morton C, Puchalski J. The utility of bronchoscopy in immunocompromised patients: a review. J Thorac Dis 2019;11(12):5603–12.

7. Rosenstengel A. Pleural infection-current diagnosis and management. J Thorac Dis 2012;4(2):186–93.

8. Kim J, Lee KH, Cho JY, et al. Usefulness of CT-guided percutaneous transthoracic needle lung biopsies in patients with suspected pulmonary infection. Korean J Radiol 2020;21(5):526–36.

9. Walter JM, Wunderink RG. Testing for respiratory viruses in adults with severe lower respiratory infection. Chest 2018;154(5):1213–22.

10. Zhang N, Wang L, Deng X, et al. Recent advances in the detection of respiratory virus infection in humans. J Med Virol 2020;92(4):408–17.

11. Couturier MR, Graf EH, Griffin AT. Urine antigen tests for the diagnosis of respiratory infections: legionellosis, histoplasmosis, pneumococcal pneumonia. Clin Lab Med 2014;34(2):219–36.

12. Almirall J, Bolibar I, Toran P, et al. Contribution of C-reactive protein to the diagnosis and assessment of severity of community-acquired pneumonia. Chest 2004;125(4):1335–42.

13. Gardner JG, Bhamidipati DR, Rueda AM, et al. The white blood cell count and prognosis in pneumococcal pneumonia. New Orleans, Louisiana: Infectious Diseases Society of America; 2016. p. 1245.

14. Jain S, Self WH, Wunderink RG, et al. Community-acquired pneumonia requiring hospitalization among U.S. adults. N Engl J Med 2015;373(5):415–27.

15. Musher DM, Montoya R, Wanahita A. Diagnostic value of microscopic examination of Gram-stained sputum and sputum cultures in patients with bacteremic pneumococcal pneumonia. Clin Infect Dis 2004;39(2):165–9.

16. Said MA, Johnson HL, Nonyane BA, et al. Estimating the burden of pneumococcal pneumonia among adults: a systematic review and meta-analysis of diagnostic techniques. PLoS One 2013;8(4):e60273.

17. Giancola SE, Nguyen AT, Le B, et al. Clinical utility of a nasal swab methicillin-resistant Staphylococcus aureus polymerase chain reaction test in intensive and intermediate care unit patients with pneumonia. Diagn Microbiol Infect Dis 2016;86(3):307–10.

18. Parente DM, Cunha CB, Mylonakis E, et al. The clinical utility of methicillin-resistant staphylococcus aureus (MRSA) nasal screening to rule Out MRSA Pneumonia: a diagnostic meta-analysis with antimicrobial stewardship implications. Clin Infect Dis 2018;67(1):1–7.

19. Shimada T, Noguchi Y, Jackson JL, et al. Systematic review and metaanalysis: urinary antigen tests for Legionellosis. Chest 2009;136(6):1576–85.

20. Peci A, Winter AL, Gubbay JB. Evaluation and comparison of multiple test methods, including real-time PCR, for Legionella detection in clinical specimens. Front Public Health 2016;4:175.

21. Wassilew N, Hoffmann H, Andrejak C, et al. Pulmonary disease caused by non-tuberculous mycobacteria. Respiration 2016;91(5):386–402.

22. Pfyffer GE, Wittwer F. Incubation time of mycobacterial cultures: how long is long enough to issue a final negative report to the clinician? J Clin Microbiol 2012;50(12):4188–9.

23. Richardson ET, Samson D, Banaei N. Rapid Identification of Mycobacterium tuberculosis and nontuberculous mycobacteria by multiplex, real-time PCR. J Clin Microbiol 2009;47(5):1497–502.

24. Beaman BL, Beaman L. Nocardia species: host-parasite relationships. Clin Microbiol Rev 1994; 7(2):213–64.

25. Paige EK, Spelman D. Nocardiosis: 7-year experience at an Australian tertiary hospital. Intern Med J 2019;49(3):373–9.

26. Georghiou PR, Blacklock ZM. Infection with Nocardia species in Queensland. A review of 102 clinical isolates. Med J Aust 1992;156(10):692–7.

27. Baptista-Rosas RC, Hinojosa A, Riquelme M. Ecological niche modeling of Coccidioides spp. in western North American deserts. Ann N Y Acad Sci 2007;1111:35–46.

28. Valdivia L, Nix D, Wright M, et al. Coccidioidomycosis as a common cause of community-acquired pneumonia. Emerg Infect Dis 2006;12(6):958–62.

29. Blair JE, Coakley B, Santelli AC, et al. Serologic testing for symptomatic coccidioidomycosis in immunocompetent and immunosuppressed hosts. Mycopathologia 2006;162(5):317–24.

30. Crum NF, Lederman ER, Stafford CM, et al. Coccidioidomycosis: a descriptive survey of a reemerging disease. Clinical characteristics and current controversies. Medicine (Baltimore) 2004;83(3):149–75.

31. Blair JE, Mendoza N, Force S, et al. Clinical specificity of the enzyme immunoassay test for coccidioidomycosis varies according to the reason for its performance. Clin Vaccine Immunol 2013;20(1):95–8.

32. Mendoza N, Blair JE. The utility of diagnostic testing for active coccidioidomycosis in solid organ

transplant recipients. Am J Transplant 2013;13(4): 1034–9.

33. Mendoza N, Noel P, Blair JE. Diagnosis, treatment, and outcomes of coccidioidomycosis in allogeneic stem cell transplantation. Transpl Infect Dis 2015; 17(3):380–8.

34. Durkin M, Connolly P, Kuberski T, et al. Diagnosis of coccidioidomycosis with use of the Coccidioides antigen enzyme immunoassay. Clin Infect Dis 2008; 47(8):e69–73.

35. Durkin M, Estok L, Hospenthal D, et al. Detection of Coccidioides antigenemia following dissociation of immune complexes. Clin Vaccin Immunol 2009; 16(10):1453–6.

36. Hage CA, Carmona EM, Epelbaum O, et al. Microbiological laboratory testing in the diagnosis of fungal infections in pulmonary and critical care practice. An official american thoracic society clinical practice guideline. Am J Respir Crit Care Med 2019;200(5): 535–50.

37. Kaufman L, Sekhon AS, Moledina N, et al. Comparative evaluation of commercial Premier EIA and microimmunodiffusion and complement fixation tests for Coccidioides immitis antibodies. J Clin Microbiol 1995;33(3):618–9.

38. Harris JR, Lockhart SR, Debess E, et al. Cryptococcus gattii in the United States: clinical aspects of infection with an emerging pathogen. Clin Infect Dis 2011;53(12):1188–95.

39. Kiertiburanakul S, Wirojtananugoon S, Pracharktam R, et al. Cryptococcosis in human immunodeficiency virus-negative patients. Int J Infect Dis 2006;10(1):72–8.

40. Setianingrum F, Rautemaa-Richardson R, Denning DW. Pulmonary cryptococcosis: a review of pathobiology and clinical aspects. Med Mycol 2019;57(2):133–50.

41. Singh N, Alexander BD, Lortholary O, et al. Pulmonary cryptococcosis in solid organ transplant recipients: clinical relevance of serum cryptococcal antigen. Clin Infect Dis 2008;46(2):e12–8.

42. Meyohas MC, Roux P, Bollens D, et al. Pulmonary cryptococcosis: localized and disseminated infections in 27 patients with AIDS. Clin Infect Dis 1995; 21(3):628–33.

43. Koczula KM, Gallotta A. Lateral flow assays. Essays Biochem 2016;60(1):111–20.

44. Jarvis JN, Percival A, Bauman S, et al. Evaluation of a novel point-of-care cryptococcal antigen test on serum, plasma, and urine from patients with HIV-associated cryptococcal meningitis. Clin Infect Dis 2011;53(10):1019–23.

45. Fandino-Devia E, Rodriguez-Echeverri C, Cardona-Arias J, et al. Antigen Detection in the Diagnosis of Histoplasmosis: A Meta-analysis of Diagnostic Performance. Mycopathologia 2016;181(3–4): 197–205.

46. Swartzentruber S, Rhodes L, Kurkjian K, et al. Diagnosis of acute pulmonary histoplasmosis by antigen detection. Clin Infect Dis 2009;49(12):1878–82.

47. Hage CA, Ribes JA, Wengenack NL, et al. A multicenter evaluation of tests for diagnosis of histoplasmosis. Clin Infect Dis 2011;53(5):448–54.

48. Arango-Bustamante K, Restrepo A, Cano LE, et al. Diagnostic value of culture and serological tests in the diagnosis of histoplasmosis in HIV and non-HIV Colombian patients. Am J Trop Med Hyg 2013; 89(5):937–42.

49. Durkin M, Witt J, Lemonte A, et al. Antigen assay with the potential to aid in diagnosis of blastomycosis. J Clin Microbiol 2004;42(10):4873–5.

50. Frost HM, Novicki TJ. Blastomyces antigen detection for diagnosis and management of blastomycosis. J Clin Microbiol 2015;53(11):3660–2.

51. Richer SM, Smedema ML, Durkin MM, et al. Development of a highly sensitive and specific blastomycosis antibody enzyme immunoassay using Blastomyces dermatitidis surface protein BAD-1. Clin Vaccin Immunol 2014;21(2):143–6.

52. Martynowicz MA, Prakash UB. Pulmonary blastomycosis: an appraisal of diagnostic techniques. Chest 2002;121(3):768–73.

53. Yale SH, Limper AH. Pneumocystis carinii pneumonia in patients without acquired immunodeficiency syndrome: associated illness and prior corticosteroid therapy. Mayo Clin Proc 1996;71(1):5–13.

54. Kanne JP, Yandow DR, Meyer CA. Pneumocystis jiroveci pneumonia: high-resolution CT findings in patients with and without HIV infection. AJR Am J Roentgenol 2012;198(6):W555–61.

55. Tasaka S, Hasegawa N, Kobayashi S, et al. Serum indicators for the diagnosis of pneumocystis pneumonia. Chest 2007;131(4):1173–80.

56. Zaman MK, White DA. Serum lactate dehydrogenase levels and Pneumocystis carinii pneumonia. Diagnostic and prognostic significance. Am Rev Respir Dis 1988;137(4):796–800.

57. Desmet S, Van Wijngaerden E, Maertens J, et al. Serum (1-3)-beta-D-glucan as a tool for diagnosis of Pneumocystis jirovecii pneumonia in patients with human immunodeficiency virus infection or hematological malignancy. J Clin Microbiol 2009; 47(12):3871–4.

58. Azoulay E, Bergeron A, Chevret S, et al. Polymerase chain reaction for diagnosing pneumocystis pneumonia in non-HIV immunocompromised patients with pulmonary infiltrates. Chest 2009;135(3): 655–61.

59. Pagano L, Fianchi L, Mele L, et al. Pneumocystis carinii pneumonia in patients with malignant haematological diseases: 10 years' experience of infection in GIMEMA centres. Br J Haematol 2002;117(2):379–86.

60. LaRocque RC, Katz JT, Perruzzi P, et al. The utility of sputum induction for diagnosis of Pneumocystis

pneumonia in immunocompromised patients without human immunodeficiency virus. Clin Infect Dis 2003; 37(10):1380–3.

61. Silva RM, Bazzo ML, Borges AA. Induced sputum versus bronchoalveolar lavage in the diagnosis of pneumocystis jiroveci pneumonia in human immuno-deficiency virus-positive patients. Braz J Infect Dis 2007;11(6):549–53.

62. Morjaria S, Frame J, Franco-Garcia A, et al. Clinical Performance of (1,3) Beta-D Glucan for the Diagnosis of Pneumocystis Pneumonia (PCP) in Cancer Patients Tested With PCP Polymerase Chain Reaction. Clin Infect Dis 2019;69(8):1303–9.

63. Marr KA, Carter RA, Boeckh M, et al. Invasive aspergillosis in allogeneic stem cell transplant recipients: changes in epidemiology and risk factors. Blood 2002;100(13):4358–66.

64. Haydour Q, Hage CA, Carmona EM, et al. Diagnosis of fungal infections. A systematic review and meta-analysis supporting american thoracic society practice guideline. Ann Am Thorac Soc 2019;16(9): 1179–88.

65. Huang YT, Hung CC, Hsueh PR. Aspergillus galactomannan antigenemia in penicilliosis marneffei. AIDS 2007;21(14):1990–1.

66. Lamoth F, Cruciani M, Mengoli C, et al. beta-Glucan antigenemia assay for the diagnosis of invasive fungal infections in patients with hematological malignancies: a systematic review and meta-analysis of cohort studies from the Third European Conference on Infections in Leukemia (ECIL-3). Clin Infect Dis 2012;54(5):633–43.

67. Mennink-Kersten MA, Ruegebrink D, Verweij PE. Pseudomonas aeruginosa as a cause of 1,3-beta-D-glucan assay reactivity. Clin Infect Dis 2008; 46(12):1930–1.

68. Avni T, Levy I, Sprecher H, et al. Diagnostic accuracy of PCR alone compared to galactomannan in bronchoalveolar lavage fluid for diagnosis of invasive pulmonary aspergillosis: a systematic review. J Clin Microbiol 2012;50(11):3652–8.

69. Cruciani M, Mengoli C, Barnes R, et al. Polymerase chain reaction blood tests for the diagnosis of invasive aspergillosis in immunocompromised people. Cochrane Database Syst Rev 2019;9: CD009551.

70. Neofytos D, Horn D, Anaissie E, et al. Epidemiology and outcome of invasive fungal infection in adult hematopoietic stem cell transplant recipients: analysis of Multicenter Prospective Antifungal Therapy (PATH) Alliance registry. Clin Infect Dis 2009;48(3): 265–73.

71. Roden MM, Zaoutis TE, Buchanan WL, et al. Epidemiology and outcome of zygomycosis: a review of 929 reported cases. Clin Infect Dis 2005;41(5): 634–53.

72. Guarner J, Brandt ME. Histopathologic diagnosis of fungal infections in the 21st century. Clin Microbiol Rev 2011;24(2):247–80.

73. Cornely OA, Alastruey-Izquierdo A, Arenz D, et al. Global guideline for the diagnosis and management of mucormycosis: an initiative of the European Confederation of Medical Mycology in cooperation with the Mycoses Study Group Education and Research Consortium. Lancet Infect Dis 2019; 19(12):e405–21.

74. Machouart M, Larche J, Burton K, et al. Genetic identification of the main opportunistic Mucorales by PCR-restriction fragment length polymorphism. J Clin Microbiol 2006;44(3):805–10.

75. Hammond SP, Bialek R, Milner DA, et al. Molecular methods to improve diagnosis and identification of mucormycosis. J Clin Microbiol 2011;49(6): 2151–3.

76. Dandachi D, Rodriguez-Barradas MC. Viral pneumonia: etiologies and treatment. J Investig Med 2018;66(6):957–65.

77. La Marca A, Capuzzo M, Paglia T, et al. Testing for SARS-CoV-2 (COVID-19): a systematic review and clinical guide to molecular and serological in-vitro diagnostic assays. Reprod Biomed Online 2020; 41(3):483–99.

78. To KK, Tsang OT, Leung WS, et al. Temporal profiles of viral load in posterior oropharyngeal saliva samples and serum antibody responses during infection by SARS-CoV-2: an observational cohort study. Lancet Infect Dis 2020;20(5):565–74.

79. Sauerbrei A. Diagnosis, antiviral therapy, and prophylaxis of varicella-zoster virus infections. Eur J Clin Microbiol Infect Dis 2016;35(5):723–34.

80. Lee HY, Rhee CK, Choi JY, et al. Diagnosis of cytomegalovirus pneumonia by quantitative polymerase chain reaction using bronchial washing fluid from patients with hematologic malignancies. Oncotarget 2017;8(24):39736–45.

81. Shah J, Chemaly R. In: Azoulay E, editor. Herpes simplex virus pneumonia in patients with hematologic malignancies. Berlin: Springer; 2010.

82. Russell ES, Gray EB, Marshall RE, et al. Prevalence of Strongyloides stercoralis antibodies among a rural Appalachian population–Kentucky, 2013. Am J Trop Med Hyg 2014;91(5):1000–1.

83. Shamsuzzaman SM, Hashiguchi Y. Thoracic amebiasis. Clin Chest Med 2002;23(2):479–92.

84. Katzenstein D, Rickerson V, Braude A. New concepts of amebic liver abscess derived from hepatic imaging, serodiagnosis, and hepatic enzymes in 67 consecutive cases in San Diego. Medicine (Baltimore) 1982;61(4):237–46.

85. Jones ME, Mitchell RG, Leen CL. Long seronegative window in schistosoma infection. Lancet 1992; 340(8834–8835):1549–50.

86. Cnops L, Tannich E, Polman K, et al. Schistosoma real-time PCR as diagnostic tool for international travellers and migrants. Trop Med Int Health 2012; 17(10):1208–16.

87. Kinkel HF, Dittrich S, Baumer B, et al. Evaluation of eight serological tests for diagnosis of imported schistosomiasis. Clin Vaccin Immunol 2012;19(6): 948–53.

88. Salam R, Sharaan A, Jackson SM, et al. Strongyloides hyperinfection syndrome: a curious case of asthma worsened by systemic corticosteroids. Am J Case Rep 2020;21:e925221.

89. Ming DK, Armstrong M, Lowe P, et al. Clinical and diagnostic features of 413 patients treated for imported strongyloidiasis at the hospital for tropical diseases, London. Am J Trop Med Hyg 2019; 101(2):428–31.

90. Campo Polanco L, Gutierrez LA, Cardona Arias J. [Diagnosis of Strongyloides Stercoralis infection: meta-analysis on evaluation of conventional parasitological methods (1980-2013)]. Rev Esp Salud Publica 2014;88(5):581–600.

Moving?

Make sure your subscription moves with you!

To notify us of your new address, find your **Clinics Account Number** (located on your mailing label above your name), and contact customer service at:

Email: **journalscustomerservice-usa@elsevier.com**

800-654-2452 (subscribers in the U.S. & Canada)
314-447-8871 (subscribers outside of the U.S. & Canada)

Fax number: **314-447-8029**

Elsevier Health Sciences Division
Subscription Customer Service
3251 Riverport Lane
Maryland Heights, MO 63043

ELSEVIER

Moving?

Make sure your subscription moves with you!

To notify us of your new address, find your Clinics Account number (located on your mailing label above your name), and contact customer service at:

email: journalscustomerservice-usa@elsevier.com

800-654-2452 (subscribers in the U.S. & Canada)
314-447-8871 (subscribers outside of the U.S. & Canada)

Fax number: 314-447-8029

Elsevier Health Sciences Division
Subscription Customer Service
3251 Riverport Lane
Maryland Heights, MO 63043

To ensure uninterrupted delivery of your subscription, please notify us at least 4 weeks in advance of move.

Printed and bound by CPI Group (UK) Ltd, Croydon, CR0 4YY

08/05/2025

01864714-0001